Human Spermatozoa in
Assisted Reproduction

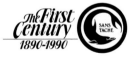

Human Spermatozoa in Assisted Reproduction

EDITORS

Anibal A. Acosta, M.D.*
R. James Swanson, M.D.*
Steven B. Ackerman, Ph.D.*

Thinus F. Kruger, M.D.**
Johannes A. van Zyl, M.D.**
Roelof Menkveld, Ph.D.**

WITH SPECIAL SECTIONS
  Reproductive Immunology: **Nancy J. Alexander, Ph.D.**
  Research Aspects: **Gary D. Hodgen, Ph.D.**

EDITORIAL ADVISOR
  Charlotte Schrader, Ph.D.

*Jones Institute for Reproductive Medicine, Andrology Section, Eastern Virginia Medical School, Medical College of Hampton Roads, Norfolk, Virginia

**University of Stellenbosch, Tygerberg Hospital, Infertility Clinic, Tygerberg, South Africa

WILLIAMS & WILKINS
Baltimore • Hong Kong • London • Sydney

Editor: Carol-Lynn Brown
Associate Editor: Victoria M. Vaughn
Design: Wilma Rosenberger
Illustration Planning: Wayne Hubbel
Production: Anne G. Seitz

Copyright © 1990
Williams & Wilkins
428 East Preston Street
Baltimore, Maryland 21202, USA

Accurate indications, adverse reactions, and dosage schedules for drugs are provided in this book, but it is possible that they may change. The reader is urged to review the package information data of the manufacturers of the medications mentioned.

Printed in the United States of America

Library of Congress Cataloging in Publication Data

Human spermatozoa in assisted reproduction / editors. Anibal A. Acosta
. . . [et al.].
    p.   cm.
  Includes index.
  ISBN 0-683-0049-7
  1. Fertilization in vitro. Human. 2. Spermatozoa. I. Acosta,
Anibal A.
  [DNLM: 1. Fertilization in Vitro. 2. Spermatozoa. WJ 834 H918]
RG135.H87 1990
612.6′1—dc20
DNLM/DLC
for Library of Congress
                        89-5730
                          CIP
          89 90 91 92 93
      1 2 3 4 5 6 7 8 9 10

Foreword

In vitro fertilization (IVF) was originally devised to bypass the reproductive disability which resulted from diseased fallopian tubes. However, with experience it became evident that the new process made it possible to study and understand disorders which, prior to IVF, were hidden from investigation. In some circumstances IVF was even found to be a successful therapeutic modality for infertility other than that caused by tubal pathology. Infertility of the male falls into both the investigative and therapeutic categories.

Andrology, the study of the reproductive capability of the male, is not a new discipline. However, during the twentieth century, progress in the diagnosis and therapy of human male infertility had been extremely modest.

IVF opened a window of opportunity in this area. At one stroke it removed the confounding factors associated with the deposition of the sperm in the vagina some 10 cm from the site of fertilizing action in the ampulla of the tube, and it furnished us an intermediate endpoint—fertilization—on the way to the ultimate endpoint—a viable pregnancy. IVF made it possible to study the correlates of successful fertilization at the level of the egg and sperm without wondering whether the sperm had, in fact, arrived at the site of fertilization or whether the fertilized egg could progress to implantation and development. Many of these new diagnostic correlations at the sperm-egg interface are already becoming available and are described in this book.

But who is the andrologist, and where is the andrologist's workshop?

It is noteworthy that this book—a synthesis of current knowledge about human andrology—comes from two departments of obstetrics and gynecology, where it was realized before the era of IVF that a new perspective was required if true progress was to be made in solving the problems of male infertility. It was this new perspective, obtained by establishing an andrology unit in the departments of obstetrics and gynecology, which revitalized the andrological field.

In the 1960s, during the chairmanship of Professor Willem A. van Niekirk, a unit of andrology was started in the Department of Obstetrics and Gynecology at Tygerberg Hospital, the University of Stellenbosch, in South Africa. This unit was under the leadership of J. A. van Zyl, a gynecologist-turned-andrologist. A similar unit was established in the 1970s at the Eastern Virginia Medical School and Old Dominion University in Norfolk, Virginia, under the chairmanship of Mason C. Andrews, by Anibal A. Acosta, a gynecologist who early understood the essential requirement for new information about the male in overcoming the general problem of infertility. These two units were poised for the new opportunities provided by IVF. The organization of andrology units within departments of obstetrics and gynecology was unique and is, even today, little imitated.

It would be a mistake to think of andrology as a mature discipline, for its personnel, its niche, and its location are all in a state of rapid evolution. This book is an elegant statement of the current understanding of the art and science of this dynamic speciality—andrology.

Howard W. Jones, Jr., M.D.
Georgeanna Seegar Jones, M.D.

Preface

The field of andrology as a discipline moved and developed slowly and laboriously from its inception in 1891, in spite of tremendous efforts made by many excellent basic and clinical investigators. During all these years, the final judgment on sperm quality and the determination of normality in sperm parameters in the various tests depended on the ability of the patient to establish a pregnancy in his partner. That was the only available yardstick. There are significant drawbacks to this approach. On the one hand, female fertility is not always easy to determine. On the other hand, unless artificial insemination is used, the quality of the sperm which established the pregnancy is, for the most part, unknown. Therefore, this end-point by which sperm is judged—the ability to produce a gestation—is quite unreliable, particularly when conception is not achieved.

The situation changed dramatically in the late 1970s when in vitro fertilization and embryo transfer came into being, followed by other methods of assisted reproduction. For the first time, investigators interested in male infertility were able to judge human oocyte-sperm interaction. Regardless of whether or not pregnancy was established, the capability of normal or abnormal sperm to fertilize the female gamete could be readily determined. A new and more reliable end-point was now at our disposal. New approaches to diagnosis and treatment of male factors, and also new procedures for sperm evaluation, manipulation, and preparation were designed. Interest began to drift away from pregnancy as a yardstick by which to measure sperm quality, and the evaluation of the many sperm tests was done by comparing their results with the results of IVF in the human system. The era of using animals for that purpose was ending. Clinicians began to look for new criteria to predict results in IVF and to develop guidelines for the acceptability of male factors into the rapidly moving field of assisted reproduction.

In spite of all efforts, a group of patients were still unable to achieve fertilization in vitro. The interest of scientists shifted once again to developing methods to allow abnormal sperm to fertilize, and a new field—assisted fertilization—emerged.

With these new developments in the area of andrology because of assisted reproduction and assisted fertilization, it seems timely to compile, summarize, critically review, and set forth this knowledge for gynecologists, urologists, andrologists, reproductive endocrinologists, basic scientists, and laboratory technologists. Such a book may be crucial for consolidating information and establishing a platform for future explorations in the field.

The collective experience of the Andrology Laboratories of Eastern Virginia Medical School and Old Dominion University, the program of assisted reproduction at the Jones Institute for Reproductive Medicine, the Tygerberg Clinic at the University of Stellenbosch, and many outstanding clinicians and researchers from other institutions who generously contributed to this book has been compiled to update the knowledge in the field and to describe the diagnostic and therapeutic tests now in use. This collaborative effort stresses the need for a multidisciplinary-multicenter approach to solve the intricacies of the male infertility problem.

We have come a long way since sperm was discovered as one of the main elements of human reproduction, but we still have a long way to go to unveil all the scientific facts of sperm function. Past and future, ignorance and knowledge, despair and hope, faith and skepticism, empiricism and science have been the extremes through which we have moved in this very delicate area of reproduction and perhaps represent the extremes through which we will continue to move, at least in the near future. To make these efforts worthwhile, this work was conceived and published.

A. A. Acosta   T. F. Kruger
R. J. Swanson   J. A. van Zyl
S. B. Ackerman   R. Menkveld

Acknowledgments

The authors wish to thank the following members of the Jones Institute: Dr. Mason C. Andrews, Chairman of the Department of Obstetrics and Gynecology, for continued support and encouragement; Myra Waters for secretarial assistance; Debi Jones for data processing; Anne Cromwell, Mindy Spicer, Clay Camp, and Carol Afflerbach of the Andrology Laboratory; Beverly Cox, Shirley Robinson, and Ruth Shaw of the Endocrinology Laboratory; Nurses Catherine Kruithoff, Carol Lundquist, Doris Gentilini, Kerry Castillo, and Terri Capps, and medical assistant Sharon Everett.

The authors also wish to thank the following staff of the Tygerberg Hospital: Professor H. J. Odendaal, Head of the Department of Obstetrics and Gynecology, for administrative support; Sisters J. Joubert, M. Silvis, and M. Verwey, and Nurses E. Janse van Rensburg and J. Geldenhuys for patient care and retrieval of clinical data; Mrs. E. Conradie and Mr. P. Afrika for the high standard of the laboratory work; Mrs. M. Van Deventer, L. Do Bruyn, and M. Steenkamp for administrative work and retrieval of data; Mrs. C. Viljeer for illustrations; Mrs. J. Husselman for manuscript preparation; and Mrs. Helena Kruger for editorial and secretarial assistance.

Research by Lourens J. D. Zaneveld and Patricia Pleban in Chapters 4 and 5 was partially supported by National Institutes of Health grant no. HD 19555.

Contributors

ACKERMAN, Steven B., Ph.D., Andrology Laboratory, Jones Institute for Reproductive Medicine, Eastern Virginia Medical School, Norfolk, Virginia

ACOSTA, Anibal A., M.D., Professor of Obstetrics and Gynecology, Jones Institute for Reproductive Medicine, Eastern Virginia Medical School, Norfolk, Virginia

ACOSTA, Maria Rosa, B.S., Andrology Laboratory, Jones Institute for Reproductive Medicine, Eastern Virginia Medical School, Norfolk, Virginia

ALEXANDER, Nancy J., Ph.D., Chief of Reproductive Immunology, Division of Basic Research, Professor of Obstetrics and Gynecology, Jones Institute for Reproductive Medicine, Eastern Virginia Medical School, Norfolk, Virginia

AMUNDSON, Cathy H., B.S., Embryology Laboratory, Jones Institute for Reproductive Medicine, Eastern Virginia Medical School, Norfolk, Virginia

AUSTIN, Ramona, B.S., Department of Biology, Old Dominion University, Norfolk, Virginia

BOCCA, Silvina, M.S., Cryobiology Laboratory, Jones Institute for Reproductive Medicine, Eastern Virginia Medical School, Norfolk, Virginia

BROTHMAN, Lisa J., B.S., Embryology Laboratory, Jones Institute for Reproductive Medicine, Eastern Virginia Medical School, Norfolk, Virginia

BRUCKER, Cosima, M.D., Reproductive Immunology, Jones Institute for Reproductive Medicine, Eastern Virginia Medical School, Norfolk, Virginia

BRUGO-OLMEDO, Santiago, M.D., Chief, In Vitro Fertilization Laboratory and Department of Andrology, Centro de Ginecologia y Reproduccion, Buenos Aires, Argentina

BURKMAN, Lani J., Ph.D., Andrology Laboratory, Jones Institute for Reproductive Medicine, Eastern Virginia Medical School, Norfolk, Virginia

CLAASSENS, Weldi, B.S., Reproductive Biology Unit, Department of Obstetrics and Gynecology, Tygerberg Hospital, Tygerberg, South Africa

CLAEYS, Geert, M.D., Department of Bacteriology, State University of Ghent, Ghent, Belgium

CODDINGTON, Charles C., M.D., Department of Obstetrics and Gynecology, Portsmouth Naval Medical Center, Portsmouth, Virginia

COETZEE, Kevin, M.S., Reproductive Biology Unit, Department of Obstetrics and Gynecology, Tygerberg Hospital and University of Stellenbosch, Tygerberg, South Africa

COMHAIRE, Frank H., M.D., Doctor in Andrology and Endocrinology, State University of Ghent, Ghent, Belgium

DELLENBACH, Pierre, M.D., Professor of Obstetrics and Gynecology, Louis Pasteur University, Strasbourg, France

DE VILLIERS, Amanda, M.C.T., Andrology Laboratory, Department of Obstetrics and Gynecology, Tygerberg Hospital and University of Stellenbosch, Tygerberg, South Africa

DE VILLIERS, Tobie J., M.D., Reproductive Biology Unit, Department of Obstetrics and Gynecology, Tygerberg Hospital and University of Stellenbosch, Tygerberg, South Africa

ERASMUS, Evelyn, M.S., Reproductive Biology Unit, Department of Obstetrics and Gynecology, Tygerberg Hospital and University of Stellenbosch, Tygerberg, South Africa

FAGLA, Blayse, B.S., State University of Ghent, Ghent, Belgium

FRANKEN, Daniel R., Ph.D., Infertility Laboratory, Department of Obstetrics and Gynecology, University of the Orange Free State, Bloemfontein, South Africa

FULGHAM, David L., B.A., Reproductive Immunology, Jones Institute for Reproductive Medicine, Eastern Virginia Medical School, Norfolk, Virgina

GROBLER, Greg M., M.D., Reproductive Biology Unit, Department of Obstetrics and Gynecology, Tygerberg Hospital and University of Stellenbosch, Tygerberg, South Africa

HINTING, Auk, M.D., Ph.D., Second Chair of Medicine, Department of Biological Medicine, Airlangga University, Suraba, Indonesia

HODGEN, Gary D., Ph.D., Chief of Pregnancy Research, Jones Institute Research Labortories, Professor of Obstetrics and Gynecology, Jones Institute for Reproductive Medicine, Eastern Virginia Medical School, Norfolk, Virginia

HULME, Victor, M.D., Reproductive Biology Unit, Department of Obstetrics and Gynecology, Tygerberg Hospital and University of Stellenbosch, Tygerberg, South Africa

IRIANNI, Francisco, M.D., Newport News, Virginia

JEYENDRAN, Rajasingam S., D.V.M., Ph.D., Department of Obstetrics and Gynecology, College of Medicine, Rush University, Rush-Presbyterian-St. Luke's Medical Center and Institute for Reproductive Medicine, Chicago, Illinois

JONES, Georgeanna Seegar, M.D., Vice President, Jones Institute for Reproductive Medicine, Professor of Obstetrics and Gynecology, Eastern Virginia Medical School, Norfolk, Virginia; Professor Emeritus of Gynecology and Obstetrics, The Johns Hopkins University School of Medicine, Baltimore, Maryland

JONES, Howard W., Jr., M.D., President, Jones Institute for Reproductive Medicine, Professor of Obstetrics and Gynecology, Eastern Virginia Medical School, Norfolk, Virginia; Professor Emeritus of Gynecology and Obstetrics, The John Hopkins University School of Medicine, Baltimore, Maryland

KAMINSKI, Joanne M., Ph.D., Department of Obstetrics and Gynecology, College of Medicine, Rush University, Rush-Presbyterian-St. Luke's Medical Center, Chicago, Illinois

KOTZE, Theuns J. van W., Ph.D., Institute for Biostatistics, Medical Research Council, Tygerberg, South Africa

KRAJESKI, Patricia, B.S.N., Rush-Presbyterian-St. Luke's Medical Center, Chicago, Illinois

KREINER, David, M.D., Director, Long Island In Vitro Fertilization Program, Mather Memorial Hospital, Port Jefferson, New York

KRUGER, Thinus F., M.D., Reproductive Biology Unit, Department of Obstetrics and Gynecology, Tygerberg Hospital and University of Stellenbosch, Tygerberg, South Africa

LANZENDORF, Susan E., Ph.D., Oregon Regional Primate Center, Beaverton, Oregon

LOMBARD, Carl J., Ph.D., Institute for Biostatistics, Medical Research Council, Tygerberg, South Africa

MAHONY, Mary Condon, M.S., Division of Reproductive Immunology, Jones Institute for Reproductive Medicine, Eastern Virginia Medical School, Norfolk, Virginia

MENARD, Agnes, M.D., Department of Obstetrics and Gynecology, Louis Pasteur University, Strasbourg, France

MENKVELD, Roelof, Ph.D., Andrology Laboratory, Department of Obstetrics and Gynecology, Tygerberg Hospital and University of Stellenbosch, Tygerberg, South Africa

MOREAU, Laurence, M.D., Department of Obstetrics and Gynecology, Louis Pasteur University, Strasbourg, France

MORSHEDI, Mahmood, Ph.D., Director, Cryobiology Laboratory, Jones Institute for Reproductive Medicine, Eastern Virginia Medical School, Norfolk, Virginia

MUASHER, Suheil J., M.D., Director of In Vitro Fertilization, Jones Institute for Reproductive Medicine, Associate Professor of Obstetrics and Gynecology, Eastern Virginia Medical School, Norfolk, Virginia

OEHNINGER, Sergio, M.D., Department of Obstetrics and Gynecology, Jones Institute for Reproductive Medicine, Eastern Virginia Medical School, Norfolk, Virginia

PLEBAN, Patricia, Ph.D., Department of Chemical Sciences, Old Dominion University, Norfolk, Virginia

PRETORIUS, Elize, M.S., Reproductive Biology Unit, Department of Obstetrics and Gynecology, Tygerberg Hospital and University of Stellenbosch, Tygerberg, South Africa

RODRIGUEZ-RIGAU, Luis J., M.D., Texas Institute for Reproductive Medicine and Endocrinology, Houston, Texas

ROSENWAKS, Zev, M.D., Director of In Vitro Fertilization, Professor of Obstetrics and Gynecology, Cornell University Medical Center, The New York Hospital, New York, New York; formerly Professor of Obstetrics and Gynecology, Jones Institute for Reproductive Medicine, Eastern Virginia Medical School, Norfolk, Virginia

SCHOONJANS, Frank, B.S., State University of Ghent, Belgium

SCOTT, Richard T., M.D., Department of Obstetrics and Gynecology, Jones Institute for Reproductive Medicine, Eastern Virginia Medical School, Norfolk, Virginia

SIMMONS, Kathryn, M.S., Department of Andrology, Jones Institute for Reproductive Medicine, Eastern Virginia Medical School, Norfolk, Virginia

SIMONETTI, Simonetta, M.S., Embryology Laboratory, Jones Institute for Reproductive Medicine, Eastern Virginia Medical School, Norfolk, Virginia

STANDER, Frik S. H., Chief Clinical Technician, Reproductive Biology Unit, Department of Obstetrics and Gynecology, Tygerberg Hospital, Tygerberg, South Africa

STEVENS, Ralph W. III, Ph.D., Department of Biology, Old Dominion University, Norfolk, Virginia

SWANSON, R. James, R.N., Ph.D., Director, Andrology Laboratory, Jones Institute for Reproductive Medicine, Eastern Virginia Medical School and Old Dominion University, Norfolk, Virginia

VAN DER MERWE, Jacobus P., M.D., Reproductive Biology Unit, Department of Obstetrics and Gynecology, Tygerberg Hospital and University of Stellenbosch, Tygerberg, South Africa

VAN ZYL, Johannes A., M.D., Andrology Laboratory, Department of Obstetrics and Gynecology, Tygerberg Hospital and University of Stellenbosch, Tygerberg, South Africa

VEECK, Lucinda L., M.L.T., Director, Embryology Laboratory, Jones Institute for Reproductive Medicine, Eastern Virginia Medical School, Norfolk, Virginia

VERMEULEN, Lutgarde, Industrial Engineer in Chemistry, Department of Andrology and Endocrinology, State University of Ghent, Belgium

VERSCHRAEGEN, Gerda, M.D., Department of Bacteriology, State University of Ghent, Belgium

WINDT, Marie-Lena, M.S., Reproductive Biology Unit, Department of Obstetrics and Gynecology, Tygerberg Hospital and University of Stellenbosch, Tygerberg, South Africa

WITTEMER, Christiane, Ph.D., Director, In Vitro Fertilization Laboratory, Centre Medico Chirurgical et Obstetrical, Schiltigheim, France

ZANEVELD, Lourens J. D., D.V.M., Ph.D., Department of Obstetrics and Gynecology, College of Medicine, Rush University, Rush-Presbyterian-St. Luke's Medical Center, Chicago, Illinois

Contents

Introduction

Since the original description of the sperm by van Leeuwenhoek in 1696 (Figs. i.1–i.3), there has been an enormous clinical and basic research effort to understand the physiology and pathology of the sperm and semen, and the significance of the changes observed in terms of reproduction, both in veterinary and human medicine. In spite of the advances made in those fields, the diagnosis and treatment of male infertility lags well behind the understanding of female reproductive function.

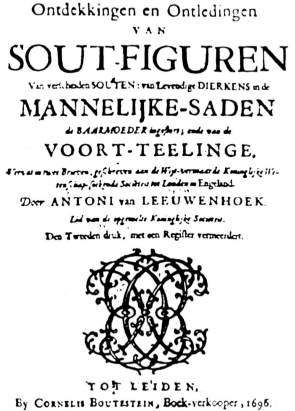

Figure i.1.

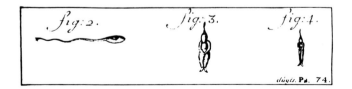

Sevende Vervolg der BRIEVEN, enz.   75

in 't werk geftelt geweeft, want laten wy eens denken,
wat een Perfoon den felven over 25. Jaren is geweeft.
   Hier hebt gy Wel Edele geftrenge Heer, het geene
ik in den Jare 1677. en in 't begin van den Jare 1678.
de KoninklijkeSocieteit hebbe toe gefonden,en fchoon
ik eLucele faaken , die onbekent waren, hebbe aan den

A. van Leeuwenhoek.

K 2   114 de. MIS-

Figure i.2.

When assisted reproduction and then assisted fertilization came into the therapeutic armamentarium for human infertility, it was assumed that male reproductive problems might be helped by those methods, but this tremendous opportunity and challenge was hampered by the lack of knowledge about human sperm when used in those areas. Then, as this knowledge developed, publications and research were widely dispersed in many different journals and books; clinicians and scientists found it difficult to gather literature pertaining to these subjects when they began working in these new fields.

The idea of trying to condense into a book the present knowledge on sperm physiology, pathology, diagnosis, and laboratory manipulation for assisted reproduction and assisted fertilization came naturally as a result of working in these areas. It was necessary to envision a book with fundamental concepts which the clinician, andrologist, urologist, gynecologist, reproductive endocrinologist, or general endocrinologist might need in his/her daily work in these areas of reproduction and would also include the principal laboratory procedures and the clinical results obtained with these techniques.

A description of basic sperm anatomy and physiology for the clinician entering the field seems to be mandatory and is presented in Chapter 1.

The andrologic consultation and the evaluation of the female have special characteristics and requirements for a couple applying for assisted reproduction or assisted fertilization; these are reviewed in Chapters 2 and 3.

Chapter 4, "Laboratory Procedures," gives a brief background and critical review of the most pertinent literature on the main diagnostic and therapeutic procedures in the evaluation and preparation of sperm. The clinician should understand the fundamental concept of each test and should realize that there are discrepancies in the literature. Much

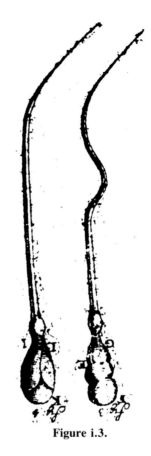

Figure i.3.

of this chapter is devoted to tests of sperm function and their relevance to assisted reproduction and assisted fertilization.

In Chapter 5, ''Evaluation and Preparation of Sperm for in Vitro Fertilization,'' the experience of the authors working with those tests in the clinical arena is emphasized. Although in some areas the reader may find repetition, this was not eliminated because, in our view, repetition is an important part of the learning process. In other areas the reader will find different opinions and results from similar diagnostic and therapeutic methods. These areas are obviously controversial, and further basic or clinical research is necessary to bring some agreement into fields that are still full of uncertainties. Most of the techniques in this chapter are relevant to in vitro fertilization and embryo transfer.

Chapters 4 and 5 are therefore the core of the book. In Chapter 6 sperm manipulation and the results with another method of assisted reproduction, gamete intrafallopian transfer (GIFT), are described and reported. GIFT is an area in which significantly more experience is needed before one reaches a conclusion, but a condition sine qua non is to unify the criteria for diagnosis and categorization of the male factor. Otherwise, the results obtained with GIFT or any other method of assisted reproduction or assisted fertilization in the male factor will be meaningless.

Chapter 7 reviews the experience in the literature and in our centers with the use of therapeutic intrauterine insemination. A similar problem can be identified in evaluating the results: the lack of uniform criteria in defining the male factor defeats the purpose of judging the reported outcomes.

Artificial insemination by donor (AID) was the first method of assisted reproduction for human infertility and has undergone radical modifications since the discovery and proliferation of acquired immune deficiency syndrome (AIDS), with its ironically similar acronym. Substantial changes have been introduced into AID because of AIDS. The use of sperm for therapeutic insemination by donor is reviewed in Chapter 8.

Another technique of insemination, direct intraperitoneal insemination (DIPI), is evaluated in Chapter 9 by the French group which originated the procedure.

Cryopreservation is now in the forefront of assisted reproduction using donor sperm, particularly since the use of fresh sperm has been banned because of AIDS. Cryopreserved sperm is also used in other modalities of assisted reproduction, such as in vitro fertilization and GIFT. Chapter 10 is devoted to these laboratory procedures.

The criteria used to evaluate sperm quality and the results of tests used to determine sperm fertilizing ability need to be reassessed from time to time, mainly by groups with long-standing experience involving a large population. Since those groups are also working in assisted reproduction, they can perform simultaneous evaluation and comparison, as reported in Chapter 11.

The donor egg program, discussed in Chapter 12, is the counterpart of the donor sperm program. Besides its therapeutic importance in solving problems of gametogenesis in females with normal uteri, it has taught us a great deal about using artificial cycles to prepare a physiologically competent endometrium, and it has helped us understand the window of transfer and the window of implantation in those patients. It has also allowed us, for the first time, to separate the maternal environment from the quality of the oocyte, which can now be measured separately.

Chapter 13, "Research on Sperm in Assisted Reproduction," addresses new techniques in the field. Sperm microinjection, for example, has been proposed as the ultimate solution to sperm problems which other procedures have failed to solve. Reservations about techniques which bypass the normal steps of sperm selection and which use sperm of doubtful or unknown quality to force fertlization must be addressed by all involved researchers to determine the place of these techniques in the treatment of severe male factor infertility.

The quantitation of sperm attachment to the zona pellucida in the human is an indirect way of measuring the quality of the sperm receptor and fills the gap in the step-by-step evaluation of sperm fertilizing potential. The hemizona assay is one way to accomplish this.

Our dream of measuring DNA content in the sperm by more accurate means has not been fulfilled. Flow cytometry, although promising, has been unable to clearly distinguish different sperm populations. Some efforts to apply this technique are described in the latter part of Chapter 13.

The fact that the skills and capabilities of many researchers and scientists were needed to create this book underscores the multidisciplinary needs and team efforts required to decipher the role of sperm in assisted reproduction and assisted fertilization. We will continue these efforts to make the present knowledge in the field easily available to the clinician. This book, even with the imperfections it may have, is our first attempt to accomplish that.

Anibal A. Acosta, M.D.
T. F. Kruger, M.D.
November 9, 1988

CHAPTER 1

Basic Spermatozoon Anatomy and Physiology for the Clinician

RALPH W. STEVENS III, PH.D.

This chapter presents the concepts and terminology related to spermatogenesis, as well as the hormonal requirements, kinetics, and morphological changes occurring as the germ cells differentiate during spermatogenesis. The morphological correlates of the differentiating germ cells are discussed at the light and electron microscopic (LM and EM) levels, and techniques for qualitative and quantitative assessments of the spermatogenic process are introduced. Comparisons of human and rodent spermatogenesis are discussed. As rodent spermatogenesis is so well understood, many of the terms and techniques were introduced describing this animal model.

Male gamete formation—spermatogenesis—occurs in the seminiferous tubules of the testis. The process is continuous in the adult male and involves mitotic and meiotic events. During embryological development, the primordial germ cells migrate from the yolk sac to the germinal (genital) ridge. Fetal testicular development requires both the primordial germ cell (gonocyte) and the somatic element of the seminiferous tubule (the Sertoli cell). During fetal development, germinal and somatic elements divide within the tubule. In this period of rapid cellular division, characteristic intercellular junctions between Sertoli cells do not form, and there is no differentiation between the basal and adluminal compartment. During human prepubertal development, Sertoli cells no longer divide, and spermatogonial differentiation occurs with bursts of mitotic and unsuccessful meiotic activity, resulting in cell death. In rodents the situation is different, since spermatogonial development is uninterrupted, beginning late in the fetal period and leading to successful meiotic and post-meiotic development. In both humans and rodents, post-meiotic development (spermiogenesis) is a maturational event associated with characteristic morphological changes. It is followed by release of the elongated spermatid (spermiation) from the Sertoli cell, yielding spermatozoa. The sperm leave the seminiferous tubule, enter the rete testis and efferent ductules, then enter the epididymis. Leaving the epididymis, the sperm enter the ductus deferens (vas deferens), then the ampulla of the ductus deferens and the ejaculatory duct during ejaculation. The sperm exit the body via the various portions of the urethra (Fig. 1.1).

Figure 1.1. Sketch of male genital organs. *A*, Testis; *B*, head of epididymis; *C*, spermatic cord; *D*, penis; *E*, glans penis; *1*, tunica albuginea; *2* septum of testis; *3*, seminiferous tubule; *4*, mediastinum with rete testis; *5*, efferent ductules; *6*, epididymis; *7*, ductus deferens; *8*, seminal vesicle; *9*, ampulla of ductus deferens; *10*, prostate gland; *11*, ejaculatory duct; *12*, colliculus seminalis; *13*, *14*, and *16*, prostatic, membranous, and penile portions of urethra; *15*, bulb of urethra. (From Kelly DE, Wood RL, Enders AC (eds): Bailey's Textbook of Microscopic Anatomy, 18th ed. Baltimore: Williams & Wilkins, 1984, p 687.)

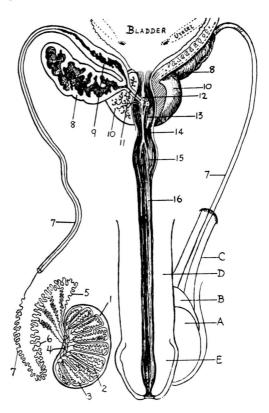

Testicular Anatomy and Physiology

ANATOMICAL ORGANIZATION

The human male gonads are paired, oval, and located in the scrotum. The testes are septated, and the tubules lie coiled in each compartment, whereas the testis of the rat is not septated and the tubules lie parallel. The average weight of the human testis is 15 to 19 g, with a specific gravity of 1.038; the right testis is usually 10% larger than the left (1). The tunic of the testis is composed of a visceral tunica vaginalis, albuginea, and vasculosa.

The scrotum is composed of an outer stratified squamous epithelium, the dartos smooth muscle layer, and a layer of loose connective tissue. Following injury or infection, fluids may accumulate there and the tissue may become edematous; blood may collect there (hematoma); or it may be filled with pus, emphasizing the delineation of the scrotum and testis. Most mammals have scrotal testes. The scrotum facilitates the maintenance of testicular and epididymal temperatures at about 33°C by promoting radiation and conduction of heat and by contraction of the dartos, in response to a cold stimulus by bringing the testes closer to the body and conserving heat. The cremaster muscle surrounds the testis with bands of skeletal muscle and is sandwiched between the external and internal spermatic fascia. It elevates the testis during sexual arousal and exposure to cold (providing a second mechanism for temperature regulation) but is not part of the scrotum (skin and dartos tunic).

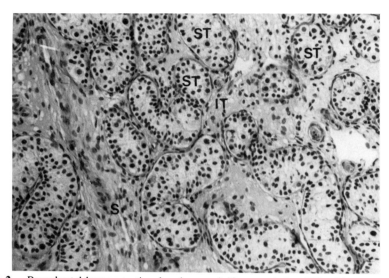

Figure 1.2.   Prepubertal human testis, showing seminiferous tubules (*ST*) without a lumen, septum (*S*), and interstitial tissue (*IT*). Hematoxylin and eosin stain, 200 ×. (From Paniagua R, Nistal M: Morphological and histometric study of human spermatogonia from birth to the onset of puberty. J Anat 139:535, 1984. Printed with permission, Drs. Richardo Paniagua and Manuel Nistal.)

The seminiferous tubules make up the greatest percentage of testicular volume. The interstitial tissue, which includes Leydig cells, stromal tissue, blood vessels, and lymphatic vessels, makes up the remaining portion of the testicular volume (Figs. 1.2 and 1.3). The interstitial tissue of the prepubertal testis represents a greater percentage of testicular volume than the adult testis. In the human adult, interstitial tissue occupies approximately 34% of the testicular volume (2), of which the Leydig cells represent 12%.

Human testicular volume remains unchanged during infancy (birth until the time of erect posture at 12 to 14 months; no longer than the first 24 months) and then increases progressively throughout childhood. The most rapid increase is during early adolescence (9 to 13 years). The seminiferous tubular diameter decreases during infancy and increases thereafter to puberty (3).

The blood-testis barrier is established during puberty (4–7). Tight junctional complexes—occluding junctions—between Sertoli cells separate the basal component (between the basement membrane an the junctional complexes) from the adluminal compartment (between the junctional complexes and the lumen) (Fig. 1.4). This physiological barrier selectively limits entry of interstitial volume into the seminiferous tubule and ensures different testicular micro-environments (8). This barrier also selectively limits the exit of sperm and related antigenic substances. The blood-testis barrier is maintained as the germ cells migrate between the basal and adluminal compartment by these tight junctional complexes forming above and below the migrating germ cell (9). Thus the Sertoli cells determine the environment for all post-mitotic cells, and the gap junctions allow intercellular communication.

ENDOCRINE AND EXOCRINE FUNCTION OF THE TESTIS

The testis is stimulated by gonadotropins, luteinizing hormone or luteotropin (LH), follicle-stimulating hormone or follitropin (FSH), and prolactin or lactotropin. When

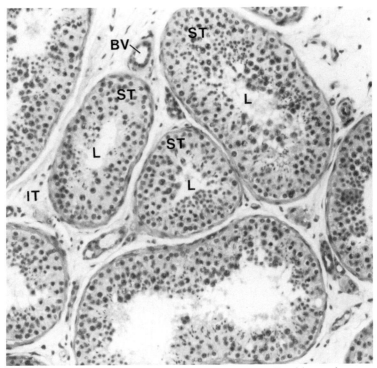

Figure 1.3.   Adult human testis, showing seminiferous tubules (*ST*) without a lumen, septum (*S*), interstitial tissue (*IT*), and blood vessels (*BV*). Hematoxylin and eosin stain, 200×. (From Paniagua R, Nistal M: Morphological and histometric study of human spermatogonia from birth to the onset of puberty. J Anat 139:535, 1984. Printed with permission, Drs. R. Paniagua and M. Nistal.)

stimulated by the gonadotropins, the interstitial compartment—specifically the Leydig cells—produce testosterone, the primary endocrine steroid (10). The Sertoli cells produce non-steroidal endocrine products: inhibin, activin, and müllerian inhibiting substance, to name a few (11, 12). The specific action of these hormones on the testis and the hypothalamic-pituitary-gonadal axis is age-dependent. Within the testes, testosterone stimulates the seminiferous tubule and the accessory sex organs, and feeds back to the hypothalamus and brain to decrease gonadotropin release (Fig. 1.5). Inhibin is involved in the feedback regulation of FSH and has documented effects on the hypothalamic-pituitary-gonadal axis (13). Activin stimulates the release of FSH from the pituitary, among other possible functions (14). The gonadotropins also stimulate the seminiferous tubule directly to produce species-specific products such as transferrin and androgen-binding protein.

The primary exocrine function of the testis is the production of sperm; its secondary exocrine function is the production of the secretions which accompany sperm. These secretions and those of the accessory sex organs are required to carry sperm into the female reproductive tract and to provide the milieu in which sperm can survive and function (15–17). The exact role of the gonadotropins in human spermatogenesis is poorly understood, yet the well-known basic mechanisms are intact. When gonadotropin levels exhibit reduced bioactivity or are non-existent, spermatogenesis is not initiated, resulting, for example, in hypothalamic hypogonadism, hypogonadotropic eunuchoidism, or Kallmann's syndrome. If spermatogenesis has been initiated and maintained,

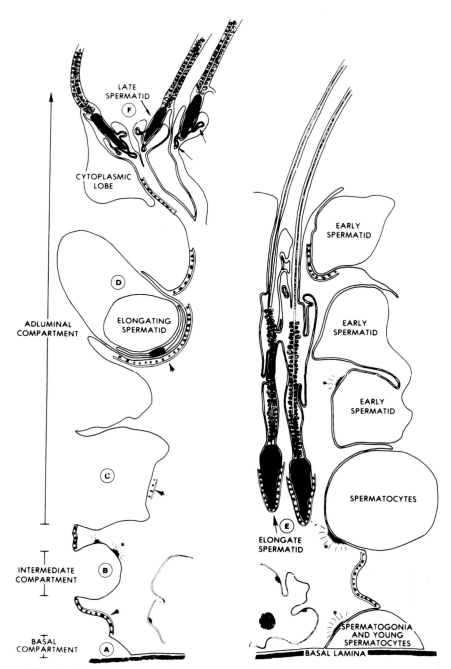

Figure 1.4. Positions of the developing spermatogenic cells in relation to the surface of a Sertoli cell. The cytoplasm of the Sertoli cell occupies the center of the figure and is split to portray its two lateral surfaces in proximity. At level *A*, spermatogonia and young spermatocytes are covered by adjacent Sertoli cells that meet above them to form occluding junctions of the blood-testis barrier. At level *B*, cells leaving the basal compartment are removed from the basal lamina, and Sertoli cells form junctional complexes below them. At level *C*, once the Sertoli junctions above the spermatocele dissociate, the germ cell is in the adluminal compartment. At level *D*, elongating spermatids become situated within a narrow recess of the Sertoli cell. At level *E*, this recess deepens as the spermatid elongates. At level *F*, the germ cell moves toward the lumen, where only its head region is related to the Sertoli cell. Specialized contacts: *arrowheads*, ectoplasmic specialization; *, desmosome-gap junctional complex. (From Kelly DE, Wood RL, Enders AC (eds): Bailey's Textbook of Microscopic Anatomy, 18th ed. Baltimore: Williams & Wilkins, 1984, p 690.)

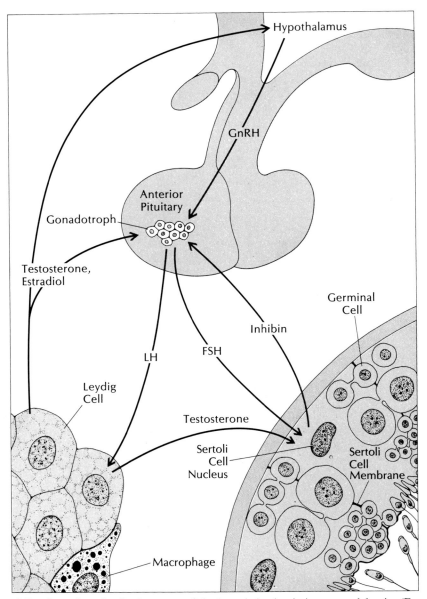

Figure 1.5. Long-loop feedback system of the hypothalamic-pituitary-gonadal axis. (From Bardin CW: Pro-opiomelanocortin peptides in reproductive physiology. Hosp Pract (Apr 15, 1988), p 111. Printed with permission of C. Wayne Bardin, The Population Council, and HP Publishing Company.)

then if there is a loss of gonadotropins due to injury or hypophysectomy, spermatogenesis ceases. The induction of spermatogenesis in many of these patients followed the classic rodent studies of Steinberger and Duckett (18), who showed different roles for FSH and LH during the initiation and maintenance of spermatogenesis. These studies have been used to explain why a patient with Kallmann's syndrome required a regimen of human chorionic gonadotropin (hCG) and human menopausal gonadotropin to initiate spermatogenesis but only hCG to maintain spermatogenesis (19). The intricacies of these feedback systems are beyond the scope of this chapter (but see 12, 13, 19–21).

Cellular Morphology

SERTOLI CELLS

Sertoli cells are the only somatic element in the seminiferous tubule (22). These cells have an irregularly shaped nucleus, a distinctive tripartite nucleolus, and volumninous cytoplasm that envelops the differentiating germ cell and extends from the basement membrane to the lumen of the seminiferous tubule (23–25). In the rat, the number of Sertoli cells per unit area of the basement membrane remains constant, regardless of the stage of the cycle of the germinal epithelium (26, 27). Similar findings have been observed in the human (28). Sertoli cells are resistant to treatments which destroy germ cells: e.g., irradiation, hypophysectomy, and elevated testicular temperature (20). In the human and other species, mitotic activity ceases after infancy (29, 30). Before puberty in the human, the immature Sertoli cells show a pseudo-stratified disposition, the nucleus is round or elongated, and a single nucleolus is close to the nuclear envelope (28). Sertoli-Sertoli junctional complexes (5) do not exist; thus the blood-testis barrier is not complete, although desmosomes are found (28).

HUMAN SPERMATOGONIA

Eight populations of spermatogonia can be described morphologically. The distinctions are not merely esoteric but assist us in understanding fetal and postpartum germ cell development. Various forms of oligospermia can be associated with failure of specific populations of spermatogonia. Radiotherapy and chemotherapy (31) (ifosfamide plus trofosfamide) and the anti-androgen cyproterone acetate selectively decrease the Ad population of cells (32). The Ap population is more sensitive to advancing age and decreases approximately 65% between the 3rd and 8th decade (33).

Gonocytes or primordial germ cells are large and light-staining. The nucleus is spherical, containing fine chromatin granules and two or more globular nucleoli (29). These cells differentiate into spermatogonia shortly before or just after birth.

Fetal spermatogonia at the LM or EM level vary in size and shape but are usually large and round with disperse chromatin and some dense chromatin around the nuclear membrane. These spermatogonia usually disappear by 6 years of age (Fig. 1.6).

Transitional spermatogonia at the LM or EM level are much like fetal spermatogonia; however, the chromatin is less dispersed. These spermatogonia also usually disappear by 6 years of age (Fig 1.7).

Type Ap (pale) spermatogonia at the LM or EM level are similar in size to the Ad spermatogonia. The cell and nucleus are round. The nucleus is pale gray, has the appearance of ground glass, and has a peripheral nucleolus. The mitochrondria are clumped (3, 34) (Figs. 1.7–1.10).

Type Ad (dark) spermatogonia at the LM or EM level are similar in size to the Ap, yet the nucleus has darker chromatin and an area that is clear or has a small region with the appearance of ground glass (3, 34). These spermatogonia are the putative resting stem cells (35) (Figs. 1.7–1.10).

Type Al (long) spermatogonia (36) are a variant of the Ad spermatogonia population which has a DNA content varying from 2N to 4N (2 copies of 2N) and is found in

Figure 1.6. Human testis (1 year) showing fetal spermatogonia (*F*). Some dark Sertoli cells are observed (*arrow*). Toluidine blue stain, 1100×. (From Paniagua R, Nistal M: Morphological and histometric study of human spermatogonia from birth to the onset of puberty. J Anat 139:540, 1984). Printed with permission, Drs. Richardo Paniagua and Manuel Nistal.)

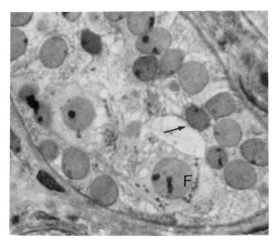

Figure 1.7. Human testis (1 year) showing transitional (star), type *Ad*, and type *Ap* spermatogonia. Some light (*LS*) and dark (*DS*) Sertoli cells are observed 2100×. (From Paniagua R, Nistal M: Morphological and histometric study of human spermatogonia from birth to the onset of puberty. J Anat 139:542, 1984. Printed with permission, Drs. Ricardo Paniagua and Manuel Nistal.)

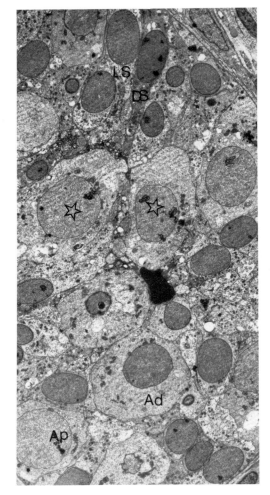

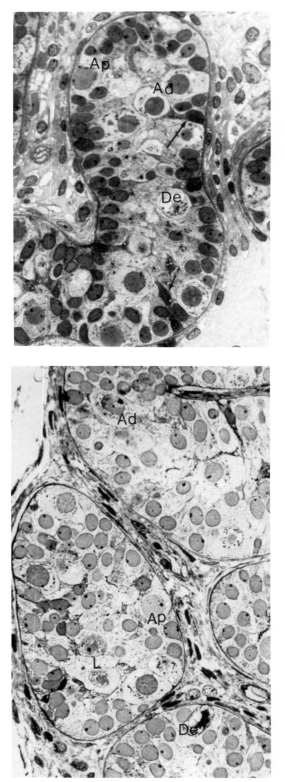

Figure 1.8. Human testis (2 years) showing both basal and adluminal spermatogonia of the *Ad* and *Ap* types, and some degenerating (*De*) spermatogonia. Some dark Sertoli cells are observed (*arrows*). 700×, hematoxylin and eosin stain. (From Paniagua R, Nistal M: Morphological and histometric study of human spermatogonia from birth to the onset of puberty. J Anat 139:540, 1984. Printed with permission, Drs. Ricardo Paniagua and Manuel Nistal.)

Figure 1.9. Human testis (7 years) showing both basal and adluminal (*L*) spermatogonia of the *Ad* and *Ap* types, and some degenerating (*De*) spermatogonia, some of which are observed in an adluminal position (*L*) 700×. (From Paniagua R, Nistal M: Morphological and histometric study of human spermatogonia from birth to the onset of puberty. J Anat 139:540, 1984. Printed with permission, Drs. Ricardo Paniagua and Manuel Nistal.)

Figure 1.10. Human testis (8 years) showing primary spermatocytes (*SPC*) and light (*S*) Sertoli cells. Unmarked luminal types Ad and Ap spermatogonia can also be observed. 700×. (From Paniagua R, Nistal M: Morphological and histometric study of human spermatogonia from birth to the onset of puberty. J Anat 139:540, 1984. Printed with permission, Drs. Richardo Paniagua and Manuel Nistal.)

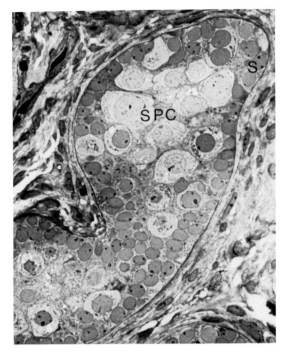

stages III to V (35). Type Al is not distinguishable from Ap at the LM level; however, the EM level shows them to be more flattened and elongated, with an irregular nucleus and trabecular nucleolus (Fig. 1.5).

Type Ac (cloudy) spermatogonia have intermingled dark and pale chromatin areas (32). This type is a variant of the Ap population, has a DNA content varying from 2N to 4N, and is found in stages III to VI (35).

Type B spermatogonia are smaller than Ap and Ad and have less intimate contact with the basal lamina. In the nucleus there are several heterochromatin masses near or attached to the nuclear membrane. At the EM level there are several differences in the cytoplasmic organelles: a more developed Golgi apparatus, and smooth and rough endoplasmic reticulum (3) (Fig. 1.11).

SPERMATOCYTES

The resulting spermatocytes from the final mitotic division of type B spermatogonia enter a resting or pre-leptotene phase. The phases of meiotic prophase follow the classic pattern as the cells leave the basal compartment. The chromatin becomes visible, and the leptotene spermatocyte has a filamentous pattern. The zygotene shows a denser, coarser, more granular chromatin pattern. The pachytene and short-lived diplotene spermatocytes possess the largest nucleus and the densest and thickest chromatin; they are the easiest cells to recognize.

SPERMATIDS

The diplotene spermatocyte undergoes diakinesis and the first meiotic reduction division in stage VI, forming a secondary spermatocyte, which is short-lived. The second meiotic division occurs and yields a round spermatid (Sa$_1$) in stage I. Using the periodic

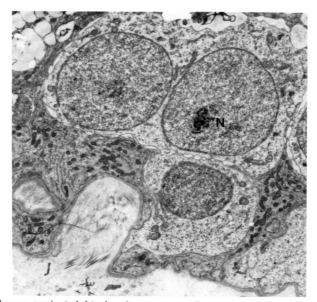

Figure 1.11. Human testis (adult) showing two type B spermatogonia. The chromatin is not homogeneously distributed and forms granules. The nucleolus (*N*) of one type B spermatogonium may be observed. 3000×. (From Paniagua R, Nistal M: Morphological and histometric study of human spermatogonia from birth to the onset of puberty. J Anat 139:546, 1984. Printed with permission, Drs. Richardo Paniagua and Manuel Nistal.)

acid-Schiff (PAS)-hematoxylin stain, Clermont and Leblond (37) described 12 steps in human spermiogenesis. Yet for most descriptions only four to eight steps are used, based on the hematoxylin and eosin (H and E) stain, resulting in six stages (Fig. 1.12). One can observe fusion of the proacrosomic granules (the idiosome is over the nuclear pole) and subsequent spreading of the acrosome over the nucleus. The spermatid in stage II (Sa_2) possesses a round nucleus and a more developed acrosome. The spermatid in stage III (Sb_1) possesses a much more developed acrosomal cap. The spermatid in stage IV (Sb_2) possesses an elongated nucleus that moves to the spermatid plasma membrane and points toward the basement membrane of the seminiferous tubule. The spermatids in stages V, VI, and I (Sc_1, Sc_2, Sd_1) undergo progressive nuclear condensation; the types are almost indistinguishable from each other. Alterations in nuclear shape can be observed during these stages and may result in many of the abnormal sperm forms. The spermatid in stage II (Sd_2) has flattened and become more oval as a result of further nuclear condensation. It has shed most of its cytoplasm and resulting residual body. These final changes and release from the Sertoli cell (spermiation) complete spermiogenesis.

SPERMATOZOA

The spermatozoon is morphologically divided into two parts—the head and tail (Fig. 1.13). The head, condensed nuclear chromatin and acrosomal cap, has a length of approximately 5 to 6 μm and a width of 2.5 to 3.5 μm. The head is divided into regions, the acrosomal and post-acrosomal (Figs. 1.13 and 1.14). The acrosomal region is covered by the plasma, outer acrosomal, inner acrosomal, and nuclear membranes. The post-acrosomal region, or neck, connects the head to the midpiece. The tail, or flagellum,

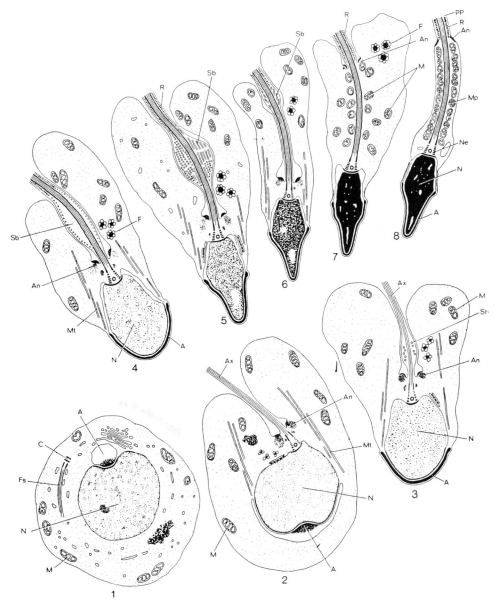

Figure 1.12.   Progressive changes in the spermatid during spermiogenesis, illustrating condensation of the nucleus (*N*), formation of the acrosome (*A*), formation of the axoneme (*Ax*), the fibrous sheath (*R*), and the association of mitochondria (*M*) in the midpiece. (From Kelly DE, Wood RL, Enders AC (eds): Bailey's Textbook of Microscopic Anatomy, 18th ed. Baltimore: Williams & Wilkins, 1984, p 697.)

allows motility in a vibratory, circular, or linear manner (Figs. 1.13, 1.15, and 1.16). The tail has three regions: a midpiece (4.7 μm long × 1 μm wide), a principal piece (50 μm long), and an endpiece of variable length, so that the spermatozoon is approximately 60 μm long (38). The midpiece has a core of the flagellum, surrounded by mitochondria. In cross section the flagellum has an axoneme, a central pair of single microtubules surrounded by nine doublets and the associated dense fibers (Fig. 1.17). The endpiece is

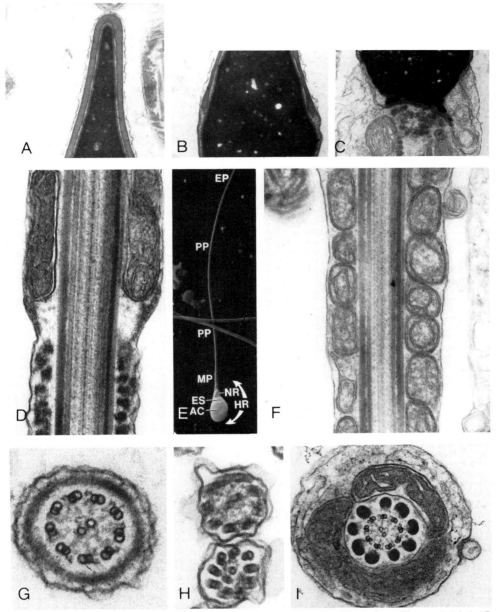

Figure 1.13. A composite of transmission electron micrographs (TEM) from Figures 1.14–1.17 and a scanning electron micrograph (SEM) of a sperm in the center. TEM of the acrosomal cap (*AC*), equatorial segment (*ES*) of the acrosome, and neck region (*NR*), all from the head region (*HR*); midpiece (*MP*) in longitudinal section, midpiece in cross section, endpiece in cross section, principal piece in cross section, and junction of the midpiece and principal piece from the tail section. (Printed with permission of Dr. D. M. Phillips, The Population Council.)

a short segment that lacks any components other than the microtubules of the axoneme and the plasma membrane.

Examination of the spermatozoon at the EM level (Figs. 1.13–1.17) reveals four membranes covering the nuclear material: the cell or plasma membrane, the outer and

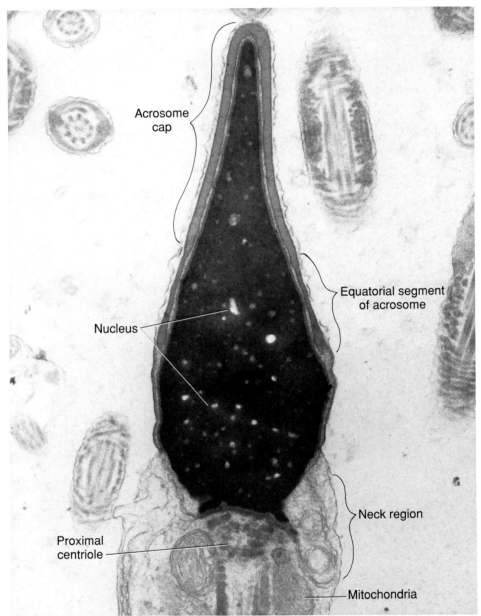

Figure 1.14.   TEM of a longitudinal section of the human sperm head. $54,000 \times$. (Printed with permission of Dr. D. M. Phillips, The Population Council.)

inner acrosomal membranes (which enclose the acrosome), and the clearly visible nuclear membrane covering the head. Fusion of the plasma and outer acrosomal membrane—the acrosome reaction—releases the lytic enzymes. The apical, principal, and equatorial segments make up the acrosomal portion of the head (39, 40). The equatorial segment of the acrosomal region is the initial region of sperm-egg fusion.

At the end of differentiation, the spermatid is freed proximally from its close contact with the Sertoli cell and is released into the tubular lumen. The cytoplasmic tag is

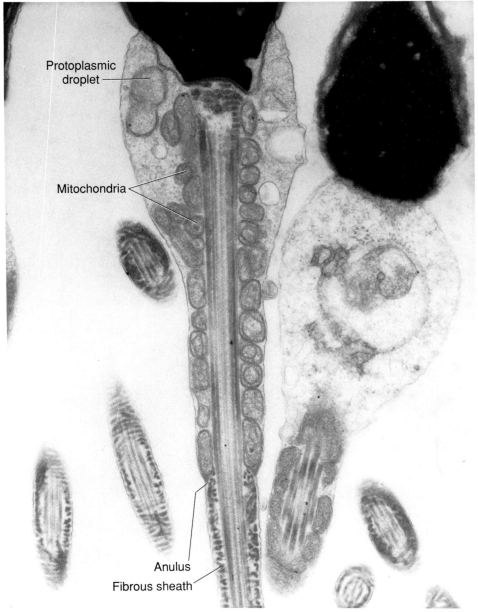

Protoplasmic droplet

Mitochondria

Anulus

Fibrous sheath

Figure 1.15. TEM of a longitudinal section through the midpiece of a human sperm. $32{,}000 \times$. (Printed with permission of Dr. D. M. Phillips, The Population Council.)

divided into two unequal parts. The smaller one, the cytoplasmic droplet, remains with the spermatozoon. The larger part is gradually separated; the residual body can remain attached by narrow cytoplasmic bridges (41). Failure in these final steps of spermiogenesis can result in abnormal forms in the ejaculate.

EM studies have shown that the division of all male germ cells except the most undifferentiated spermatogonia differs from somatic cell division. Following division of the nucleus (karyokinesis), the division of the cell body (cytokinesis) is incomplete, and

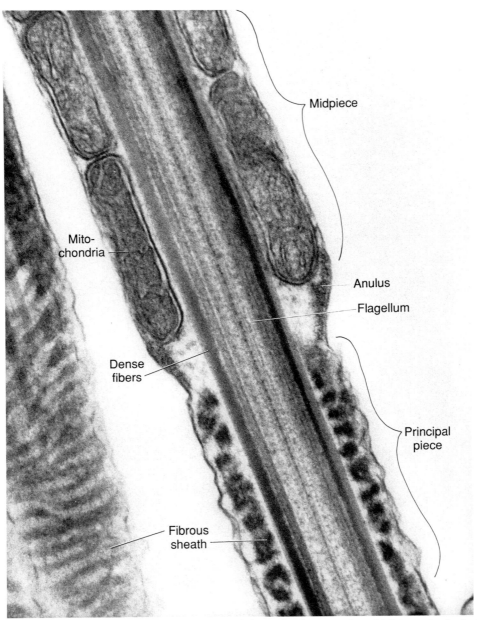

Figure 1.16. TEM of a longitudinal section of the region between the midpiece and principal piece of a human sperm. 140,000×. (Printed with permission of Dr. D. M. Phillips, The Population Council.)

the daughter cells remain connected by protoplasmic, intracellular bridges (42). Thus all type B spermatogonia resulting from the divisions of specific Ap/Ac spermatogonia remain attached and develop in synchrony. These data were incorporated into the clonal concept of Chowdhury and Steinberger) (43) and may explain the synchronized development of large numbers of germ cells, as well as the frequency of double sperm in the ejaculate. When cell death occurs in rodents, all interconnected cells die (44). This has not been documented in the human.

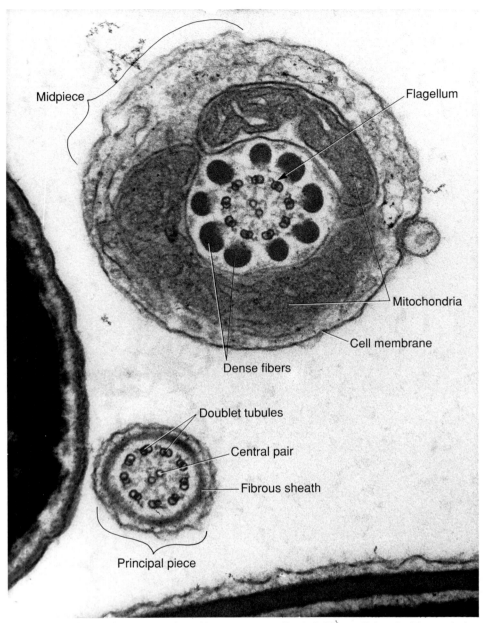

Figure 1.17. TEM of a cross section of human sperm tails. 160,000×. (Printed with permission of Dr. D. M. Phillips, The Population Council.)

Cellular Associations

The classic definition of a stage is the characteristic cellular association discernible in a histological cross section of a seminiferous tubule. In the human, one would observe many

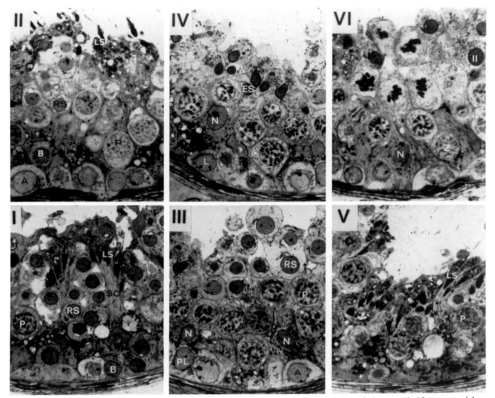

Figure 1.18.   Testis from a normal man. The six stages of the cycle of the seminiferous epithelium are shown. Note the Sertoli cells (*SC*) and the various classes of germ cells: *B*, type B spermatogonium; *P*, pachytene spermatocyte; *RS*, round spermatid; *LS*, late spermatid; *L*, leptotene spermatocyte; *N*, Sertoli cell nucleus; *ES*, early spermatid; *II*, secondary spermatocyte; *PL* preleptotene spermatocyte; *Z*, zygotene spermatocyte. (From Holstein AF, Koerner F: Light and electron microscopic analysis of cell types in human seminoma. Path Anat Histol 363:97, 1974. Printed with permission, Dr. A. F. Holstein.)

different stages of development, due in part to the clonal development of human germ cells. A histological preparation stops development at one moment, analogous to a photo finish in a race. If the photo had been taken about 4 days later, the cells that made up the cellular associations of stage I would have differentiated into the cells of stage II (Fig. 1.18). Figure 1.19 is a series of photomicrographs depicting the classic cellular associations described by Clermont (34) (Table 1.1); stages, I, II, V, and VI stand out. Stages I and II are both round and elongated because of two generations of spermatid, stage IV because of spermatid elongation, and stage VI because of the diplotene spermatocyte and the cells associated with meiotic reduction division. When one analyzes the spermatid population, the notations of Sa, Sb, Sc, and Sd may be confusing. In the Sd population, the loss of spermatid cytoplasm is dramatic, as is the obvious elongation in the Sc population, thus warranting the distinction. The morphological differences in the Sa_1, Sa_2, Sc_1, and Sc_2 populations are less obvious with the H and E stain and, for the most part, represent changes in time which are evident because of morphological changes in other germ cells.

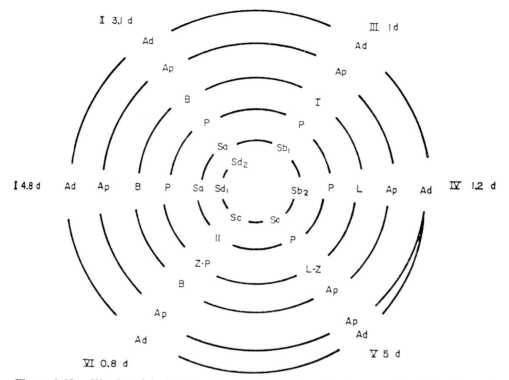

Figure 1.19. Kinetics of the human spermatogenic 16-day cycle shown as cells differentiate and move toward the lumen. (From Paniagua R, Nistal M: Morphological and histometric study of human spermatogonia from birth to the onset of puberty. J Anat 139:535, 1984. Printed with permission, Drs. Ricardo Paniagua and Manuel Nistal.)

Development of Spermatogenesis in Man

KINETICS OF SPERMATOGENESIS DURING DEVELOPMENT

Kinetics, the timing of cellular change or differentiation, is critical to an understanding of spermatogenesis. During human prepubertal development, the Sertoli cells no longer divide, and eight populations of spermatogonia can be described morphologically. Even though the exact lineage of spermatogonia (stem cell progression) is not completely understood, the following progression is a logical representation: gonadocyte[a] → fetal spermatogonia[b] → transitional spermatogonia[b] → Ad spermatogonia[c] to the Al variant → Ap spermatogonia[c] to the Ac variant → type B spermatogonia.[d] During the prepubertal years, spermatogonial differentiation occurs in bursts of mitotic and meiotic activity. The spermatocyte and spermatid progeny of these divisions do not continue to differentiate and die (45–47).

---

[a]Not observable at birth.
[b]Not observable after 6 years of age.
[c]Observable in increasing numbers from birth to adulthood.
[d]Observable after the age of 4 years and throughout adulthood.

Table 1.1.
Cellular Associations[a]

Stage	Spermatogonia	Spermatocyte	Spermatid
1	Ad, Ap type A; type B	Pachytene	Sa_1, Sd_1
2	Ad, Ap type A; type B	Pachytene	Sa_2, Sd_2
3	Ad, Ap,[b] Al, Ac type A	Resting, pachytene	Sb_1
4	Ad, Ap,[b], Al, Ac type A	Leptotene, pachytene	Sb_2
5	Ad, Ap,[b], Al, Ac type A	Leptotene, pachytene	Sc_1
6	Ad, Ap,[b], Ac type A	Zytogene, diplotene	Sc_2

[a] Adapted from Clermont Y: The cycle of the seminiferous epithelium in man. Am J Anat 112:35, 1963.
[b] This somewhat new addendum to Clermont's scheme by Paniagua (34) is an attempt to better explain and correlate the morphological changes observed at the LM and EM levels to aspects of stem cell renewal and differentiation. In addition to the Ap and Ad type A spermatogonia, Al-type spermatogonia are found in stages III to V, and Ac spermatogonia are found in stages III to VI.

KINETICS OF SPERMATOGENESIS DURING ADULTHOOD

When one discusses the kinetics of spermatogenesis in adulthood, one must establish a point of reference, a specific cell type, for example. Different cell types may differentiate at varying rates (stem cells, months to years; spermatogonia, days; pre- and post-meiotic cellular events, weeks). Heller and Clermont (48) used a classic technique of intratesticular titrated thymidine injections and found stage III preleptotene spermatocytes labeled hours after the injection. Sixteen days later, stage II pachytene spermatocytes were found labeled. Thus one cycle was 16 days. The initial 64-day duration of spermatogenesis was based on the assumption that we were dealing with committed, differentiating cells and that only four cycles were needed for spermatogenesis. This scheme did not allow any time for stem cell recruitment. The total maturation time in the human more realistically encompasses 70.4 days, or 4.5 cycles. This time does not allow for epididymal transit or for prolonged inactivity due to the action of cytotoxic agents on stem cell populations. Once a germ cell is committed to differentiate, it has only two options—to become a mature spermatozoon or to die. In human and other species, there is no evidence that age, hormonal deprivation, heat, or cytotoxic agents alter duration; however, these can alter efficiency.

Degeneration of differentiating germ cells is not abnormal unless it renders the patient oligospermic or azoospermic. Multi-nucleated spermatogonia, spermatocytes, or spermatids are thought to be due to incomplete cytokinesis, which can contribute to the abnormal sperm forms in human ejaculate.

Clinical Evaluation of Spermatogenesis

NON-INVASIVE TECHNIQUES

In comparing non-invasive and invasive techniques to evaluate spermatogenesis, one must weigh the information which is needed against the technique necessary to procure it. Non-invasive techniques can analyze the ejaculate, which consists of seminal plasma and sperm. However, the cellular portion may include more than sperm: e.g., sloughed germinal epithelium, abnormal forms of spermatids, macrophages, leukocytes, and urinary tract epithelial cells. The quality of semen depends on the exocrine function of the seminiferous tubules, epididymides, vas deferens, seminal vesicle, prostate, and bulbourethral gland. Analysis of seminal plasma for acid phosphatase, zinc, fructose, citric acid, and a host of other exocrine products gives an indication of accessory sex organ function (15–17). Analysis of semen for sperm-related parameters gives an indication of seminiferous tubular and testicular function. From the quantitative values of sperm number and volume, one can derive sperm density. Qualitative assessment of motility, viability, and directional swimming pattern are highly subjective. With the advent of computer-assisted microscopic semen analysis, many of these qualitative parameters become less subjective, more reliable, and comparable among laboratories. The parameter of abnormal morphology takes on additional meaning as ''normal'' is better defined. Semen can also be analyzed for antisperm antibodies, which may compromise fertility yet have no microscopic correlate other than agglutination.

INVASIVE TECHNIQUES

Invasive techniques include everything from testicular biopsy and orchiectomy to blood samples for antisperm antibody tests. Orchiectomy is reserved for cancer therapy and research purposes. For example, the Heller-Clermont protocol (48) requires intratesticular injection and subsequent orchiectomy. Biopsies may be used to determine the efficacy of a vasovasostomy, to explain azoospermia, to rule out tubular blockage, and to determine age-related differences in germ cell degeneration.

Invasive studies, however, provide unique clinical information. Daily sperm production can be evaluated from ejaculates per milliliter or homogenate testicular tissue per gram of testicular parenchyma. These can then be compared to histological assessments. Daily sperm production is comparable in the right and left testis (49). The homogenate method reveals that there is almost 100% survival of differentiating spermatids as they go from early to late forms (50); 50% of potential sperm production is lost during the prophase of meiosis (51). The age-related differences in germ cell degeneration which result in lower rates of sperm production in older men occur in meiotic prophase during the transition from early (leptotene) to late (pachytene) spermatocytes or among the late spermatocytes (52).

Toxicity

The cytotoxic effects of drugs, pesticides, and other xenobiotics have been associated with decreasing sperm counts. The effects may be on the central nervous system, the hypothalamic-pituitary-gonadal axis, or directly on the testis. The collective impact of xenobiotics may result in decreased sperm count, increased abnormal forms, or azoospermia (53). Cell-specific cytotoxic effects were first described in rats: type A spermatogonial cytotoxicity by triethylenemelamine (54). Hypothalamic-pituitary-gonadal axis disruption was shown to affect specific spermatogonial, spermatocyte, and spermatid populations (55). In the human, radiotherapy and chemotherapy and the antiandrogen cyproterone acetate selectively decrease the Ad spermatogonial population of cells (31). In rats, δ-9-tetrahydrocannabinol (THC) has a direct effect on the Sertoli cells (56); 1,2,dibromo-3-chloropropane (DBCP), chlordecone (kepone), THC, and other xenobiotics also have direct and indirect effects (57).

References

1. Handelsman DJ, Stara S: Testicular size: the effects of aging, malnutrition, and illness. J Androl 6:144, 1985
2. Christensen AK: Leydig cells. In Hamilton DW, Greep RO (eds): Handbook of Physiology, vol 5, sec 7. Washington, DC: American Physiological Society, 1975, p 57
3. Paniagua R, Nistal M: Morphological and histometric study of human spermatogonia from birth to the onset of puberty. J Anat 139:535, 1984
4. Dym M, Fawcett DW: The blood-testis barrier in the rat and the physiological compartmentation of the seminiferous epithelium. Biol Reprod 3:308, 1970
5. Fawcett DW: The mammalian spermatozoa. Dev Biol 44:394, 1975
6. Setchell BP, Waites GMH: The blood-testis barrier. In Hamilton DW, Greep RO (eds): Handbook of Physiology. Williams & Wilkins, 1975, vol 5, p 143
7. Russell LD: The blood-testis barrier and its formation relative to spermatocyte maturation in the adult rat: a lanthanum tracer study. Anat Rec 190:99, 1978
8. Christensen AK, Komorowski TE, Wilson B, Ma S-F, Stevens RW: The distribution of serum albumin in the rat testis, studied by electron microscopic immunocytochemistry on ultrathin frozen sections. Endocrinology 116:1983, 1985
9. Dym M: The fine structure of the monkey (Macaca) Sertoli cell and its role in maintaining the blood-testis barrier. Anat Rec 175:639, 1973
10. Eik-Nes KB: Biosynthesis and secretion of testicular steroids. In Hamilton DW, Greep RO, (eds): Handbook of Physiology. Baltimore: Williams & Wilkins, 1975, vol 5, p 95
11. Mason AJ, Hayflick JS, Ling N, Esch F, Ueno N, Ying S, Guillemin R, Niall H, Seeburg PH: Complementary DNA sequences of ovarian follicular fluid inhibin show precursor structure and homology with transforming growth factor-B. Nature 318:659, 1985
12. Josso N: Antimullerian hormone: new perspective for a sexist molecule. Endocr Rev 7: 421, 1986
13. Steinberger A: Testicular inhibin. Sem Reprod Endocrin 1:357, 1983
14. Ling N, Ying S, Ueno N, Shinaski S, Esch F, Hotta M, Guillemin R: Pituitary FSH is released by a heterodimer of the β-subunits from the two forms of inhibin. Nature 321:779, 1986
15. Yeung CH, Cooper TG, Waites GMH: Carnitine transport into perfused epididymis of the rat: regional differences, stereospecificity, stimulation by choline and other luminal factors. Biol Reprod 23:294, 1980
16. Mann T, Lutwak-Mann C: Male Reproductive Function and Semen. Berlin: Springer-Verlag, 1981
17. Zaneveld LJD, Chatterton RT: Biochemistry of Male Reproduction. New York: John Wiley & Sons, 1982
18. Steinberger E, Duckett GE: The effect of estrogen or testosterone on initiation and maintenance of spermatogenesis in the rat. Endocrinology 76:1184, 1965
19. Matsumoto AM, Bremner WJ: Endocrinology of the hypothalamic-pituitary-testicular axis with particular references to the hormonal control of spermatogenesis. Clin Endocrinol Metab 1:71, 1987
20. Steinberger E: Hormonal control of mammalian spermatogenesis. Physiol Rev 51:1, 1971
21. Rich KA, de Kretser DM: Spermatogenesis and the Sertoli cell. Monogr Endocrinol 25:84, 1983
22. Elftman H: Sertoli cells and testis structure. Am J Anat 113:25, 1963
23. Wong V, Russell LD: Three-dimensional reconstruction of a rat stage V Sertoli cell. I. Methods, basic configuration, and dimensions. Am J Anat 167:143, 1983
24. Webber JE, Russell LD, Wong V, Peterson RW: Three-dimensional reconstruction of a rat stage V Sertoli cell. II. Morphometry of Sertoli-Sertoli and Sertoli-germ cell relationships. Am J Anat 167:163, 1983
25. Russell LD, Tallon-Doran M, Weber JE, Wong V, Peterson RN: Three-dimensional reconstruction of a rat stage V Sertoli cell. III. A study of specific cellular relationships. Am J Anat 167:181, 1983
26. Bustos-Obregon E: On Sertoli cell number and distribution in the rat testis. Arch Biol (Liege) 81:99, 1970
27. Wing T-Y, Christensen AK: Morphometric studies on rat seminiferous tubules. Am J Anat 165:13, 1982
28. Nistal M, Abaurrea MA, Paniagua R: Morphological and histometric study on the human Sertoli cell from birth to the onset of puberty. J Anat 14:351, 1982
29. Clermont Y, Perey B: Quantitative study of the cell population of the seminiferous tubules in immature rats. Am J Anat 100:241, 1957
30. Steinberger A, Steinberger E: The Sertoli cells. In Johnson AD, Gomes R (eds): The Testis. New York: Academic Press, 1978, vol 4, p 371
31. Schulze C: Morphological characteristics of the spermatogonial stem cell in man. Cell Tissue Res 198:191, 1979
32. Schulze W: Leicht- und elektronenmikroskopische studien an de A Spermatogonien von männern mit intakter spermatogenese und bei patienten nach behandlung mit antiandrogenen. Andrologia 10:307, 1978

33. Nistal M, Codesal J, Paniagua R, Santamaria L: Decrease in the number of human Ap and Ad spermatogonia and in the Ap/Ad ratio with advancing age. J Androl 8:64, 1987

34. Clermont Y: The cycle of the seminiferous epithelium in man. Am J Anat 112:35, 1963

35. Paniagua R, Codesal J, Nistal M, Rodriguez MC, Santamaria L: Quantification of cell types throughout the cycle of the human seminiferous epithelium and their DNA content: a new approach to the spermatogonial stem cell in man. Anat Embryol 176:225, 1987

36. Rowley MJ, Berlin J.D., Heller CG: The ultrastructure of four types of human spermatogonia. Zeitschr Zellfor Mikroskop Anat 112:139, 1971

37. Clermont Y, Leblond CP: Spermatogenesis of man, monkey, ram, and other mammals as shown by the 'Periodic Acid-Schiff' technique. Am. J. Anat. 96:229, 1955

38. Cummins JM, Woodall P.F: On mammalian sperm dimensions. J. Reprod. Fert. 75:153, 1985

39. Yanagimachii R: Mechanisms of fertilization in mammals. In Mastroianni L Jr, Biggers JD (eds): Fertilization and Embryonic Development in Vitro. New York: Plenum Press, 1981, p 81

40. Langlais J, Roberts KD: A molecular membrane model of sperm capacitation and acrosome reaction of mammalian spermatozoa. Gam Res 12:183, 1986

41. Breucker H, Schafer E, Holstein A-F: Morphogenesis and fate of the residual body in human spermiogenesis. Cell Tissue Res. 240:303, 1985

42. Dym M, Fawcett DW: Further observations on the number of spermatogonia, spermatocytes, and spermatids connected by intercellular bridges in the mammalian testis. Biol Reprod 4:195, 1971

43. Chowdhury AK, Steinberger E: In vitro ^{3}H-thymidine labeling pattern and topographic distribution of spermatogonia in human seminiferous tubules. In Troen P, Nankin HR (eds): The Testis in Normal and Infertile Men. New York: Raven Press, 1977, p 69

44. Huckins C: The morphology and kinetics of spermatogonial degeneration in normal adult rats: An analysis using a simplified classification of the germinal epithelium. Anat Rec 190:905, 1978

45. Holstein AF, Koerner F: Light and electron microscopic analysis of cell types in human seminoma. Path Anat Histol 363:97, 1974

46. Bustos-Obregon E, Courot M., Flechon JE, Hochereau-de-Reviers MT, Holstein AF: Morphologic appraisal of gametogenesis: spermatogenetic processes in mammals with particular reference to man. Andrologia 7:141, 1975

47. Schulze C: Morphological characteristics of the spermatogonial stem cell in man. Cell Tissue Res 198:191, 1981

48. Heller CG, Clermont Y: Kinetics of the germinal epithelium in man. Recent Prog Horm Res 20:545, 1964

49. Johnson L, Petty CS, Neaves WB: The relationship of biopsy evaluations and testicular measurements to over-all daily sperm production in human testes. Fertil Steril 34:36, 1980

50. Johnson L, Petty CS, Neaves WB: A new approach to quantification of spermatogenesis and its application to germinal cell attrition during human spermiogenesis. Biol Reprod 25:217, 1981

51. Johnson L, Petty CS, Neaves WB: Further quantification of human spermatogenesis: germ cell loss during postprophase of Meiosis and its relationship to daily sperm production. Biol Reprod 29:207, 1983

52. Johnson L, Nguyen H-B, Petty CS, Neaves WB: Quantification of human spermatogenesis: germ cell degeneration during spermatocytogenesis and meiosis in testes from younger and older adult men. Biol Reprod 37:739, 1987

53. Wyrobek AJ: Identifying agents that damage human spermatogenesis: abnormalities in sperm concentration and morphology. IARC Sci Pub. 59:387, 1984

54. Steinberger E: A quantitative study of the effects of an alkylating agent (triethylenemelamine) on the seminiferous epithelium of rates. J Reprod Fertil 3:250, 1962

55. Russell LD, Malone JP, Karpas SL: Morphological pattern elicited by agents affecting spermatogenesis by disruption of its hormonal stimulation. Tissue Cell 13:369, 1981

56. Heindel TJ, Heindel JJ, Keith WB: Delta-9-tetrahydrocannabinol inhibtion of c-AMP accumulation in cultured Sertoli cells from immature rats. Ann NY Acad Sci 513:503, 1987.

57. Foster PMD, Lamb JC: Physiology and Toxicology of Male Reproduction. New York: Academic Press, 1988, pp 1, 7, 137

CHAPTER 2

Andrological Consultation

SANTIAGO BRUGO-OLMEDO, M.D., JOHANNES A. VAN ZYL, M.D., AND SERGIO OEHNINGER, M.D.

Infertility, defined as the inability to produce a pregnancy within a 1-year period of sexual intercourse without contraceptive measures, affects approximately 15% of married couples (1, 2). In addition, probably 10% to 15% of couples have fewer children than they desire. It is estimated that in 40% to 50% of infertile couples the man is infertile, which in the general population equals about 5% to 10% of married men (3, 4). However, infertility should not be viewed as solely male-related or female-related but as relative to varying degrees of fertility potential in both conjugal partners. Marginal male fertility can often be offset by excellent female fertility and vice versa. Therefore, it is strongly advised that both partners undergo simultaneous fertility evaluation.

Causes of Male Infertility

Male infertility can be categorized into five etiological groups: (*a*) testicular causes (factors affecting spermatogenesis); (*b*) post-testicular causes (ductal factors and sexual dysfunctions); (*c*) pretesticular causes (hypothalamic-pituitary disorders and other endocrinopathies); (*d*) genitourinary infections; and (*e*) immunological causes. Defects in spermatogenesis may be associated with primary testicular diseases due to genetic abnormalities (Klinefelter's or Down's syndrome); non-genetic disorders of gonadal development (cryptorchidism, testicular atrophy, germ cell aplasia, Sertoli cell-only syndrome, or even anorchism); varicocele; environmental factors (such as heat); mumps; autoimmune orchitis; certain drugs; radiation orchitis; etc. Malformations or obstructions in the excretory ducts or accessory sex gland dysfunctions may result in oligozoospermia or azoospermia. This may be due to congenital abnormalities (absence of the vas deferens or stenosis of the ejaculatory ducts), post-infectious conditions (epididymitis or prostatitis), or post-surgical causes (vasectomy). Retrograde ejaculation is another relatively infrequent cause, usually as a consequence of diabetic neuropathy, sympathectomy, or injury to the sympathetic nerves, not uncommonly following retroperitoneal node dissection for cancer therapy.

Endocrinopathies associated with male infertility include hypopituitarism, other specific gonadotropin disorders such as Kallmann's syndrome and fertile eunuch syndrome, prolactinomas, and androgen insensitivity states (testicular feminization, androgen resistance), or defective androgen production (congenital adrenal hyperplasia).

Sexual dysfunctions include coital factors or problems in delivery of semen into the vagina (impotence, ejaculatory incompetence, hypospadias, improper coital technique, abnormally long or short abstinence intervals, or improper use of lubricants with spermicidal effects). Although some authors have presented evidence that infection with *Ureaplasma urealyticum, Chlamydia trachomatis*, and other common gram-negative bacteria can cause both male and female infertility, the relationship between genitourinary infections and inability to conceive is still controversial (2). Sperm antibodies, particularly when the sperm antibody level in serum or semen is high, are an accepted cause of infertility. Finally, in a relatively large proportion of patients, no obvious factor can be detected as the cause of infertility; thus these patients are included in an ''idiopathic'' category. Efforts should be made to perform exhaustive and thorough diagnostic tests to categorize these patients adequately.

Clinical History

The cornerstone of the andrological evaluation is the history and physical examination. Although the history is frequently unremarkable in most infertile males, a careful review is still important, since occasionally it will suggest a cause of infertility. As in any other medical specialty, an andrological evaluation must begin with the patient's family history, followed by the personal history, social and sexual history, and finally a physical examination before the semen analysis is performed. In the authors' clinical practice, various questionnaires are used to gather this essential information and to facilitate retrospective studies (Appendices 2.1 and 2.2). Table 2.1 shows the schedule used for serial consultations in the management of the infertile couple, as currently practiced at the Tygerberg Clinic in South Africa.

The duration of the sexual relationship, with and without birth control, should be established, as well as the previous marital history of both partners, including pregnancies.

A patient's occupation may be important, since it is known that several kinds of activity may lead to testicular disorders. There is much speculation that environmental agents and workplace toxins can cause infertility. The only industrial agents now known to cause male infertility are dibromochloropropane, toluenediamine, ethylene dibromide, and lead (5). Pesticides have also been shown to affect gonadal function (6). Because spermatogenesis is heat-sensitive, exposure to excessive heat is thought to reduce sperm production (7). In the human, hyperthermia has been recognized since the time of Hippocrates to be injurious to spermatozoa (8). Numerous clinical observations have linked testicular hyperthermia with reduced spermatogenesis. These observations include the suppression of spermatogenesis in disorders such as cryptorchidism (9, 10), retractile testes (11), and acute febrile diseases (12); oligospermia in men wearing tight jockey shorts and suspensories (13, 14); and reduced conception rates in hot weather and among men who work in environments with high temperatures (15, 16). These observations confirm previous animal studies showing damage to the spermatogenic function of the testes by way of artificial cryptorchidism, acute febrile illness, raised ambient tempera-

Table 2.1.
Schedule for Serial Consultations in the Management of the Infertile Couple

Consultation 1 (Husband and Wife)
1. Interaction: doctor-patients
2. Explanation: history and special investigations
3. BBT[a] charts (3)
4. Spermiograms (4)

Consultation 2 (Husband)
1. History and physical examination
2. Psychosexual history
3. X-ray: skull and chest (when indicated)
4. Serological tests

Probably Fertile
1. Immunological tests
2. Test for genital tract infection

Probably Infertile
1. Same as "probably fertile" 1 and 2
2. Plasma hormones (serial):
   FSH
   LH
   Testosterone
   Estrogen (E_2)
   Prolactin
3. Thyroid function
4. Adrenal function
5. Liver function
6. Hematogram

Test for retrograde ejaculation

Oligozoospermia
1. Same as "probably infertile" 1–6
2. Chromosomal analysis
3. Follow-up semen examinations

Azoospermia
1. Same as "probably infertile" 1–6
2. Same as "oligozoospermia" 2 and 3
3. Testicular biopsy (when indicated)

Aspermia
Test for retrograde ejaculation

Consultation 2 (Wife)
1. History and physical examination
2. Psychosexual history
3. X-ray: skull and chest (when indicated)
4. Serological tests
5. 6–10 menstrual blood specimens (TB culture)
6. Fertility index[b]
7. Immunological tests
8. EUA, D&C, laparoscopy and salpingography simultaneously

Consultation 3 (Husband and Wife)
1. Discussion of factors: male, female, and combined
2. Diagnosis

Consultation 4 (Husband and Wife)
Psychoanalytic consultations
Medical treatment and surgical procedures
Adoption
Artificial insemination

[a]Abbreviations: BBT, basal body temperature; FSH, follicle-stimulating hormone; LH, luteinizing hormone; FSH, follicle-stimulating hormone; EUA, examination under anesthesia; D&C, dilatation and curettage.

ture, and experimental varicocele in various species (7). The bulk of available evidence suggests that spermatozoal damage after heat exposure is related to (*a*) the effects on the early and mature stages of spermatogenesis, (*b*) the location of spermatozoa in the excretory system (seminiferous tubules to the vas deferens), (*c*) species susceptibility to the effect of heat, and (*d*) degree and duration of heat exposure (7). Younger spermatozoa present in the terminal portion of seminiferous tubules and the head of the epididymis are more susceptible to the injurious effect of heat than those spermatozoa present in the tail of the epididymis or in the vas deferens (7). The effect of heat exposure on mature spermatozoa also depends on the temperature obtained and the duration of heat exposure. This is exemplified by studies in boars in which short-term local or whole-body heating that increased testicular temperature by 2° to 7°C adversely affected the structure and function of spermatozoa stored in the epididymis, whereas long-term breeding of cold-climate animals at a higher ambient temperature failed to do so (17). The deleterious effect of short-term high temperature on relatively heat-resistant sperm (from the tail of the epididymis) was also illustrated in in vitro experiments (18). In the rat, scrotal temperature was shown to be a major determinant of the sperm storage capacity of the cauda epididymis (19). The function of young and mature spermatozoa can also be affected by heat, even in the absence of significant morphological changes. Loss of spermatozoa-fertilizing capacity occurs in rabbits 3 days after experimental cryptorchidism (20). Other investigators have shown a reduced survival rate of embryos produced by heat-exposed spermatozoa (21). In the human, studies in patients with varicocele provide most of the available information (7). Morphological abnormalities of spermatozoa (fewer normal oval forms, increased numbers of tapered forms and immature sperm) are frequently found in these patients (22). However, semen analysis findings in patients with varicocele do not always correlate with morphological changes in their testicular tissue, and the same morphological alterations may be present in the semen of other subfertile men without varicocele (23). In paraplegic men with a significantly higher mean testicular temperature after spinal cord injuries, a significant association between high scrotal temperature and lack of motile sperm has been described (14). Heat exposure probably also determines metabolic changes in testicular tissue. In the rabbit, an increase in testicular oxygenation in response to heat application has been found (24). The exact significance of this and other circulatory factors in the genesis of testicular damage remains to be determined (7). In addition, there appears to be a decrease in protein synthesis by sperm exposed to increased temperature, probably due to a fall in the ribosomal activity perhaps resulting from disaggregation of polysomes (25). Other in vitro studies with rat testicular tissue have shown increased permeability of spermatocyte and spermatid membranes and leakage of cytoplasmic constituents when incubated at 37°C (26). A concurrent release of hydrolytic enzymes from the lysosomal membranes has also been observed.

Electromagnetic and ultrasound waves have been shown to impair and compromise testicular function (7). They appear to involve mechanisms of altering testicular tissue metabolism other than those attributed to heat. For example, application of ultrasound alters the charge of proteins and the isoelectric point of the cell membrane and also generates free radicals and peroxides (27). The synergistic effect of heat and these physicochemical changes leads to disruption of spermatogenetic cells at a temperature lower than is necessary for heat alone to cause an equal degree of damage. However, the detrimental dosage and duration of exposure to these agents have not been identified (7).

Table 2.2.
Physical Examination Findings and Semen Analysis Results in Patients with Unilateral Cryptorchidism Treated Surgically or with Gonadotropins at a Prepubertal Age[a]

	Treated Surgically (no. of cases (%); N = 19)	Treated with Gonadotropins (no. cases (%); N = 19)
Physical Examination		
Normal	6 (31.57%)	5 (29.41%)
Unilateral hypotrophy	4 (21.05%)	4 (23.52%)
Bilateral hypotrophy	5 (26.31%)	6 (35.29%)
Unilateral atrophy	3 (15.78%)	2 (11.76%)
Unilateral anorchism	1 (5.26%)	—
Semen Analysis		
Normospermia	2 (10.52%)	2 (11.76%)
Asthenozoospermia	3 (15.78%)	3 (17.64%)
Oligoasthenozoospermia	10 (52.63%)	10 (58.82%)
Azoospermia	3 (15.78%)	2 (11.76%)
Polyzoospermia	1 (5.26%)	—

[a] Data from Centro de Ginecologia y Reproduccion, Buenos Aires, Argentina.

A history of childhood diseases may be an important element in the evaluation of an infertile man. It has been shown that in the male born with a unilateral undescended testis, regardless of the age of orchiopexy, the overall semen quality is considerably poorer than that of normal men (28). Despite this impairment in gonadal function, many men with one undescended testis are able to initiate a pregnancy without difficulty (29). The history of testicular dystopia, however, remains important. Thus it is of great value to indicate whether cryptorchidism has been unilateral or bilateral, at what age the patient was treated, and whether treatment was medical or surgical. Previous studies have shown that in unilateral cryptorchidism, fertility is higher in patients treated with human chorionic gonadotropin (hCG) than in those treated by surgery (30). Bilateral cryptorchidism, regardless of treatment, seriously affects fertility. Tables 2.2 and 2.3 present results from the Centro de Ginecologia y Reproduccion (CEGYR), Buenos Aires, Argentina, after 91 patients (out of 1225 andrological consultations) with a history of unilateral or bilateral cryptorchidism were treated medically (doses of hCG ranging from 6,000 to 45,000 IU) or surgically.

Equally important in the childhood history is a finding of post-pubertal mumps orchitis. Mumps, when experienced pre-pubertally, does not appear to affect the testes. However, after the age of 11 or 12 years, unilateral mumps orchitis is seen in 30% of males affected, and bilateral orchitis in approximately 10% (31). Furthermore, the testicular damage can be quite severe and should be readily seen on physical examination, since the involved gonad will be markedly atrophic (29). In the data from CEGYR, 56 of 1225 patients had post-pubertal mumps. Of these, 18 patients (32%) had subsequent unilateral or bilateral orchitis leading to testicular hypotrophy or atrophy; 10 of them had azoospermia and eight had severe oligo-asthenozoospermia. Of the 10 azoospermic patients, nine had both serum gonadotropin levels increased, while the remaining patient showed normal values but had an abnormal follicle-stimulating hormone (FSH) response to the acute gonadotropin hormone-releasing hormone (GnRH) test.

Table 2.3.
Physical Examination Findings and Semen Analysis Results in Patients with Bilateral Cryptorchidism Treated Surgically or with Gonadotropins at a Prepubertal Age[a]

	Treated Surgically (no. of cases (%), N = 9)	Treated with Gonadotropins (no. of cases (%); N = 8)
Physical Examination		
Normal	2 (22.22%)	5 (62.5%)
Unilateral hypotrophy	2 (22.22%)	—
Bilateral hypotrophy	4 (44.44%)	1 (12.5%)
Unilateral atrophy	—	1 (12.5%)
Bilateral atrophy	1 (11.11%)	1 (12.5%)
Semen Analysis		
Normospermia	1 (11.11%)	1 (12.5%)
Asthenozoospermia	2 (22.22%)	3 (37.5%)
Oligoasthenozoospermia	4 (44.44%)	3 (37.5%)
Azoospermia	2 (22.22%)	1 (12.5%)

[a] Data from Centro de Ginecologia y Reproduccion, Buenos Aires, Argentina.

Other abnormalities in developmental milestones, such as delayed onset of puberty or gynecomastia, may indicate problems with the hypothalamic-pituitary-gonadal axis.

Venereal disease, especially if it is recurrent and improperly treated, has been suggested as another major cause of infertility. Damage to the seminal tract may occur, followed by alterations in seminal plasma constituents, causing asthenozoospermia or other spermatic disorders. Gonococcal and gram-negative epididymitis, if untreated, may result in ductal obstruction (32). Tuberculous infection of the genitalia is uncommon, and appropriate anti-tuberculous therapy usually prevents epididymal occlusion. On the other hand, active urinary tract infections, including non-specific urethritis or chlamydia infection, may influence sperm motility. It is also important to investigate the patient's urinary habits in terms of daily frequency, characteristics of the stream, dysuria, hematuria, prostatorrhea, urinary burning or itching, final dripping, etc., which could indicate a prostatic dysfunction with a subsequent alteration of seminal plasma.

Systemic illnesses may affect semen parameters. As mentioned above, fever can damage the spermatocytes and possibly mature sperm, and oligospermia can appear within 3 weeks of the febrile episode and can last approximately 2 months. Uremia can be associated with impotence and infertility, probably related to a decrease in plasma testosterone. Dialysis does not correct a low count, but successful renal transplantation will. Diabetes mellitus may also result in organic impotence and/or retrograde ejaculation (32).

A history of scrotal trauma is important if it was associated with testicular inflammation or orchitis.

A patient's surgical history is of interest particularly because of the possibility of procedures such as herniorrhaphy causing accidental ligation of the vas deferens, or interference with testicular blood supply resulting in testicular atrophy (32). In addition, urethral surgery may result in strictures impeding the flow of semen. Two new groups of patients are now emerging whose previous diseases render them very likely to be infertile (29). The first group are those who have had operative correction of the bladder neck during childhood concurrent with ureteral reimplantation (33). As a consequence of surgery, these individuals often have retrograde ejaculation, which should be suspected in the man who gives a history of bladder surgery and whose ejaculate is less than 1 ml in volume, oligozoospermic, and abnormally alkaline. The correct diagnosis can be made by finding large numbers of sperm cells in the post-ejaculation urine. The second group requiring urological care for infertility are those with testicular cancer who are now surviving their disease (more than 85% of those treated) (34). These patients experience the sequelae of chemotherapy, radiotherapy, retroperitoneal lymph node dissection, or a combination of these. It also appears that these patients may often have impaired function in their contralateral testis (29). Their semen quality should be viewed with a cautious prognosis if fewer than 5 years have elapsed since treatment, because the return of sperm from the irradiated or chemotherapeutically treated gonad may take 4 or 5 years (35). A patient who has had retroperitoneal lymph node dissection with interruption of the sympathetic nodal chains or the peripheral long nerves may show either aspermia or, less frequently, retrograde ejaculation (36). Some of these patients can be effectively treated pharmacologically with sympathomimetic drugs.

Radiation has its greatest effect on the less differentiated cells (spermatogonia), with relative preservation of the more mature spermatids and spermatozoa (35). A patient who has undergone radiotherapy remains fertile until these mature cells undergo a period of maturation depletion. Although post-meiotic cells survive, they probably have radiation-induced chromosomal abnormalities, and conception during this early post-radiation period is associated with a high risk of lethal or serious non-lethal abnormalities in the fetus (37). This would be manifested by an increasing incidence of spontaneous abortions, stillbirths, or gross congenital abnormalities. After that, the patient undergoes a period of relative sterility or subfertility, which may last from 12 months to 3 or 4 years and is the result of depopulation of the radiosensitive spermatogenic epithelium (38). However, the early type A spermatogonia slowly regenerate. These cells are believed to emanate from a few sluggish type A spermatogonia that have long intermitotic periods and a different sensitivity to radiation (39). With a slow regeneration of the spermatogonia, spermatogenesis recurs and almost always returns to pretreatment levels. This post-radiation fertility probably carries a lower risk of abortion or fetal abnormality because (*a*) many primitive germ cells damaged during radiation die in their attempts at meiosis, and (*b*) many surviving radiated cells subsequently recover as they mature.

The amount of radiation necessary to induce this sequence of events or to produce aspermic sterility is not clear, since no controlled studies in man have been reported. However, experimental data and scattered reports of accidental radiation exposure in men indicate that 600 rads in a single dose usually causes permanent sterility, and 250 rads causes sterility for at least 12 months (37). The bulk of the evidence suggests that radiation has no long-term effect on fertility or progeny (35). It is true that there is a period when fertility should not and often cannot occur. However, since the prognosis may often be poor for patients who have, for example, testicular tumors, it seems prudent to recommend contraception during this period. Apparently, the data suggest that the risk in these patients of having abnormal children is no greater than in the general population, but it is advisable for them to wait at least 18 months before attempting conception.

On the other hand, the potential fertility of men evaluated in terms of semen quality after accidental exposure to nuclear radiation is initially impaired, but a reasonably good level of potential usually is attained at least 40 to 41 months after exposure (38). Acute radiation (200 to 360 rads) determines virtual sterility within 4 months after exposure, ranging to at least 21 months. Oligospermia, azoospermia, and abnormalities in sperm morphology are present in the ejaculate during this time. Ultimately, recovery of some degree of fertility is possible in most published cases.

Any generalized insult (viremia, for example) can cause impaired testicular function, and the effects may not appear in the ejaculate for 1 to 3 months after the gonadotoxic event. This is based on the fact that spermatogenesis takes approximately 72 to 74 days, from the initiation of the type B spermatogonia until the appearance of the mature spermatozoa in the ejaculate (40). Including transit time through the ductal system, the entire spermatogenic process takes approximately 3 months. The actual time lapse between the injurious event and the appearance of abnormal cells in the ejaculate varies depending upon what stage of spermatogenesis is affected. For that reason, if a patient gives a history of medical problems in the 3 months before his first office visit and if the analysis shows subnormal semen, it should be repeated at monthly intervals for 3 to 6 months before a decision is made regarding the quality of sperm production.

The history should also include a detailed inquiry into medication used. Medications such as sulfasalazines (41), cimetidine (42), colchicine (43), and nitrofurantoin (2), as well as ingestants such as caffeine, nicotine, alcohol (2), and marijuana (44) have been implicated as gonadotoxic agents. Withdrawal from some of these substances should effect return of normal spermatogenesis. Finally, the use of exogenous androgenic steroids, while mistakenly thought by some clinicians to improve gonadal function, actually acts as a male contraceptive, depressing gonadotropin secretion and interfering with normal spermatogenesis (45). Many anti-cancer agents produce oligozoospermia or azoospermia; prominent among these are anti-metabolites and alkylating agents such as cyclophosphamide, methotrexate, doxorubicin, and chlorambucil (2, 29). These agents deplete the germinal epithelium in a dose-dependent fashion, and the interval required for repletion is also dose-dependent. Fetal anomalies and irreversible germinal cell aplasia may result from long-term use of these agents (35, 46). Several amebicides can cause reversible depletion in germ cell numbers. The ingestion of alcohol may reduce serum testosterone, and chronic alcoholism associated with hepatic fibrosis and cirrhosis can lead to testicular atrophy with gonadal failure (47, 48). Propranolol, an anti-hypertensive drug, has occasionally been shown to be associated with asthenospermia. This drug has been tested as an efficacious spermicidal agent when used in vaginal tablets (49).

An association between cigarette smoking and testicular dysfunction has been documented (50, 51). Cigarette smokers have been shown to have an increase in abnormal spermatozoa compared to non-smokers (52). Furthermore, a solid body of experimental evidence suggests that exposure to nicotine, cigarette smoke, and/or polycyclic aromatic hydrocarbons can cause testicular atrophy, blocked spermatogenesis, altered sperm morphological features, and DNA mutations in animals (53). Acute and chronic adverse effects of smoking on the hypothalamic-pituitary-testicular axis have been reported (54). In addition to teratozoospermia, sperm density and the percentage of motile sperm have been found to be decreased in smokers compared to non-smokers (52).

Animal studies (55, 56) and data from marijuana users (57) are consistent in showing decreased sperm function following chronic marijuana use. Marijuana causes decreased testicular size, degenerative changes in spermatogenesis, and abnormal sperm morphology (teratozoospermia). In rodents and dogs, marijuana also inhibits the secretion of pituitary luteinizing hormone (LH), FSH, and prolactin. Although no clinical studies have evaluated the effects of marijuana on infertility in men, it is clear from current evidence that marijuana should be considered as a factor contributing to unexplained infertility in men (57, 58).

A number of central nervous system agents, including drugs of abuse (cocaine, narcotics), can inhibit reproductive function (57). These chemically diverse drugs show an important pharmacological property: they are highly potent neuroactive drugs that can disrupt the hypothalamic-pituitary-gonadal function. Most of these neuroactive drugs produce only transient effects on the central nervous pathways necessary for gonadotropin secretion. The disruptive effects of these drugs are likely to be transient; complete reversal and tolerance to the inhibitory drug effects may occur even with continued use (57). Under these circumstances, normal adults may experience only subtle changes in sexual function. However, individuals with compromised reproductive function may exhibit major problems. It is also likely that adolescents may be at substantial risk for reproductive damage from these neuroactive drugs, since the endocrine events associated with puberty are dependent on the normal development of the hypothalamic-pituitary axis (57).

The roles of stress and nutrition in male infertility are largely unknown (2). Although severe stress has been associated with reduced spermatogenesis, there is no evidence that the normal stress level in Western culture is responsible for reduced fertility. No specific nutritional factors have been related to male infertility.

Finally, the subject of sexual habits must be addressed during the initial history. Sexual problems have been suggested as common causes of male infertility, mainly too frequent or too infrequent intercourse. It is important to discuss with the couple coital techniques and the use of lubricants; they should be instructed on the proper timing of intercourse. In the CEGYR study, only nine patients (0.7% of the total group) presented with sexual dysfunction.

Physical Examination

The physical examination of a patient who consults for infertility should be thorough and complete, with emphasis on the external genitalia. He should be examined naked, first while he stands erect, then while he lies on the examining couch. General examination should include habitus and distribution of body hair, which, if abnormal, may suggest endocrine or chromosomal abnormalities. The thyroid gland should be carefully palpated, and the breast inspected for gynecomastia. Although it is uncommon in infertile males, inspection of the mammary glands for gynecomastia is essential because hyperprolactinemia may lead to gynecomastia associated with loss of libido, lack of erection, hypospermia, and oligozoospermia. The incidence of hyperprolactinemia varies according to the patient selection procedure, ranging from 2.9% in hypogonadal males to 3.6% to 9.0% in oligospermic patients without endocrine abnormalities (59).

External genitalia should be carefully examined, with inspection and palpation of the penis, followed by testicular evaluation. Testicular size and consistency are of utmost interest, and a Prader orchidometer or a special ruler may be used. Standard testicular measurements have been established for the normal population (60, 61). Since testicular volume is determined mainly by the seminiferous tubules and the amount of germ cells within them, a lack of these cells would diminish volume, leading to hypotrophy or atrophy. Therefore, both testicular volume and consistency provide an approximation of the state of spermatogenesis. Testicular consistency can also be a clue to underlying pathology; a testis that has experienced orchitis episodes will present an atrophic size and a decreased consistency, whereas a testis of Klinefelter's syndrome would be more consistent although also atrophic.

The epididymides are perfectly palpable adjacent to the testes. Abnormalities include cysts attached to the head of the epididymis (appendix epididymis) and a hard, rosary-like appearance, which probably indicates a previous infection with an obstructive sequel. It is important to define the presence and state of the head, corpus, and tail of the epididymis. The vasa deferentiae are also readily palpable, and it should be verified that there are no irregularities or nodularities anywhere on their course.

In approximately 10% of azoospermic patients, a bilateral agenesis of the vasa deferentiae has been found. Unilateral agenesis, usually on the right side, is rarer than bilateral agenesis and is often associated with congenital renal abnormalities. Therefore, if the vasa deferentiae are absent, it would be important to perform an intravenous pyelogram to verify any possible urological abnormality.

Prostate examination is also important, although there are many cases in which pathological findings may not be demonstrable. Together with the genitourinary questionnaire, palpation of the prostate may suggest prostatitis, which may (not) be confirmed by bacteriological studies of semen and urine. Such pathologies may cause semen abnormalities such as asthenozoospermia.

Varicocele is one of the most important and most controversial causes of male infertility. Examination for varicocele is essential for the patient's diagnosis and prognosis. The patient should be examined first while he is lying on the examining couch, then while he is standing. He should be asked to perform the Valsalva maneuver so that the scrotal varicosities that form the venous system will dilate. In typical cases, the scrotum will feel like a bag of worms. Since there are cases in which the varicocele is not so evident, other tests and analyses can contribute to the clinical examination: Doppler investigation, blood-pooling radioisotope, spermatic phlebography, scrotal thermography, etc. The Doppler investigation is one of the simplest; however, its usefulness is limited by false positives. Scrotal thermography provides a measure of scrotal temperature, taking into account the absence of subcutaneous fat to assess the temperature of the testis. A direct correlation between the spermatic vein reflux demonstrated by retrograde caval venography and abnormalities in the thermographic evaluation have been reported (62). Spermatic phlebography, although invasive, is also an important diagnostic method, mainly since a vein catheterization, followed by radiologically guided vein occlusion, can be used for treatment.

Diagnostic Methodologies for Infertile Patients

The semen analysis is the mainstay of the evaluation of the infertile male. If abnormalities are noted, multiple collections over a 4- to 6-month period may be necessary. If persistent abnormalities are found, endocrine evaluations in the form of serum FSH, LH, prolactin, estradiol, and testosterone determinations are obtained.

The evaluation and treatment of the infertile male with abnormal semen analysis can be divided into two groups: those with no sperm (azoospermia) and those with other abnormalities such as low sperm count, low sperm motility, increased morphological abnormalities, alteration in semen volume, and presence of antisperm antibodies. In both groups, evaluation of the hypothalamic-pituitary-testicular axis, as measured by FSH and LH, is paramount. FSH and LH respectively indicate indirectly the function of the Sertoli

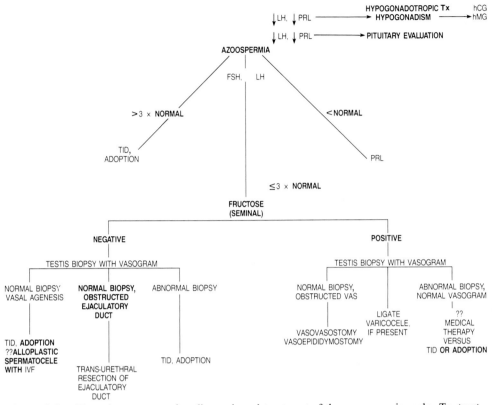

Figure 2.1. Flow sheet representing diagnosis and treatment of the azoospermic male. *Tx,* treatment. (From Acosta AA, Van Uem J, Ackerman SB, Mayer JF, Stecker JF, Swanson RJ, Pleban PP, Yuan J, Chillick C, Brugo S: Estimation of male fertility by examination and testing of spermatozoa. In Jones HW Jr et al. (eds): In Vitro Fertilization—Norfolk. Baltimore: Williams & Wilkins, 1986, p 130. Originally adapted from Lipschultz L: Lectures in Urology. Vail Urologic Conference, 1985.)

and Leydig cells because of their negative-feedback action and indicate directly the possibility of primary hypothalamic-pituitary abnormalities.

The next step in evaluating azoospermic patients is the measurement of seminal fructose in combination with testicular biopsy and vasograms. It is necessary to look for surgically correctable causes of azoospermia such as varicocele and obstructed vas deferens. In patients with vasal agenesis but with some remaining epididymis, the use of an alloplastic spermatocele surgically attached to the epididymis remnant may provide a means of collecting enough semen for in vitro fertilization (IVF) (32). In patients with abnormal semen parameters other than azoospermia, surgically correctable causes are again searched for. Approximately 37% of infertile males have a varicocele, and internal spermatic vein ligation will result in subsequent pregnancy rates of 40% to 50%. Whenever a varicocele is found, treatment is individualized according to the type of semen abnormality. In patients with retrograde ejaculation, where collection of an adequate number of sperm is a problem, and in those with severe oligospermia unresponsive to medical therapy, IVF can play an important role (Figs. 2.1 and 2.2).

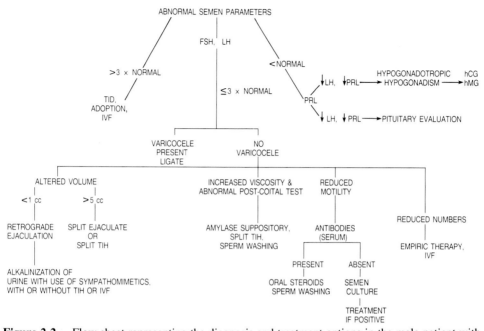

Figure 2.2.   Flow sheet representing the diagnosis and treatment options in the male patient with abnormal semen parameters. (From Acosta AA, Van Uem J, Ackerman SB, Mayer JF, Stecker JF, Swanson RJ, Pleban PP, Yuan J, Chillick C, Brugo S: Estimation of male fertility by examination and testing of spermatozoa. In Jones HW Jr et al. (eds): In Vitro Ferilization—Norfolk. Baltimore: Williams & Wilkins, 1986, p 131. Originally adapted from Lipschultz L: Lectures in Urology. Vail Urologic Conference, 1985.)

As mentioned above, it is useful to approach oligospermic patients considering the cause of infertility as pre-testicular, testicular, or post-testicular factors. Pretesticular factors consist of hypothalamic-pituitary lesions or abnormal gonadotropins, with subsequent gonadal dysfunction. The diagnosis should be ascertained by (*a*) the pituitary response of FSH and LH after GnRH infusion (GnRH test); (*b*) pituitary and testicular response to clomiphene citrate (clomiphene test); and (*c*) a study of prolactin secretion.

The testicular factor, the most common cause of consultation, should be evaluated in three aspects: (*a*) hormonal profile, as described above; (*b*) genetic studies (karyotype); and (*c*) histological studies (testicular biopsy). It is essential in this case to look for absence or atrophy of the germinal epithelium, spermatogenesis blockage, absence of germinal cells, hypospermatogenesis, tubal wall lesions, etc.

Post-testicular factors should be evaluated by (*a*) biochemical studies of the seminal plasma (pH, semen fructose, carnitine, phosphoglyceryl choline, and zinc levels); (*b*) tests for obstruction (vasography with bilateral testicular biopsy when indicated); (*c*) tests for antisperm antibodies in serum and in seminal plasma; and (*d*) bacteriological studies, as discussed in Chapters 4 and 5.

References

1. Menning BE: The emotional needs of infertile couples. Fertil Steril 34:313, 1980
2. Sharlip ID: Clinical andrology. In Smith DR (ed): General Urology. Los Altos, CA: Lange Medical Publications, 1984, p 608
3. MacLeod J: Human male infertility. Obstet Gynecol Surv 26:325, 1971

4. Simmonds FA: Human infertility. N Engl J Med 255: 1140, 1956
5. Whorton MD: Male occupational reproductive hazards. West J Med 137:521, 1982
6. Lipshultz LI, Ross CE, Whorton D: Dibromochloropropane and its effect on testicular function in man. J Urol 124:464, 1980
7. Kandeel FR, Swerdloff RS: Role of temperature in regulation of spermatogenesis and the use of heating as a method for contraception. Fertil Steril 49:1, 1988
8. Hippocrates: Aphorisms. In Adams FI (trans): The Genuine Work of Hippocrates. Baltimore: Williams & Wilkins, 1939, p 312
9. Weisman AI: Azoospermia due to testicular non-descent (semen studies on occult cryptorchids) Hum Fertil 6:45, 1941
10. Lipshultz LI: Cryptorchidism in the subfertile male. Fertil Steril 27:609, 1976
11. Nistal M, Paniagua R: Infertility in adult males with retractile testes. Fertil Steril 41:395, 1984
12. MacLeod J: Effect of chicken pox and pneumonia on semen quality. Fertil Steril 2:523, 1951
13. Kapadia RM, Phadke AM: Scrotal suspenders and subfertility. J Fam Welf 2:27, 1955
14. Brindley GS: Deep scrotal temperature and the effect on it of clothing, air temperature, activity, posture and paraplegia. Br J Urol 54:49, 1982
15. Lamar NJ, Rodger R: Season and human fertility in Galveston, Texas. Anat Rec 87:453, 1943
16. Levine RJ, Bordson BL, Mathew RM, Brown MH, Stanley JM, Starr TB: Deterioration of semen quality during summer in New Orleans. Fertil Steril 49:900, 1988
17. Egbunke GN, Elemo AO: Testicular and epididymal sperm reserves of cross bred European boars raised and maintained in the humid tropics. J Reprod Fertil 54:245, 1978
18. Young WC: The influence of high temperature on the guinea pig testes. J Exp Zool 49:459, 1927
19. Foldesy RG, Bedford JM: Biology of the scrotum. I. Temperature and androgen as the determinants of the sperm storage capacity of the rat cauda epididymis. Biol Reprod 26:673, 1982
20. Kraus H: Zur physiologie der spermatozoer. Arch Gynaek 151:302, 1932
21. Burfening RJ, Ulberg LC: Embryonic survival subsequent to culture of rabbit spermatozoa at 38 and 40°C. Reprod Fertil 15:87, 1968
22. MacLeod J: Further observations on the role of varicocele in human male infertility. Fertil Steril 20:545, 1969
23. Rodriguez-Rigau LJ, Smith KD, Steinberger E: Varicocele and the morphology of spermatozoa. Fertil Steril 35:54, 1981
24. Cross BA, Silver IA: Neurovascular control of oxygen tension in the testes and epididymis. J Reprod Fertil 3:377, 1962
25. Kakamura M, Hall PF: The influence of temperature upon polysomes of spermatids of rat testis. Biochem Biophys Res Commun 85:756, 1978
26. Lee LPK: Temperature effect on the permeability of plasma membranes of advanced germinal cells of the rat testis. Can J Biochem 52:586, 1974
27. Lehmann JF, Biegler R: Changes of potentials and temperature gradients in membranes caused by ultrasounds. Arch Phys Med Rehab 35:287, 1954
28. Lipshultz LI: Cryptorchidism in the subfertile male. Fertil Steril 27:609, 1979
29. Lipshultz LI, Howards SS: Evaluation of the subfertile man. In Lipshultz LI, Howards SS (eds): Infertility in the Male. NY: Churchill Livingstone, 1983, p 187
30. Zamudio Albsecu J, Bergada C, Cullen M: Male fertility in patients treated for cryptorchidism before puberty. Fertil Steril 22:829, 1971
31. Werner C: Mumps, orchiditis, and testicular atrophy. Ann Intern Med 32:1066, 1950
32. Acosta AA, van Uem J, Ackerman SB, Meyer JF, Stecker JF, Swanson RJ, Pleban PP, Yuan J, Chillik C, Brugo S: Estimation of male fertility by examination and testing of spermatozoa. In Jones HW Jr, Jones GS, Hodgen GD, Rosenwaks Z (eds): In Vitro Fertilization—Norfolk. Baltimore: Williams & Wilkins, 1986, p 126
33. Smith DR: Critique on the concept of vertical neck obstruction in children. JAMA 207:1686, 1969
34. Donohue JP, Perez JM, Einhorn LH: Improved management of nonseminomatous testis tumors. J Urol 121:425, 1979
35. Orecklin JR, Kaufman JT, Thompson RW: Fertility in patients treated for testicular tumors. J Urol 109:293, 1973
36. Kedia KR, Marbland C, Fraley EE: Sexual function following high retroperitoneal lymphadenectomy. J Urol 114:237, 1955
37. Rubin P, Casarett GW: The male genital tract. In: Clinical Radiation Pathology. Philadelphia: WB Saunders, 1968, p 378

38. MacLeod J, Hotchkiss RS, Sitterson BW: Recovery of male fertility after sterilization by nuclear radiation. JAMA 187:77, 1964

39. LeGrande CE: Radiation effects. In Johnson AD, Gomes WR, van Demak NL (eds): The Testis, Influencing Factors, vol 3. NY: Academic Press, 1970, p 337

40. Heller CB, Clermont Y: Kinetics of the germinal epithelium in men. Recent Prog Horm Res 20:545, 1964

41. Toovey S, Hudson E, Hendry WF, Levi AJ: Sulphasalazine and male infertility: reversibility and possible mechanism. Gut 22:452, 1981

42. Van Thiel DH, Gavalet JS, Smith WI, Gwendolyn P: Hypothalamic-pituitary-gonadal dysfunction in men using cimetidine. N Engl J Med 300:1012, 1979

43. Merlin HE: Azoospermia caused by colchicine: a case report. Fertil Steril 23:180, 1972

44. Kolodny RC, Masters WH, Kolodny RM, Toro G: Depression of plasma testosterone levels after chronic intensive marijuana use. N Engl J Med 290: 872, 1974

45. McClure RD, Palacios A, Brosman SA, Swerdloff RS: Suppression of spermatogenesis in normal subjects with testosterone enanthate. Clin Res 25:149A, 1977

46. Karnofsky DA: Late effects of immunosuppressive anti-cancer drugs. Fed Proc 261:925, 1967

47. Van Thiel DH, Gavalet JS, Lester R: Alcohol-induced testicular atrophy. Gastroenterology 69:326, 1975

48. Ylikahri R, Huttunen M, Harkonem M: Low plasma testosterone values in men during hangover. J Steroid Biochem 5:655, 1974

49. Zipper J, Wheeler RG, Potts DM, Rivera M: Propranolol as a novel, effective spermicide: preliminary findings. Br Med J 287:1245, 1983

50. Viczian M: Ergebnisse mit spermauntersuchungen bei zigarettenrauchern. Z Hautkr 48:181, 1969

51. Evans HJ, Fletcher J, Torrance M, Hargreave TB: Sperm abnormalities in cigarette smoking. Lancet 1:627, 1981

52. Stillman RJ, Rosenberg MJ, Sachs BP: Smoking and reproduction. Fertil Steril 46:545, 1986

53. Mattison DR: The effects of smoking on fertility from gametogenesis to implantation. Environ Res 28:410, 1982

54. Shaarawy M, Mahmoud KZ: Endocrine profile and semen characteristics in male smokers. Fertil Steril 38:255, 1982

55. Zimmerman AM, Zimmerman S, Raj AY: Effects of cannabinoids on sperm morphology. Pharmacology 18:143, 1979

56. Dixit VP, Gupta CL, Agrawal M: Testicular degeneration and necrosis induced by chronic administration of cannabis extract in dogs. Endokrinologie 69:299, 1977

57. Smith CG, Asch RH: Drug abuse and reproduction. Fertil Steril 48:355, 1987

58. Maugh TH: Marijuana: new support for immune and reproductive hazards. Science 190:865, 1975

59. Del Pozo E: Hyperprolactinemia in male infertility: treatment with bromocriptine. In Bain J, Schill WB, Schwarzstein L (eds): Treatment of male infertility. Berlin: Springer-Verlag, 1982, p 71

60. Charny CW: The spermatogenic potential of the undescended testis before and after treatment. J Urol 83:697, 1960

61. Lubs HA Jr: Testicular size in Klinefelter's syndrome in men over fifty. N Engl J Med 267:326, 1962

62. Comhaire F, Montyene R, Kunnen M: The value of scrotal thermography as compared with selective retrograde venography of the internal spermatic vein for the diagnosis of ''subclinical'' varicocele. Fertil Steril 27: 694, 1976

Appendix 2.1.
Tygerberg Hospital History and Examination Forms

TYGERBERG—HOSPITAL
DEPARTMENT OF ANDROLOGY
HISTORY AND EXAMINATION OF MALE PATIENTS

NB: These questions form part of the history of all male patients and must be answered in print-hand by the *wife* in cooperation with her husband, as male patients usually can not give all of the required detail. Unfortunately, male patients can not be examined unless these questions are *fully answered.*

Surname: _____ Initials: husband: _____ wife: _____
Address: _____
_____ Post code: _____
Phone: husband (work): _____ wife (work:) _____ home: _____
Age: husband: _____ wife: _____
Date of birth: husband: _____ wife: _____
Date of marriage: _____
Date of first appointment at clinic: _____
Married for _____ years and _____ months at time of first appointment
Referred by (Dr.) _____

Profession: husband: _____ wife: _____
Employer: husband: _____ wife: _____
Denomination: husband: _____ wife: _____

Highest school standard achieved: husband: _____ wife: _____
Academic qualifications: husband: _____ wife: _____
Degree obtained: husband: _____ wife: _____
Technical training: husband: _____ wife: _____

WIFE

Have you ever used contraceptives after marriage?   yes   no   (encircle).
Name, type, or method of contraceptive and state period of use:
_____
_____

Have you had previous pregnancy *during this marriage?*   yes   no   (encircle).
Children: date of birth: 1. _____ weight: _____ sex: _____
                         2. _____ weight: _____ sex: _____
Method of delivery:
Child no. 1.: _____
Child no. 2.: _____
Have you had any miscarriages?   yes   no   (encircle).
Date of miscarriage: 1. _____ duration of pregnancy: _____
                     2. _____ duration of pregnancy: _____
                     3. _____ duration of pregnancy: _____
Have you had a tubal pregnancy?   yes   no   (encircle).
Left tube or right tube? _____
Date on which this tubal pregnancy was terminated: _____
Have you used any contraception *after* these conceptions? State type of contraceptive and period used:
_____
_____

Have you been married previously?   yes   no   (encircle). How many times? _____
Children from *previous* marriages of the *wife:*
1. Date of birth: _____ weight: _____ sex: _____
   Method of delivery: _____
2. Date of birth: _____ weight: _____ sex: _____
   Method of delivery: _____
3. Date of birth: _____ weight: _____ sex: _____
   Method of delivery: _____

HUSBAND

Have you been married previously?   yes   no   (encircle).   How many times?
_____

Do you have any children from previous marriages?   yes   no   (encircle).
Children from *previous* marriages of the *husband*:
1. Date of birth _____ weight: _____ sex: _____
2. Date of birth _____ weight: _____ sex: _____
3. Date of birth _____ weight: _____ sex: _____

Did you have any previous tests (except semen tests) with regard to infertility?   yes   no   (encircle).
Describe these tests in your own words:
_____
_____

Have you had previous *semen* examinations?   yes   no   (encircle).
Describe in your own words the results of these examinations:
_____
_____

Did you have any operations of your genital organs?   yes   no   (encircle).
Describe these operations in your own words:
_____
_____

Any other remarks:
_____
_____
_____

NOTE: Should you not have enough space for your answers, please continue overleaf.

Infertility
   Have you ever conceived? Yes _____ If "yes," how many times? _____
                            No _____
   Have you got any children? Yes _____ If "yes," how many? _____
                            No _____
   Have you got any twins or triplets etc? Yes _____ No _____ If
   "Yes," describe: _____

Do you work with any of the following: (yes or no)
   Poisonous gas: _____
   Poisonous spray: _____
   Lead: _____
   Welding: _____
   X-rays: _____
   Other: (Describe) _____
   _____

Have you had any of the following infections? (Give date and if patient received complete treatment)
Malaria: _____
Bilharzia: _____
Frequent infections of the tonsils: _____
Frequent sinusitis: _____
Tuberculosis: _____
Bladder and kidney infections: _____
Have you ever had any infections as a result of intercourse with other women?
Prostate: _____
Virus: _____
Any other infections: _____
Have you ever noticed blood in your urine? _____
Have you ever noticed blood in your sperm? _____
Have you ever noticed a yellow discharge from your penis? _____
Have you ever felt an itch from your penis after intercourse? _____

Have you ever noticed that your penis flakes after intercourse? _____
Are your teeth healthy? _____
Any illnesses:

Childhood diseases:

Previous operations:

Is your vision good? _____
Do you frequently get headaches? _____
Mention anything you are allergic to? _____

Are you on any diet? _____
Do you use appetite suppressants? _____
How much do you weigh? _____
Does your weight remain constant? _____
Do you smoke? _____ If "yes," how many? _____
What type of cigarettes do you smoke? _____
From which age did you begin to smoke? _____
Do you use alcohol in excess? _____
How do you like your bath water: Cold   _____
                                 Lukewarm   _____
                                 Warm   _____
                                 Very warm   _____
Do you stay in the bath longer than 10 minutes? _____
Are your underclothes made of cotton or synthetic material? _____

Do you use any tranquilizers? _____
Do you use any habit-forming drugs or tablets? _____
Do you take any other medicine or tablets regularly?
Yes _____ No _____ If "yes," how often? _____
Describe: _____

Is there anything else you wish to mention in connection with your emotional condition? _____

FAMILY HISTORY

Are you an adopted child?   Yes _____   No _____
Have your parents ever had any problems with infertility?
Yes _____ No _____ (If "yes," describe overleaf)

_____

Father
   Living: _____
   Age: _____
   Deceased: _____ Reason: _____
   Height: Short _____
         Average _____
         Tall _____

Mother
   Living: _____
   Age: _____
   Deceased: _____ Reason: _____
   Height: Short _____
         Average _____
         Tall _____
Has your mother ever had a miscarriage? Yes _____ No _____
If "yes," how many? _____
Has your mother ever had a stillborn baby? Yes _____ No _____
If "yes," how many? _____
Has any of your brothers or sisters died within their first year of life?
Yes _____ No _____ If "yes," give reason: _____
_____

Are your father and mother related to each other? Yes _____ No _____
If "yes," describe: _____
_____

Are you and your spouse related to each other? Yes _____ No _____
If "yes," describe: _____
How many children are there in your family? (Do *not* include adopted children.)
_____

How many brothers or sisters are there in your family that are deceased?
Brothers: _____ Reason: _____
_____

Sisters: _____ Reason: _____
_____

How many of your *brothers* have children? _____ How many children: _____
How many of your *married brothers* have not got children? _____
How many of your *brothers* are not yet married? _____ Ages: _____

How many of your *sisters* have children? _____ How many children: _____
How many of your *married sisters* have not got children? _____
How many of your *sisters* are not yet married? _____ Ages: _____

Has any of your brothers or sisters any problems or had any problems regarding infertility? Yes
_____ No _____ Describe: _____
_____

FAMILY TREE

Include own blood family, e.g., parents, brothers, sisters, cousins, and grandparents. In case of abnormalities, please describe each instance in detail on overleaf.

Has anyone in your family ever had the following problems (please specify if on mother's or father's side):

1. A baby born with hereditary abnormality: Yes _____ No _____ If "yes," explain: _____
_____

2. A baby with Down's syndrome: Yes _____ No _____ If "yes," explain: _____

3. A mentally retarded child: Yes _____ No _____ If "yes," explain: _____

4. Diabetes: Yes _____ No _____ If "yes," explain: _____
_____

5. Tuberculosis: Yes _____ No _____ If "yes," explain:_____
_____

6. Blood disease (bleeding tendency, leukemia, purpura, thrombosis, etc.): Yes _____
_____ No _____ If "yes," explain: _____
_____

7. Porphyry: Yes _____ No _____ If "yes," explain: _____
_____

8. Carcinoma (cancer): Yes _____ No _____ If "yes," explain: ___
_____

9. Hypertension: Yes _____ No _____ If "yes," explain: _____
_____

10. Heart disease: Yes _____ No _____ If "yes," explain: _____
_____

11. Kidney disease: Yes _____ No _____ If "yes," explain: _____
_____

12. Multiple pregnancies: Yes _____ No _____ If "yes," explain: __
_____

13. Epilepsy: Yes _____ No _____ If "yes," explain: _____
_____

Have you ever considered adoption? _____
What are your views on adoption? _____

Are you familiar with artificial insemination? _____
What are your views on artificial insemination using:
Husband's semen? _____

Donor's semen? _____

SEX AND MARRIAGE

How often do you have intercourse? Per week: _____
Per month: _____
Other: _____
Are you happy with your sex life? Yes _____ No _____
(If "no," this section must be completed in detail by the *consultant*.)

_____
_____
_____

CLINICAL EXAMINATION

General appearance: Healthy: _____
Unhealthy: _____
Feminine: _____
Masculine: _____

Weight: _____
Height: _____
Arm span: _____
Vision: _____

Ears, nose, and throat: _____

Thyroid: _____

Blood pressure: _____

Pulse rate: _____

Heart: _____

Lungs: _____

Abdomen: _____

Extremities: _____

Secondary sex attributes
Facial hair: _____
Body hair: _____
Pubic hair: _____
Mammary development: _____
Muscle development: _____
Habits: _____
Voice: _____
Excess pigmentation and nevi: _____

Genitals
Penis: Length in cm: _____
Hypospadias: Yes _____ No _____

Epispadias: Yes _____ No _____

Phimosis: Yes _____ No _____

Circumcision: Yes _____ No _____

Scrotum: Eczema: _____

Thickness of skin: _____

Abnormalities: _____

Testicles:

Right Testicle	Left Testicle
Length: _____	Length: _____
Width: _____	Width: _____
Thickness: _____	Thickness: _____
Hard: _____	Hard: _____
Soft: _____	Soft: _____
Soft-hard: _____	Soft-hard: _____
Undescended: _____	Undescended: _____
Low in scrotum: _____	Low in scrotum: _____

Epididymides

Right Epididymis	Left Epididymis
Caput: _____	Caput: _____
Corpus:_____	Corpus: _____
Cauda: _____	Cauda: _____
Joining of testicles: _____	Joining of testicles: _____

Vas Deferens Blood Veins (circle):

Right Vas Deferens	Left Vas Deferens
Normal Yes _____	Normal Yes _____
No _____	No _____
Varicocele (right) Small: _____	Varicocele (left) Small: _____
Average: _____	Average: _____
Large: _____	Large: _____
None: _____	None: _____
Hydrocele (right) Small: _____	Hydrocele (left) Small: _____
Average: _____	Average: _____
Large: _____	Large: _____
None: _____	None: _____
Hernia indirect (right) Small _____	Hernia Indirect (left) Small: _____
Average: _____	Average: _____
Large: _____	Large: _____
None: _____	None: _____

Other abnormalities of genitals (describe): _____

_____

Prostate: Enlarged: Slight: _____

Average: _____

Severe: _____

None: _____

Tender—painful: Yes _____ No _____
Seminal vesicles: Enlarged—tender: _____
                Normal: _____
                  (Note: Normal = not touchable)

Clinical diagnosis: Normal: _____ Abnormal (give reasons):
_____
_____

THE HISTORY OF THIS PATIENT WAS
TAKEN BY:
_____

THE PATIENT WAS EXAMINED BY:
_____

(Please Print—Initials and surname must be legible).

Appendix 2.2.
Eastern Virginia Medical School Andrology History Form

EASTERN VIRGINIA MEDICAL SCHOOL
DEPARTMENT OF OBSTETRICS AND GYNECOLOGY
DIVISION OF REPRODUCTIVE ENDOCRINOLOGY
ANDROLOGY HISTORY FORM

Name: _____ Date of first visit: _____

Wife's name: _____ Physician: _____

Patient's age: _____ Race _____ Referring physician: _____

Home address: _____

Office address: _____

Home telephone: _____ Office telephone: _____

1. *Chief complaint:* _____
_____

2. *Family history*

Family Hx.	Living	Dead	Cause of Death	Number of Children
Father				
Mother				
Brothers				
Sisters				

Illnesses:
    Tumors: _____
    Thyroid diseases: _____
    Tuberculosis: _____
    Congenital anomalies: _____
    Diabetes: _____
    Genetic disorders: _____
    Infertility: _____
    Others: _____

3. *Past history*
Childhood diseases (mumps, virus, etc): _____
Chronic illnesses (diabetes mellitus, arthritis, chronic infections): _____
_____
Venereal disease (type, treatments, dates): _____
Tuberculosis: _____
Diabetes: _____
Thyroid diseases: _____
Kidney diseases: _____
Prostate diseases: _____
Testicular problems and treatment (give details): _____
_____
Breast enlargement: _____
Surgical procedures (include doctor's name, hospital, dates): _____
_____
X-ray therapy: _____
Illness during last week (cold, flu, ?): _____
Actual medications: _____
Vitamins: _____

Others: _____

4. *Developmental history*
   Date of birth: _____ Birth weight: _____
   History of mother's hormone treatment during pregnancy: _____
   Paternal age at patient's birth: _____ Maternal age at patient's birth: _____
   Abnormalities during pregnancy: _____ Delivery: _____
   Age at puberty: _____ Pubertal development: _____
5. *Social history*
   Tobacco: _____ Others: _____
   Alcohol: _____ Drugs: _____
6. *Employment and environmental history*
   Toxic substances: _____ Heat: _____
   X-ray exposure: _____ Other: _____
7. *Allergies:* _____
8. *Marital history:* Sexual life started: _____
   Age at first marriage: _____ Wife's age: _____
   Age at second marriage: _____ Wife's age: _____

Number of Marriages	1	2	3	Husband	1	2	3	
Duration								
Number of pregnancies								

Sexual intercourse (per week):   1   2   3   4   −   +

Contraception: _____

Do you usually have morning erections?   Yes   No

Have you ever had difficulties in   (circle):
    Obtaining an erection?
    Maintaining an erection?
    Ejaculation (pain)?
    Masturbation?
    Penetrating into the vagina?
    Ejaculation into the vagina?
    Bringing about lubrication of your partner?

Has inability to conceive changed sexual frequency or enjoyment?   Yes   No

Has it altered your desire for intercourse?   Yes   No

Do you feel your sexual drive satisfied by actual frequency of intercourse?   Yes   No

Do you feel your partner's sexual drive is satisfied by actual frequency of
    intercourse?   Yes   No

Have you noticed any change in sexual drive?   Increase?   Decrease?   Yes   No

Have you ever visited a marital/sexual counselor?   Yes   No

9. *History of present illness:*

10. *Physical Examination:* Height: _____ Weight: _____ Span: _____
   BP:[a] _____ Pulse: _____ Resp: _____
   Habitus: Normal: _____ Emaciated: _____ Android: _____
   Obesity: _____ General: _____ Cushingoid: _____
   Hair (shaves): _____ Baldness: _____
   Head and neck: _____
       Thyroid: _____
   Thorax: _____
       Lungs: _____
       Cardiovascular: _____
       Breast: _____
   Abdomen: _____
   Genital exam:
       Pubic hair: _____
       Penis: _____
       Scrotum: _____
       Testis: _____
           Right: _____ Left: _____
       Spermatic cord: _____
           Right: _____ Left: _____
       Inguinal areas: _____
           Right: _____ Left: _____
       Rectal examination: _____
           Prostate: _____
Impression: _____ *Etiology:* _____
Instructions: _____ *Recommendation:* _____
Physician's signature: _____

---

[a]Abbreviations: BP, blood pressure; Resp, respiration; EEG, electroencephalogram; IVP, intravenous pyelogram; CBC, complete blood cell count; SR, sedimentation rate; STS, serologic test for syphilis; FSH, follicle-stimulating hormone; RIA, radioimmunoassay; LH, luteinizing hormone; TSH, thyroid-stimulating hormone; PBI, protein-bound iodine; BMR, basal metabolic rate; T_3, triodothyronine; T_4, thyroxine; GTT, glucose tolerance test; 17 KS, 17-ketosteroid; 17 OH Cs, 17-hydroxy corticosteroids; DHT, dihydrotestosterone; E_1, estrone; E_2, 17β-estradiol; DHEA, dehydroepiandrosterone; DHEA-S, dehydroepiandrosterone sulfate. 17αOH-P, 17α-hydroxyprogesterone; AIH, artificial insemination by husband; IVF, in vitro fertilization; EM, electron microscopy.

INVESTIGATIVE PROCEDURES

Psychiatric evaluation: _____

Neurological investigation
   EEG: _____
   Visual fields: _____
   Others: _____

X-ray examination
   Chest: _____
   Skull (sella turcica): _____
   Venogram: _____
   Vasogram: _____
   IVP: _____
   Others: _____

Blood Analysis
   Hematocrit: _____
   CBC: _____
   SR: _____
   Platelets: _____
   Clotting time: _____
   Bleeding time: _____
   Prothrombin time: _____
   Blood glucose: _____
   Serum cholesterol: _____
   Capillary fragility test: _____
   STS: _____
   Brucella test: _____
   Huddlesson test: _____
   Liver function test: _____
   Kidney function test: _____

Endocrine function tests
   Total urinary gonadotropins: _____
   FSH (RIA): _____ LH (RIA): _____
   Hypothalamic reserve function test: _____
   Pituitary reserve function test: _____
   Prolactin (RIA): _____ L-dopa test: _____ PBI _____ TSH (RIA) _____ BMR _____
   I uptake: _____ T_3, T_4 (RIA) _____ Others _____
   GTT: _____
   Total urinary 17-Ks: _____ Fractionation: _____ Suppression: _____
   Total Urinary 17 OH Cs: _____ Fractionation: _____ Stimulation: _____
   Testosterone (RIA): _____ Androstenedione (RIA): _____
   DHT (RIA): _____ Free T (RIA): _____
   Total urinary estrogens: _____ Fractionation: _____
   H chorionic gonadotropin stimulation test: _____
   Plasma E_2 (RIA): _____ Plasma E_1 (RIA): _____
   Plasma progesterone (RIA): _____ Pregnanediol: _____
   Pregnanetriol: _____ DHEA: _____ DHEA-S: _____
   17αOH-P: _____
   Others: _____

SEMEN EVALUATION—SPERM FUNCTION—I

Name: _____ Date: _____

Previous evaluations: Yes _____ No _____ Dates: _____

Last emission: _____ Days (2–7 days)[b]

Semen volume: _____ ml (2–6 ml)

Semen viscosity: _____

pH: _____ (7.1–7.8) Time: _____

Liquefaction: _____ minutes (complete by 30 min)

Sperm concentration: _____ $(20–250 \times 10^6/\text{ml})$

Sperm agglutination: _____ None: _____ 1+ _____ 2+ _____

Motility

    Percentage motile: _____% at _____ hours (>40%)

    Mean swimming speed: _____ μm/sec (>25 μm/sec)

    Sperm with motility ≥25 μm/sec: _____% (>50%)

Morphology

    Normal: _____%   (>14%)   Other: _____

    Abnormal: _____%   Comments: _____

Microbiology

    Ureaplasma urealyticum: _____

    Gonococcus: _____

    Chlamydia: _____

Sperm Immunology

    Serum immobilizing antibodies (Isojima): _____

    Serum macro-agglutinating antibodies (Kibrick): _____

    Serum micro-agglutinating antibodies (Franklin-Dukes): _____

    Comments: _____

Semen biochemistry

Total proteins: _____ mg/ml (21–66)

Fructose: _____ mg/ml (0.7–5.0)

Citric acid: _____ mg/ml (1.8–8.4)

Acid phosphatase: _____ IU/dl (88–979)

Glycerylphosphorylcholine: _____ μmol/ml (0.85)

Carnitine: _____ mg/100 ml (11.5–53.5)

Zinc: _____ mg/liter (103–178)

Copper: _____ mg/liter (50–150)

Selenium: _____

Cadmium: _____

Other: _____

Sperm-cervical mucus assay

Postcoital: _____ Comments: _____

Contact: _____

Penetration: _____

SEMEN EVALUATION—SPERM FUNCTION—II

Preparation of sperm for AIH or IVF

---

[b]Values in parentheses represent normal range.

Hamster ova/human sperm penetration assay

_____% penetrated
_____% attached

Human zona/human sperm penetration test

_____

Sperm EM

_____

CHAPTER 3

Evaluation of the Female for Assisted Reproduction

SUHEIL J. MUASHER, M.D.

The evaluation of the female partner for methods of assisted reproduction should be the same as the workup for infertility. Patients who are referred for in vitro fertilization (IVF) and embryo transfer, gamete intrafallopian transfer (GIFT), or any other method of assisted reproduction usually have undergone all the diagnostic procedures to determine the cause of infertility. The objective of this chapter is to review the various steps in the infertility workup of the female partner, with special emphasis on areas of particular importance for assisted reproduction.

Definition

Infertility is usually defined as failure to conceive after 12 months of unprotected intercourse. Primary infertility refers to a patient who has never been pregnant. Secondary infertility refers to a patient with a history of one or more pregnancies, regardless of viable or non-viable outcome, the latter including spontaneous or induced miscarriage and/or ectopic gestation. The workup in the female is the same for primary and secondary infertility.

The Initial Visit

The infertility workup begins with the initial interview. Patients referred for assisted reproduction have usually had most of the workup completed by one or more physicians. Nevertheless, it is the duty of the infertility specialist to review with the patient the previous workup to evaluate it critically and to repeat or order any tests that are questionable or have not been performed. During this interview, the physician should seek to accomplish the following:

1. Get to know the husband and wife and learn what their goals and objectives are;

2. Take a thorough medical, personal, and social history, which should include questions about the couple's sexual habits;
3. Perform a complete physical examination, with special emphasis on breast, abdominal, and pelvic examination;
4. Explain the diagnostic procedures that have been or will be performed;
5. Educate the couple regarding the evaluation, emphasizing the importance of the diagnostic steps and dispelling any fears or misconceptions that they may have;
6. Provide adequate time to answer their questions about the evaluation or previous investigations.

The goals of the infertility evaluation are twofold: to establish the etiology of the infertility and to give a prognosis for future fertility. Establishing the etiology for infertility is possible in approximately 90% of infertile couples and is largely dependent on the expertise of the clinician performing the evaluation, the availability of up-to-date laboratory facilities, and the perseverance of the couple. Three major areas of consideration can affect the prognosis:

1. *Age of the woman:* Fertility in women usually declines after the age of 30 years with a significant difference observed after the age of 35. It is extremely important to institute an infertility evaluation without delay in women over the age of 30 and to proceed with therapy as expeditiously as possible.
2. *Duration of infertility:* The longer the history of infertility, the more significant is the factor causing the infertility.
3. *Medical factor(s) causing infertility:* A medical factor causing infertility in the female obviously has a tremendous effect on the prognosis. Idiopathic infertility, ovulatory disturbances, luteal phase defect, and cervical factors carry a favorable prognosis with treatment, while severe tubal damage and/or severe endometriosis carries a less favorable prognosis.

Basic Infertility Investigation of the Female

There are five major areas in the infertility evaluation of the female: the ovulatory factor, the cervical factor, the uterine and tubal factor, the endometrial factor, and the peritoneal factor. Patients who are referred for assisted reproduction usually have been evaluated for all of these factors, probably several times and by several physicians. It is the physician's duty to evaluate thoroughly the previous investigative procedures to be sure that they were complete and in accord with modern standards. The physician should repeat or perform any test that is questionable or has not been done.

In the female, unlike the male, most of the investigative procedures must be performed at certain times during the menstrual cycle. It is very helpful if the patient keeps a basal body temperature (BBT) chart throughout the investigation. This will help the physician to interpret the diagnostic procedures. It is also helpful for the physician to look at the patient's previous BBT charts when interpreting tests that were performed, such as a postcoital test or an endometrial biopsy.

OVULATORY FACTOR

Ovulation usually occurs about 2 weeks before the onset of the next menstrual period. The detection and precise timing of ovulation requires careful monitoring of clinical and laboratory parameters. Ovulatory menstrual cycles, however, can usually be distinguished easily from anovulatory cycles with simple tools such as clinical history, pelvic examination, and unsophisticated diagnostic testing. Most of these simple tools provide indirect evidence of ovulation. The only direct evidence is the establishment of a pregnancy in the cycle of study, the observance of an ovulatory stigma at laparoscopy or laparotomy, and the recovery of a metaphase II oocyte from the peritoneal cavity or the fallopian tube. The indirect (presumptive) methods of ovulation detection are these:

1. *History:* Regularly occurring menstrual periods, especially those associated with cramping and premenstrual symptoms, are usually indicative of ovulatory cycles. The occurrence of midcycle abdominal pain (mittelschmerz) is usually indicative of impending ovulation.
2. *BBT graph:* The BBT graph is the simplest and most frequently used method for ovulation detection. Progesterone (P) is a thermogenic hormone. With ovulation, a corpus luteum is formed concomitant with P production, and the BBT rises by 0.5°F or more from its level in the follicular phase. This temperature elevation lasts for 12 to 14 days, after which it drops because of corpus luteum demise, unless pregnancy intervenes. Proper instructions and patient motivation are essential for the reliability of this method.
3. *Cervical mucus index:* Cervical mucus and vaginal cytology change with an increase in the level of circulating estradiol (E_2) in the few days preceding ovulation. Production of abundant, clear, and markedly stretchable mucus occurs along with dilatation of the external cervical os. After ovulation, due to P production, the cervical mucus become scanty, thick, highly cellular, viscous, and diminished in stretchability. After ovulation, the percentage of superficial and pyknotic cells in a vaginal smear is markedly decreased; these cells are replaced with intermediate cells.
4. *Laboratory assays of E_2, luteinizing hormone (LH), and P:* A sustained elevation of E_2 in the preovulatory period (usually ≥ 200 pg/ml for 50 hours or more) exerts a positive feedback stimulus which induces the preovulatory LH surge leading to ovulation 28 to 36 hours after the onset of the surge. The detection of the onset requires frequent monitoring of immunoreactive LH in the blood or urine. (Recently developed urinary LH assays for home monitoring are less accurate and provide only an estimation of ovulation timing.) A shift in steroidogenesis in favor of P over E_2 by the dominant follicle occurs even before the LH surge. Serum P levels increase significantly about 12 hours before the onset of the LH surge (1). A level of $P \geq 3$ ng/ml is usually indicative of ovulation.
5. *Endometrial biopsy:* Secretory endometrium by histology is another indirect evidence of ovulation.
6. *Ultrasonography:* High-resolution real-time ultrasound probes allow us to examine cycle changes in the ovary and endometrium. The availability of vaginal probes in particular makes ultrasonography an invaluable tool for the infertility specialist. The dominant follicle can be distinguished from its cohort of follicles 3 to 5 days before ovulation. During this time, the dominant follicle grows in a linear manner by approximately 2 to 3 mm a day, reaching a mean diameter of 19 to 26 mm by the time of ovulation. Several studies (2, 3) have demonstrated a good correlation between the dominant follicular diameter and peripheral E_2 levels, lending proof to the argument that the dominant follicle is the major source of circulating E_2 in the late follicular phase. After ovulation there is usually a collapse of the dominant follicle, with the absence of clear edges and the appearance of intrafollicular echoes representing blood clot formation. Free fluid can often be observed in the pouch of Douglas.

    Cyclic changes in the endometrium can also be detected by ultrasonography (4). The endometrial lining changes from a thin, homogeneous echo in the early follicular phase to a thick, bright echo in the late follicular phase, with the appearance of a sonolucent rim around the canal before ovulation, caused by stromal edema. Following ovulation, the edema disappears and the endometrium shrinks in thickness, often giving the appearance of a ring-like echo in the canal similar to that of an early gestational sac or a decidual cast in ectopic pregnancy.

The differential diagnosis of anovulatory conditions is listed in Table 3.1. The workup of anovulatory status involves the following steps and guidelines:

1. The physician should evaluate the biological estrogen status to determine whether the patient is hypoestrogenic or hyperestrogenic. This can be done in the office by observing the quality of the cervical mucus and by performing a maturation index of the vaginal cells.

Table 3.1.
Differential Diagnosis of Anovulatory Status and/or Amenorrhea

I.   Disorders of the central nervous system
    A.   Hypothalamic amenorrhea
        1.   Nutritional, anorexia nervosa
        2.   Exercise-related
        3.   Stress-related
        4.   Combination of the above
    B.   Pituitary tumor or lesion
    C.   Polycystic ovarian disease (PCOD)
    D.   Hyperprolactinemia
II. Disorders of ovarian etiology
    A.   Congenital defects
        1.   Gonadal dysgenesis
        2.   Turner's syndrome
        3.   Hermaphroditism
    B.   Tumors
    C.   Premature ovarian failure
        1.   Iatrogenic: drugs, irradiation
        2.   Autoimmune disease
        3.   Chromosomal defects
        4.   Polyendocrinopathic conditions
        5.   Idiopathic
    D.   Insensitive ovary syndrome
III. Disorders of intermediate metabolism
    A.   Thyroid: hyperthyroidism, hypothyroidism
    B.   Pancreas: diabetes mellitus
    C.   Adrenal
        1.   Enzyme defects
            a.   Congenital (classic) adrenal hyperplasia
            b.   Adult-onset (non-classic) adrenal hyperplasia
        2.   Tumors
        3.   Cushing's syndrome

2. Serum should be measured for LH, follicle-stimulating hormone (FSH), and prolactin. High FSH indicates ovarian failure. (The workup of ovarian failure is presented in Chapter 12). An LH:FSH ratio $\geq 2:1$ is usually indicative of polycystic ovarian disease (PCOD). Patients with elevated serum prolactin levels should be investigated for hyperprolactinemic conditions, and macro- or microadenoma of the pituitary should be ruled out when suspected.

3. Every attempt should be made to establish the etiology of the anovulatory status. Hyperandrogenic states should be properly investigated to rule out Cushing's syndrome, adrenal or ovarian tumors, and non-classic adrenal hyperplasia. Such investigation should include total serum testosterone, serum diehydroepiandrosterone sulfate (DHEAS), serum 17-hydroxyprogesterone (17-OHP), and total urinary free cortisol or early morning serum cortisol after an overnight dexamethasone (DXM) suppression test (1 mg orally at 11 PM). Thyroid function tests can be ordered when disorders of the thyroid metabolism are suspected. Elevated serum thyroid-stimulating hormone (TSH) is a sensitive indicator of primary hypothyroidism.

4. Patients should be properly counseled about exercise and stress. Disorders of nutrition, whether obesity or underweight, should be corrected before ovulation induction for assisted reproduction is begun.

Table 3.2.
Causes of an Abnormal Postcoital Test (PCT)

I. With abnormal cervical mucus
    A. Poor timing: too early in the follicular phase or after ovulation
    B. Poor quality of mucus
        1. Infection: cervicitis, mycoplasma or chlamydia
        2. Prior cervical conization, cauterization, or cryotherapy
        3. Anatomical defects, in utero exposure to diethylstilbestrol (DES)
    C. Poor quality and quantity of mucus
        1. All of the above
        2. Clomiphene citrate therapy for induction of ovulation
II. With normal cervical mucus
    A. Faulty coital technique
    B. Oligospermia or asthenospermia
    C. Low semen volume (≤ 1 ml)
    D. Antisperm antibodies

CERVICAL FACTOR

The sperm-cervical mucus interaction in vivo is evaluated by the Sims-Huhner test, better known as the postcoital test (PCT). This test should be performed when the cervical mucus is most estrogenic, in the 2 to 3 days before ovulation. The timing and interpretation of the test is variable among investigators. In my practice, the couple are instructed to have intercourse 12 to 14 hours before the office visit, usually on the night before. This is certainly more convenient than instructing them to have intercourse on command a few hours before the visit.

The physician performing the test should record the quantity and quality of the cervical mucus. The test is usually considered normal if there are at least five actively motile sperm per high-power field and the mucus is estrogenic. A normal PCT is reassuring and implies that the couple have satisfactory coital habits, that the mucus is estrogenic in the preovulatory period, reflecting adequate function of the dominant follicle, and that there is a likelihood of normal male fertility.

The value of one abnormal PCT is not clear, and repeat examinations should be performed. One should remember that the test may not reflect the adequacy of sperm concentration at the site of fertilization, in the ampullary portion of the fallopian tube. Laparoscopic sperm recovery from the peritoneal cavity after intercourse or homologous artificial insemination in the preovulatory period correlates poorly with the PCT.

The PCT is particularly important when an infertile female is considering intrauterine insemination or the GIFT procedure. The causes of an abnormal PCT are listed in Table 3.2.

UTERINE AND TUBAL FACTOR

Evaluation of the uterine cavity and tubal patency is usually done by hysterosalpingography (HSG), which should be performed after cessation of menses but before ovulation (cycle days 8 to 10). Performance of the procedure at this time assures that the patient is not pregnant and the endometrium is not thick, which would render a low, false-positive result. Both oil-based and water-soluble media have been used as contrast material. The oil-based medium provides a sharper image, is usually less painful, and has

Table 3.3.
Uterine Abnormalities Detected by Hysterosalpingography

   I. Double uterus: didelphic, septate, bicornuate
  II. Submucus myoma(s)
 III. T-shaped configuration due to in-utero exposure to diethylstilbestrol (DES)
  IV. Endometrial polyp(s)
   V. Intrauterine synechiae (Asherman's disease)

been associated more often with an increased incidence of conception within a few months after the test. The main advantages of the water-soluble medium are the reduced risk of embolization, the better appearance of intratubal rugae, and the greater convenience of obtaining the delayed film when necessary (after 15 minutes versus after 24 hours with oil-based medium).

Uterine abnormalities that can be detected by HSG are listed in Table 3.3. Tubal abnormalities detected by HSG are listed in Table 3.4. HSG should not be the definitive test of tubal patency or disease. Rather, HSG findings should always be confirmed by laparoscopy. False positive results can be obtained because of cornual spasm; false negative results are mostly found in conjunction with peritubal adhesions. HSG is absolutely contraindicated if the patient has a history of allergy to the contrast material, if acute pelvic inflammatory disease is present, or if the patient is pregnant. Complications and adverse effects of HSG include allergic reaction, uterine perforation and bleeding, and development of acute pelvic inflammatory disease. The incidence of infectious complications is probably less than 1%. A history of pelvic inflammatory disease predisposes to this complication (5). Almost all women who develop pelvic inflammatory disease after HSG have distal tubal obstruction. The value of prophylactic antibiotics in preventing infectious complications is highly controversial (6).

Hysteroscopy has also been used to detect intrauterine pathology. Hysteroscopy complements HSG in the infertility investigation but does not replace it. Hysteroscopy is best performed in the immediate postmenstrual period, when the endometrium is thinnest; it is often combined with laparoscopy. The distending medium most commonly used is 32% dextran 70, especially when operative procedures are contemplated. Discrepancies can exist between findings obtained by HSG and hysteroscopy (7). When the uterine cavity is normal by HSG, there is usually little to be gained by performing hysteroscopy. When the uterine cavity is abnormal by HSG, however, hysteroscopy should be performed to confirm the findings and often to correct the abnormality. Complications of hysteroscopy include bleeding (cervical laceration, uterine perforation), infection, and adverse effects of low-molecular-weight dextran (allergic reaction, cardiovascular overload, and coagulopathy).

ENDOMETRIAL FACTOR

Deficiency in corpus luteum function is manifested clinically as a luteal phase defect defined as a corpus luteum defective in P production. This defect was described by Georgeanna Seegar Jones in 1949; since then, it has been recognized as accounting for approximately 5% of cases of infertility and up to 35% of cases with repeated miscarriages. Multiple diagnostic modalities have been proposed to diagnose a luteal phase defect:

Table 3.4.
Tubal Abnormalities Detected by Hysterosalpingography

I.	Proximal tubal obstruction
II.	Distal tubal obstruction
III.	Peritubal and fimbrial adhesions
IV.	Salpingitis isthmica nodosa
V.	Tuberculous salpingitis
VI.	Intratubal polyp(s)

1. *BBT graph:* A luteal phase defect can be suspected if the temperature elevation after ovulation lasts less than 11 days. A normal BBT graph, however, does not rule out a luteal phase defect (8).
2. *P assays:* Measurement of serum P on three separate days between days 4 and 11 before menstruation can test for corpus luteum insufficiency (9). A single P assay in the luteal phase has no diagnostic value for this condition. However, these assays require a laboratory with adequate control values.
3. *Endometrial biopsy:* A properly performed and well-timed endometrial biopsy, in correlation with a BBT chart, is the best method for diagnosing a luteal phase defect. The biopsy should be performed 2 to 3 days before expected menstruation and is read according to the criteria of Noyes (10). The diagnosis of a luteal phase defect is establish if the biopsy is out of phase by 2 days or more in at least 2 cycles. The pathogenesis of a luteal phase defect includes multiple etiologies, which are listed in Table 3.5.

PERITONEAL FACTOR

The peritoneal factor is best evaluated by laparoscopy, which enables the physician to diagnose peritubal and ovarian adhesions and to document the presence/absence of pelvic endometriosis. Laparoscopy is an integral part of the infertility investigation and should be performed by a competent gynecologist who is experienced in the procedure. General anesthesia is recommended; often an additional suprapubic puncture is necessary to introduce ancillary instruments for complete evaluation. An adequate laparoscopic evaluation should include the following:

1. Observation of the size and shape of the uterus;
2. Examination of all pelvic peritoneal surfaces, including the anterior uterine peritoneum, bladder peritoneum, cornual ligaments, posterior cul-de-sac, and uterosacral ligaments;
3. Examination of the full length of the fallopian tubes, including adequate visualization of the fimbriated ends;
4. Examination of all ovarian surfaces for endometriosis, cysts, developing follicles, corpus luteum, and spatial relationship to the fimbria;
5. Transcervical injection of dye to check for tubal patency.

It is often helpful to draw a picture immediately after the procedure to show the normal/abnormal pelvic findings. If the patient has pelvic endometriosis, staging of the disease according to the revised American Fertility Society classification (11) should be attempted.

Unexplained Infertility

Unexplained infertility refers to the condition of an infertile couple in whom no definite cause for infertility can be identified. The incidence of this condition varies, but

Table 3.5.
Pathogenesis of the Luteal Phase Defect

    I. Defects of the central nervous system
        A. Inadequate FSH stimulation in the follicular phase
        B. Inadequate LH/FSH surge
        C. Inadequate tonic LH secretion in the luteal phase
        D. Hyperprolactinemia
    II. Ovarian defects
        A. Genetic, chromosomal
        B. Receptor
  III. Metabolic defects
  IV. Effect of drugs and hormones
        A. Progestational agents
        B. Clomiphene citrate
        C. Prostaglandins
    V. End organ endometrial defects
  VI. Hypobetalipoproteinemia

---

it should be limited to less than 10% when a thorough infertility investigation has been performed. Possible causes of unexplained infertility are listed in Table 3.6.

LUTEINIZED UNRUPTURED FOLLICLE (LUF) SYNDROME

The LUF syndrome is the absence of ovulation in women with apparently normal ovulatory cycles as judged by BBT charts, increased peripheral P in the luteal phase, and secretory endometrium by biopsy. Several methods have been proposed to diagnose LUF:

1. *Absence of an ovulatory stigma at laparoscopy:* This method is impractical and highly inaccurate because of rapid epithelialization of the stigma site and occasional difficulty in visualization of all ovarian surfaces.
2. *Peritoneal fluid E_2 and P determinations:* It has been proposed (12) that higher concentrations of E_2 and P are found in the peritoneal fluid of women with an ovulatory stigma at laparoscopy than in women without an ovulatory stigma. This method is also impractical and has a high incidence of false-positive and false-negative results.
3. *Ultrasonography:* Several studies (13, 14) have pointed to the value of serial ultrasonography in the diagnosis of the LUF syndrome. The diagnosis is made when the dominant follicle fails to collapse despite indirect evidence of ovulation (BBT chart, high serum P levels). This method is simple to perform but has not been correlated with peritoneal fluid sampling of steroid levels and the presence/absence of an ovulatory stigma by laparoscopy.

    The incidence, frequency, and repetition of the LUF syndrome in fertile and infertile women are controversial. The value of serial ultrasound in diagnosing the condition in women with unexplained infertility has not been established (15). In one diagnostic study (16) using serial ultrasound, 40 of 600 cycles in 27 of 270 infertile patients were found to have the condition. Correlation with serum hormone levels revealed significantly lower mean LH peak levels in midcycle and lower midluteal P levels in the LUF cycles than in control cycles.

UREAPLASMA INFECTIONS

Although the incidence of ureaplasma infections (in cervical mucus and/or seminal plasma) is higher in infertile couples than in fertile ones, several studies (17–19) have found no difference in the pregnancy rates of treated and untreated infertile couples.

Table 3.6.
Possible Causes of Unexplained Infertility

I.	Occult male factor
II.	Occult female factor: perimenopause
III.	Occult abnormalities of oocyte development
IV.	Luteinized unruptured follicle (LUF) syndrome
V.	Immunological factors
VI.	Occult infections (cervical or seminal): ureaplasma, chlamydia
VII.	Occult endometriosis
VIII.	Psychogenic and emotional factors

Therefore, a definitive role for ureaplasma infections in infertile couples has not been established.

OCCULT ENDOMETRIOSIS

The term refers to the presence of pelvic endometriosis despite a lack of visualization of endometrial implants by laparoscopy. In one study (20) using scanning electron microscopy, foci of endometriosis were identified in 25% of random biopsies of normal epithelium in patients with known pelvic endometriosis. The exact mechanism by which the early stages of pelvic endometriosis cause infertility remains unknown. Several theories have been suggested, including macrophage-mediated autoimmune response; increased prostaglandins in peritoneal fluid; association with the LUF syndrome; association with hyperprolactinemia and luteal phase defects; presence of constituents in peritoneal fluid that may impair sperm/oocyte interaction and early embryonic development; and recent observations of increased concentrations of interleukin-1 in peritoneal fluid in infertile women with early stages of endometriosis (21). The discussion of these theories is beyond the scope of this chapter.

Indications for Assisted Reproduction

The indications for IVF and embryo transfer are listed in Table 3.7. Most patients for whom IVF is indicated have infertility due to tubal disease and/or pelvic endometriosis. More patients with unexplained infertility are being referred for GIFT rather than IVF, although IVF in these patients serves not only as a therapeutic modality but also as a diagnostic one, providing information about the success/failure of fertilization. Pronuclear stage tubal transfer (PROST) has recently been proposed (22) for patients with unexplained infertility in order to combine the diagnostic advantages of IVF with the therapeutic advantages of GIFT. The indications for GIFT are listed in Table 3.8. The value of IVF and GIFT in patients with male factor and immunological infertility are discussed in Chapters 5 and 6.

TUBAL INFERTILITY

Most patients with tubal disease referred for IVF will have had at least one operative procedure to correct the problem. There should be no role for a repeat tuboplasty in patients with tubal infertility, since the expectancy of success is only about 5% (23). There are patients with certain forms of tubal disease who are candidates for IVF as a primary method of therapy. Such patients include those with bilaterally enlarged

Table 3.7.
Indications for In Vitro Fertilization (IVF)

I.	Tubal disease and/or obstruction
II.	Pelvic endometriosis
III.	Unexplained infertility
IV.	Male factor(s)
V.	Immunological factor(s)
VI.	Other factors
	A. Cervical factor
	B. Anovulation
	C. Luteal phase defect

hydrosalpinges that are thickened and/or fixed with adhesions, those who are candidates for tubal reanastomosis with the remaining tube less than 4 cm in length, and those with cornual obstruction requiring tubal reimplantation (24–26). In the Norfolk program, the pregnancy rate after IVF in patients with tubal disease has been slightly less than that in patients with other infertility factors, although all patients compared had had their eggs harvested by laparoscopy, which can affect the outcome, depending on ovarian accessibility (27).

In the Norfolk program, the effect on IVF outcome of the severity of tubo-ovarian disease and previous surgery was also studied (28). Results showed no correlation between the severity of tubo-ovarian disease, the number of preovulatory oocytes recovered and fertilized, and pregnancy rates. Likewise, the type of surgical procedure (salpingectomy, tuboplasty, adhesiolysis) had no effect on IVF outcome.

PELVIC ENDOMETRIOSIS

Most patients with pelvic endometriosis referred for IVF will have failed medical and/or surgical therapy for correction of infertility due to endometriosis. In the Norfolk program, the pregnancy rates after IVF are substantially higher in patients with stages 1 and 2 endometriosis than in patients with stages 3 and 4 (29). The pregnancy outcome in patients with a history of endometriosis but without evidence of active disease at laparoscopy for oocyte retrieval is similar to patients with stage 1 and 2 endometriosis at retrieval (29). The mean number of preovulatory oocytes recovered is usually less in patients with stages 3 and 4 than in patients with stages 1 and 2 (29–31). Most studies have used laparoscopic oocyte retrieval, and it remains to be seen whether the same findings will be observed with ultrasound-guided methods of retrieval. In a large series of

Table 3.8.
Indications for Gamete Intrafallopian Transfer (GIFT) in Patients with at Least One Patent Fallopian Tube

I.	Unexplained infertility
II.	Male factor(s)
III.	Pelvic endometriosis (primarily stages 1 and 2)
IV.	Cervical factor
V.	Other factors
	A. Immunological factor
	B. Anovulation
	C. Luteal phase defect

patients in the Norfolk program, we recently reported (32) a higher miscarriage rate in patients with stages 3 and 4 endometriosis than in those with stages 1 and 2. We speculate that this finding may indicate a poor embryo quality in patients with moderate or severe endometriosis. The reduced fertilization rate in patients with endometriosis, as reported by Wardle (33), has not been confirmed by other programs (29–31).

UNEXPLAINED INFERTILITY

With the availability of high-technology programs for assisted reproduction, more patients with unexplained infertility are being referred for IVF or GIFT. Prognosis for these patients, even without assisted reproduction, need not be dismal. In one study (34), it was estimated that women with unexplained infertility of 1 year's duration have a high chance of spontaneous pregnancy during the following year. The pregnancy rate is related to the age of the patient at presentation: 76% for a 20-year-old woman, 57% for a 30-year-old, and 40% for a 40-year-old. There is some merit to the notion that diagnosis of unexplained infertility should not be attempted unless all other factors have been excluded and the history of infertility is of at least 2 years' duration. In the Norfolk program, the post-IVF experience of patients with unexplained infertility has been very favorable and has yielded the best pregnancy rate among all the infertility factors (27). We recently reported (35) a comparison between IVF patients with unexplained infertility and a control group of tubal infertility patients. Although the mean number of preovulatory oocytes retrieved was higher in the tubal infertility patients (3.6 ± 2.0 versus 2.8 ± 2.1), the pregnancy rate per transfer was higher in patients with unexplained infertility (37% versus 24%). We have not found a lower fertilization rate in patients with unexplained infertility than in those with tubal infertility, as reported by Leeton (36).

GIFT was reported by Asch (37) as an alternative to IVF for patients with unexplained infertility. Other groups (38) have reported higher success rates with GIFT than with IVF in patients with unexplained infertility. One group (39) reported higher success rates in patients with unexplained infertility after tubal transfer procedures (GIFT, PROST, and tubal embryo-stage transfer) than in patients with tubal infertility after IVF.

Impact of Certain Factors on the Success or Failure of Assisted Reproduction in the Female

OVARIAN ACCESSIBILITY AND PELVIC ADHESIONS

With the introduction of ultrasound-guided oocyte retrieval, ovarian accessibility by laparoscopy is no longer a prerequisite for admitting patients into an IVF program. The main types of ultrasound-guided aspiration are percutaneous transvesical (40), transurethral (41), and transvaginal (42). In Norfolk we now use the transvaginal method exclusively, except in patients for whom a diagnostic laparoscopy is indicated. The advantages of transvaginal aspiration over laparoscopy include use of local anesthesia, less operative and recovery time, greater patient acceptability, and potentially fewer complications. We compared cycles with transvaginal aspiration to cycles with laparoscopic aspiration in women undergoing the same stimulation protocol (43). We found no significant differences in the mean numbers of follicles aspirated, preovulatory oocytes aspirated, and preovulatory oocytes transferred. With transvaginal aspiration, the need is almost eliminated for a screening laparoscopy or a laparotomy with lysis of adhesions and ovarian suspension for better ovarian accessibility before IVF (44).

The effect of ovarian adhesions on the success/failure of IVF has been studied. Diamond (45) reported no correlation between the presence of periovarian adhesions at laparoscopic retrieval and serum E_2 levels on the day of hCG administration or the day after, the total number of follicles on the day of hCG or the day after, and the number of oocytes recovered. Molloy (46) reported IVF results of a higher cancellation rate and lower rate of E_2 rise, lower peak E_2 levels, lower number of follicles by ultrasound, lower number of oocytes recovered, and lower pregnancy rate in patients with "frozen pelvis" than in patients with adhesion-free ovaries. In another study (47) using transurethral oocyte aspiration, the mean number of oocytes recovered, fertilized, and transferred was similar in patients with a frozen pelvis and in patients with adhesion-free ovaries.

PRESENCE OF ONE OR TWO OVARIES

Several studies have reported on the IVF outcome of patients with one or two ovaries. Diamond (48) compared the follicular response to ovulation induction with clomiphene citrate (CC) and with human menopausal gonadotropin (hMG) in patients with one or two ovaries. With either stimulation protocol, the number of oocytes recovered by laparoscopy was the same for both groups. With hMG stimulation, women with two ovaries developed a greater number of follicles and had a greater number of oocytes aspirated than did women stimulated with CC. In another study (49) using CC and hMG protocols, there were no statistically significant differences between the two groups in the mean numbers of hMG ampules, days of hMG stimulation, follicles ≥ 15 mm on ultrasound, mature and immature oocytes recovered, and pre-embryos transferred. Dodds (50) reported a higher pregnancy rate after IVF in patients with two ovaries than in those with one, although there were no statistically significant differences between the two groups in the mean level of E_2 on the day of hCG administration or the mean numbers of follicles ≥ 15 mm and preovulatory oocytes recovered. In Norfolk we compared our results after IVF in patients with one or two ovaries and with tubal infertility (51). Although the mean numbers of preovulatory oocytes per laparoscopy and per transfer were significantly higher in patients with two ovaries than in those with one ovary (2.33 versus 1.67; 2.28 versus 1.99, respectively), the pregnancy rates per transfer were almost identical in the two groups (24.4% with two ovaries, 23.9% with one ovary). These results were the same regardless of the stimulation protocol and patient age. Similar results (32) were found in patients with pelvic endometriosis, regardless of the stage of the disease. We concluded that patients with one ovary are not compromised in their chances to achieve a pregnancy after IVF. However, because the total number of follicles and oocytes retrieved is less in women with one ovary, surgical management of unilateral tubal pathology should not include paradoxical oophorectomy. Preservation of the ovaries at surgery also has the benefit of making oocytes or embryos available for cryopreservation.

UTERINE ANOMALIES

HSG films should be evaluated before a patient is accepted for IVF or GIFT. Uterine abnormalities such as submucous fibroids, extrinsic deformity from an intramural leiomyoma, and intrauterine adhesions should be corrected before therapy. In Norfolk we have reported (52) a favorable outcome after IVF in patients with a T-shaped uterine cavity due to diethylstilbestrol (DES) exposure in utero, and thus we continue to accept these patients into our program. The application of GIFT for patients with a T-shaped uterine cavity and patent fallopian tubes should be of concern because of the higher incidence in these patients of ectopic pregnancy due to a spontaneous gestation (53). The validity of correcting a septate anomaly of the uterus in patients with primary infertility before accepting them into an IVF program is questionable in the absence of a history of miscarriages and the lack of information on the incidence of this anomaly in patients with a normal obstetrical outcome. Hysteroscopic resection of the septum may be offered to the patient for the reduced morbidity involved (54).

AGE OF THE PATIENT

In Norfolk the IVF success rate in women aged 35 to 39 years has not been significantly different from that in younger women (27). The success rate in women ≥ 40 years of age was recently evaluated in our program (55). There were no statistically significant differences between the number of preovulatory and immature oocytes harvested, fertilized, and transferred in this group and the number in patients <40 years of age. The pregnancy rate in patients ≥ 40 years old was comparable to that in younger patients (23.4% per attempt, 27.7% per retrieval, and 29.4% per transfer). The total abortion rate (60%) was higher and the ongoing pregnancy rate per transfer (12%) was lower, however, in patients ≥ 40 years old than in patients <39 years old. These findings are in accord with those reported by Edwards (56). Patients ≥ 40 years old should be advised of the higher abortion rates and lower ongoing pregnancy rates in their age group and should be thoroughly counseled before being admitted to an IVF program. Sharma (57) reported that with increasing age there appears to be a progressive decrease in the mean numbers of total oocytes collected, fertilized oocytes, and cleaved embryos. However, this has no major impact on the pregnancy rates in women <40 years of age with normal endocrine profiles (see below).

BASAL SERUM FSH AND LH ON CYCLE DAY 3

The aim of stimulating a patient for IVF or GIFT is the recruitment of multiple fertilizable oocytes. Patients respond differently in terms of peripheral E_2; number of follicles recruited, as seen by ultrasonography; and number and quality of oocytes retrieved, even when they are stimulated with the same type and dosage of recruiting agent or hormone. Patients are classified as high, normal, or low responders according to their E_2 levels when stimulation is discontinued and hCG is administered (58). The quality and number of oocytes obtained, as well as pregnancy rates, also correlate with the E_2 response, and the least successful outcome is obtained in low responders (59).

In Norfolk we have demonstrated (60) that serum FSH and LH levels on cycle day 3, before stimulation is initiated, are predictive of the E_2 response, number of preovulatory oocytes aspirated and transferred, and pregnancy rates. Patients were classified into three groups by their basal serum levels of FSH and LH on cycle day 3: (a) patients with a higher FSH:LH ratio; (b) patients with an equal ratio of FSH:LH (usually both levels at <10 mIU/ml); and (c) patients with a higher LH:FSH ratio. Patients with a higher FSH:LH ratio (group 1) invariably had FSH levels ≥ 15 mIU/ml on cycle day 3 and responded poorly to stimulation in terms of peripheral E_2 levels, number of oocytes aspirated, and pregnancy rate. The higher the FSH level on cycle day 3, the poorer the IVF outcome. Patients with a higher LH:FSH ratio (group 3) demonstrated higher peripheral E_2 levels in response to stimulation, larger numbers of follicles recruited and oocytes retrieved, and respectable pregnancy rates ($\geq 30\%$). The miscarriage rate, however, was high in this group, demonstrating the need to administer special stimulation protocols to them to obtain a better quality of oocytes and/or more favorable conditions for implantation. Patients with normal FSH and LH levels had an intermediate peripheral E_2 response to stimulation, a respectable number (mean $= 4$) of preovulatory oocytes, and a pregnancy rate of $>30\%$ after IVF.

Alternate methods of stimulation should be investigated for patients with an elevated basal serum FSH level on cycle day 3, if they are allowed to have repeated IVF attempts. Such methods of stimulation for the high-FSH patients are under investigation in Norfolk. Similarly, patients with a high LH:FSH ratio on cycle day 3 were found to benefit from suppression with a gonadotropin-releasing hormone agonist before gonadotropin stimulation for oocyte recruitment (61).

References

1. Hoff JD, Quigley ME, Yen SSC: Hormonal dynamics at midcycle: a re-evaluation. J Clin Endocrinol Metab 57:792, 1983
2. Hackeloer BJ, Fleming R, Robinson HP: Correlation of ultrasonic and endocrinologic assessment of human follicular development. Am J Obstet Gynecol 135:122, 1979
3. Kerin JF, Edmonds DK, Warnes GM: Morphological and functional relationships of graafian follicle growth to ovulation in women using ultrasonic, laparoscopic, and biochemical measurement. Br J Obstet Gynaecol 88:81, 1981
4. Hackeloer BJ: Ultrasound scanning of the ovarian cycle. J In Vitro Fertil Embryo Trans 1:217, 1984
5. Stumpf PG, March CM: Febrile morbidity following hysterosalpingography: identification of risk factors and recommendations for prophylaxis. Fertil Steril 33:487, 1980
6. Siegler AM: Hysterosalpingography. Fertil Steril 40:139, 1983
7. Snowden EU, Jarrett JC, Dawood MY: Comparison of diagnostic accuracy of laparoscopy, hysteroscopy, and hysterosalpingography in evaluation of female infertility. Fertil Steril 41:709, 1984
8. Downs KA, Gibson M: Basal body temperature graph and the luteal phase defect. Fertil Steril 40:466, 1983
9. Abraham GE, Maroulis GB, Marshall JR: Evaluation of corpus luteum function using measurements of plasma progesterone. Obstet Gynecol 44:522, 1974
10. Noyes RW, Hertig AT, Rock J: Dating the endometrial biopsy. Fertil Steril 1:3, 1950
11. American Fertility Society: Revised American Fertility Society classification of endometriosis. Fertil Steril 44:56, 1985
12. Koninckx PR, DeMoor P, Brosens IA: Diagnosis of the luteinized unruptured follicle syndrome by steroid hormone assays on peritoneal fluid. Br J Obstet Gynaecol 87:929, 1980
13. Coulam LB, Hill LM, Breckle R: Ultrasonic evidence for luteinization of unruptured preovulatory follicles. Fertil Steril 37:524, 1982
14. Liukkonen S, Koskimies AL, Tenhunen A, Ylostalo P: Diagnosis of luteinized unruptured follicle syndrome by ultrasound. Fertil Steril 41:26, 1984
15. Daly DL, Soto-Albors C, Walters C: Ultrasonographic assessment of luteinized unruptured follicle syndrome in unexplained infertility. Fertil Steril 43:62, 1985
16. Hamilton CJ, Wetzels LC, Evers JLH, Hoogland HJ, Muijtjens A, deHaan J: Follicle growth curves and hormonal patterns in patients with the luteinized unruptured follicle syndrome. Fertil Steril 43:541, 1985
17. Harrison RF, Blades M, deLouvois J, Hurley R: Doxycycline treatment and human fertility. Lancet 1:605, 1975
18. Matthews CD, Elmslie RG, Clapp KH, Svigos JM: The frequency of genital mycoplasma infection in human fertility. Fertil Steril 26:988, 1975
19. Hinton RA, Egdell LM, Andrews BE: A double blind crossover study of the effect of doxycycline on mycoplasma infection and infertility. Br J Obstet Gynaecol 85:379, 1979
20. Murphy AA, Green WR, Bobbie D, de la Cruz ZL, Rock JA: Unsuspected endometriosis documented by scanning electron microscopy in visually normal peritoneum. Fertil Steril 46:522, 1986
21. Fakih H, Baggett B, Holtz G: Interleukin-1: a possible role in the infertility associated with endometriosis. Fertil Steril 47:213, 1987
22. Yovich JL, Blackledge DG, Richardson PA, Matson PL, Turner SR, Draper R: Pregnancies following pronuclear stage tubal transfer. Fertil Steril 48:851, 1987
23. Jones HW Jr: The impact of in vitro fertilization on the practice of gynecology and obstetrics. Int J Fertil 31:99, 1986

24. Rock JA, Jones HW Jr: Factors influencing the success of salpingostomy techniques for distal fimbrial obstruction. Obstet Gynecol 52:591, 1978
25. Rock JA, Bergquist CA, Zacur HA: Tubal anastomosis following unipolar cautery. Fertil Steril 37:613, 1982
26. Shortle B, Jewelewicz R: Uterine rupture following reimplantation: review of the literature and report of three additional cases. Obstet Gynecol Surv 39:407, 1984
27. Jones HW Jr: Indication for in vitro fertilization. In Jones HW Jr, Jones GS, Hodgen GD, Rosenwaks Z (ed): In Vitro Fertilization—Norfolk. Baltimore: Williams & Wilkins, 1986, p 3
28. Oehninger S, Scott R, Jones D, Acosta AA, Muasher SJ, Kreiner D, Rosenwaks Z: Effect of the severity of tubo-ovarian disease and previous pelvic surgery on in vitro fertilization and embryo transfer. Abstract P-033, 44th Annual Meeting of the American Fertility Society, Atlanta, GA, October 1988
29. Chillik CF, Acosta AA, Garcia JE, Perera S, Rosenwaks Z, Jones HW Jr: The role of in vitro fertilization in infertile patients with endometriosis. Fertil Steril 44:56, 1985
30. Chillik C, Rosenwaks Z: Endometriosis and in vitro fertilization. Semin Reprod Endocrinol 3:377, 1985
31. Matson PL, Yovich JL: The treatment of infertility associated with endometriosis by in vitro fertilization. Fertil Steril 46:432, 1986
32. Oehninger S, Acosta AA, Kreiner D, Muasher SJ, Jones HW Jr, Rosenwaks Z: In vitro fertilization and embryo transfer: an established and successful therapy for endometriosis. J In Vitro Fertil Embryo Trans 5:249, 1988
33. Wardle PG, McLaughlin EA, McDermott A, Mitchell JD, Ray BD, Hull MGR: Endometriosis and ovulatory disorder: reduced fertilization in vitro compared with tubal and unexplained infertility. Lancet 2:236, 1985
34. Wood C, Baker G, Trounson A: Current status and future projects. In Wood C, Trounson A (eds): Clinical In Vitro Fertilization. Berlin: Springer-Verlag, 1984, p 11
35. Navot D, Muasher SJ, Oehninger S, Liu H-C, Veeck LL, Kreiner D, Rosenwaks Z: The value of in vitro fertilization for the treatment of unexplained infertility. Fertil 49:854, 1988
36. Leeton J, Mahadevan M, Trounson A, Wood C: Unexplained infertility and the possibilities of management with in vitro fertilization and embryo transfer. Aust NZ J Obstet Gynaecol 24:131, 1984
37. Asch RH, Ellsworth LR, Balmaceda JP, Wong PC: Pregnancy after translaparoscopic gamete intrafallopian transfer. Lancet 2:1034, 1984
38. Molloy D, Speirs A, du Plessis Y, McBain J, Johnson I: A laparoscopic approach to a program of gamete intrafallopian transfer. Fertil Steril 47:289, 1987
39. Yovich JL, Yovich JM, Edirisinghe WR: The relative chance of pregnancy following tubal or uterine transfer procedures. Fertil Steril 49:858, 1988
40. Feichtinger W, Kemeter P: Laparoscopic or ultrasonically guided follicle aspiration for in vitro fertilization. J In Vitro Fertil Embryo Trans 1:244, 1984
41. Parsons J, Riddle A, Booker M: Oocyte retrieval for in vitro fertilization by ultrasonically guided needle aspiration via the urethra. Lancet 1:1076, 1985
42. Deuenbach P, Wisand I, Moreau L: Transvaginal sonographically controlled ovarian follicle puncture for egg retrieval. Lancet 1:1467, 1984
43. Flood JT, Muasher SJ, Simonetti S, Kreiner D, Acosta AA, Rosenwaks Z: Comparison between laparoscopic and ultrasonographically guided transvaginal follicular aspiration methods in an in vitro fertilization program in the same patients using the same stimulation protocol. J In Vitro Fertil Embryo Trans 6:180, 1989
44. Garcia JE, Jones HW Jr, Acosta AA, Andrews MC: Reconstructive pelvic surgery for in vitro fertilization. Am J Obstet Gynecol 153:172, 1985
45. Diamond MP, Pellicer A, Boyers SP, DeCherney AH: The effect of periovarian adhesions on follicular development in patients undergoing ovarian stimulation for in vitro fertilization-embryo transfer. Fertil Steril 49:100, 1988
46. Molloy D, Martin M, Speirs A, Lopata A, Clarke G, McBain J, Ngu A, Johnston IH: Performance of patients with a "frozen pelvis" in an in vitro fertilization program. Fertil Steril 47:450, 1987
47. Imoedemhe DAG, Wafik AH, Chan RCW: In vitro fertilization in women with "frozen pelvis": clinical outcome of treatment. Fertil Steril 49:268, 1988
48. Diamond MP, Wentz AC, Herbert CM, Pittaway DE, Maxson WS, Daniell JF: One ovary or two: differences in ovulation induction, estradiol levels, and follicular development in a program of in vitro fertilization. Fertil Steril 41:524, 1984
49. Alper MM, Seibel MM, Oskowitz SP, Smith BD, Ransil BJ, Taymor ML: Comparison of follicular response in patients with one or two ovaries in a program of in vitro fertilization. Fertil Steril 44:652, 1985

50. Dodds WG, Chin N, Awadalla SG, Miller F, Friedman C, Kim M: In vitro fertilization and embryo transfer in patients with one ovary. Fertil Steril 48:249, 1987

51. Boutteville C, Muasher SJ, Acosta AA, Jones HW Jr, Rosenwaks Z: Results of in vitro fertilization in patients with one or two ovaries. Fertil Steril 47:821, 1987

52. Muasher SJ, Garcia JE, Jones HW Jr: Experience with diethylstibestrol-exposed infertile women in a program of in vitro fertilization. Fertil Steril 42:20, 1984

53. Sandberg EC, Riffle WC, Higdon JV, Getman CE: Pregnancy outcome in women exposed to diethylstibestrol in utero. Am J Obstet Gynecol 140:194, 1981

54. Daly DC, Walters CA, Soto-Albors CE, Riddick DH: Hysteroscopic metroplasty: surgical technique and obstetric outcome. Feril Steril 39:623, 1983

55. Romeu A, Muasher SJ, Acosta AA, Veeck LL, Diaz J, Jones GS, Jones HW Jr, Rosenwaks Z: Results of in vitro fertilization attempts in women 40 years of age and older: the Norfolk experience. Fertil Steril 47:130, 1987

56. Edwards RJ, Fishel SB, Cohen J: Factors influencing the success of in vitro fertilization for alleviating human infertility. J In Vitro Fertil Embryo Trans 1:3, 1984

57. Sharma V, Riddle A, Mason BA, Pampiglione J, Campbell S: An analysis of factors infuencing the establishment of a clinical pregnancy in an ultrasound-based ambulatory in vitro fertilization program. Fertil Steril 49:468, 1988

58. Garcia JE, Jones GS, Acosta AA, Wright G: Human menopausal gonadotropin follicular maturation for oocyte aspiration: phase II, 1981. Fertil Steril 39:174, 1983

59. Jones HW Jr, Acosta AA, Andrews MC, Garcia JE, Jones GS, Mantzavinos T, McDowell J, Sandow B, Veeck L, Whibley T, Wilkes C, Wright G: The importance of the follicular phase to success and failure in vitro fertilization. Fertil Steril 40:317, 1983

60. Muasher SJ, Oehninger S, Simonetti S, Matta J, Ellis LM, Liu H-C: The value of basal and/or stimulated serum gonadotropin levels in prediction of stimulation response and in vitro fertilization outcome. Fertil Steril 50:298, 1988

61. Droesch K, Muasher SJ, Brzyski RG, Jones GS, Simonetti S, Liu H-C, Rosenwaks Z: Value of suppression with a gonadotropin-releasing hormone agonist prior to gonadotropin stimulation for in vitro fertilization. Fertil Steril 51:292, 1989

CHAPTER 4

Laboratory Procedures: Review and Background

Part One—Diagnostic Procedures

Section A:

BASIC SEMEN ANALYSIS

ROELOF MENKVELD, PH.D., AND THINUS F. KRUGER, M.D.

The scientific approach to male infertility and semen analysis started in 1677 with van Leeuwenhoek's letter to the Royal Society in London describing the discovery of the human spermatozoon by Johan Ham. According to Schirren (1), van Leeuwenhoek stated that, in the case of a sterile marriage, the microscope could solve the question of who was the responsible partner. According to Joël (2), the same statement was made about 100 years later by von Gleichen-Russworm (1717–1783). In 1866, the importance of the microscope and the presence of spermatozoa for fertilization were again stressed by Sims (3), who performed postcoital examinations of fluids of the vagina and the endocervix. He stated that spermatozoa had to be present in the endocervical mucus for conception to occur. Only since the turn of this century has a more scientific approach to semen analysis been adopted. According to Ross (4), it was only in the 1940s that Wiesman stated that a semen analysis was not complete unless the volume, motility, concentration, and morphology were determined. This was further supported by the work of Hotchkiss (5) in 1945.

Minimum requirements and standards for the performance and rating of semen analysis were established in 1951 by the American Fertility Association (6), in 1966 by Freund (7), and in 1971 by Eliasson (8) and by the World Health Organization (9). The minimum requirements for a complete semen analysis are still being expanded and today include the so-called functional tests such as the zona-free hamster ova penetration test as described by Yanagimachi (10), the triple-staining technique for the acrosome reaction (11), and the determination of the acrosin activity of the spermatozoa (12). The sperm-cervical mucus interaction test is also included by some authors (13). We feel that it is important that some type of antispermatozoa antibody test should also be included.

A complete semen analysis (for which several samples may be needed) can therefore be divided into the following five categories: (*a*) background data, (*b*) physical data, (*c*) quantitative and qualitative analysis, (*d*) biochemical analysis, and (*e*) functional tests.

Background Data

A semen analysis cannot be interpreted unless certain basic facts are known: the days of abstinence, the method by which the sample was produced, and the time lapse between production and analysis. Another important aspect is the number of semen analyses that must be performed.

METHODS FOR THE PRODUCTION OF SEMEN

The method of obtaining a semen sample has been a problem since the time of van Leeuwenhoek's research. Masturbation as a means of obtaining a sample has, until recently, been condemned; even now it may still pose a problem at times. In earlier years, the most accepted method was through use of the condom (14, 15), although samples obtained from the vagina after intercourse (15) or obtained by masturbation (16, 17) were also used sporadically. Hotchkiss (18) in 1941 and MacLeod and Hotchkiss (19) in 1946 suggested that semen samples could be obtained by masturbation or, if that was not possible, by coitus interruptus. The sample had to be brought to the laboratory as soon as possible, preferably in less than 2 hours (20, 21). Only if the sample was needed for special investigation was the patient asked to produce the sample at the laboratory (22–24).

Today it is becoming more important that the sample should be produced in a specially equipped room at the laboratory (25–28), especially when more sophisticated tests are involved (24). This method has the advantage of permitting observations of coagulation, liquefaction, etc., and of exercising control over environmental conditions. The time lapse between ejaculation and investigation, and the manner in which the sample was produced are ascertainable. Also, a relationship with the patient can be established, information is easy to obtain, and questions can be answered. If the sample is brought to the laboratory, it may be left on a counter without any information so that the results cannot be evaluated or interpreted, or patients may produce samples by coitus interruptus even though they may claim otherwise. Coitus interruptus has disadvantages: the first part of the sample may be lost, and vaginal epithelial cells may be present (28).

Patients having problems producing a semen sample by masturbation can use a vibrator (29) or a special plastic condom (Milex) (23). However, better results have been obtained with the new seminal collection device (30) (HDC Corporation, Mountain View, CA).

CONTAINERS

In the past, glass containers were used, but they must be washed and sterilized after use, and they may break (25). The ideal container is a 60- to 100-ml wide-mouth jar made of polypropylene, with a screw cap that fits tightly to prevent any loss of semen when it is transported. In our experience, some types of plastics (such as polystyrene) have disadvantages: they may cause increased viscosity, may be toxic to the spermatozoa, or may influence motility. It is therefore important to test any new type of container before it is used.

ABSTINENCE

Since the 1930s, it has been well known that the period of abstinence can have a significant effect on the semen volume and sperm concentration (22, 31–35). Since that time, the period of abstinence that should be adhered to before a semen analysis is done has remained controversial. There are two primary schools of thought. One feels that the period of abstinence should be based on the length of time from which the optimal semen potential can be expected (1, 22, 32, 36), so that the optimal sperm production capacity of the testes can be determined (8). The other group feels that the period should be determined according to the patient's normal coital frequency (37–40) or that a fixed period of 3 to 4 days of abstinence, based on the average patient's coital frequency, should be prescribed (33). Still others simply ask for a routine 3-day abstinence to ensure better uniformity of results (20, 41).

We feel that it is important for a fixed period of 3 to 4 days of abstinence to be prescribed so that the semen analyses are performed according to more standardized conditions and so that the results of different semen analyses can be compared. If this is not done, it is impossible to know whether the differences in the semen parameters of different samples from the same patient are due to a normal variation, to the variation of number of days of abstinence, or to both. In a study performed on 1808 men (42), we found that the optimal period of abstinence to obtain the best semen quality is 3 to 5 days. When the period of abstinence exceeded 10 days, motility and morphology were severely depressed. Today the most commonly prescribed period of abstinence is 3 to 4 days, although a period of 3 to 7 days is accepted by some laboratories (1, 36). However, it is important that the patient's circumstances be taken into consideration, as the prescribed period of abstinence may interfere with the marital lifestyle and can be disruptive to the couple's sex preferences. In these cases, motivation to adhere to the prescribed days of abstinence is of great importance.

NUMBER OF SAMPLES TO BE ANALYZED

Zaneveld (43) feels that if a patient produces a normal sample the first time, it is not necessary to do any further analysis. However, if the sample is borderline or classified as abnormal according to the laboratory standards, it is necessary to collect more specimens before a final diagnosis can be made. Zaneveld recommends that three semen analyses be carried out at 3- to 5-week intervals. Ross (4) stipulates that three semen samples be obtained at 2- to 6-week intervals and analyzed before a diagnosis of abnormal semen can be made. Some authors feel that there will always be some variation from sample to sample and that it is therefore necessary to perform at least two semen analyses before a final evaluation can be made (30, 44, 45). Others state that several (23) or three or four (25, 46) analyses over a period of 3 months are required to make an estimation of a patient's fertility potential.

Sherins (47) and Poland (48) both calculated that, on the average, three samples are sufficient to make a reliable estimation of a patient's fertility potential. In cases where the first analysis showed doubtful results, Sherins (47) found that it may be necessary to do six to nine analyses before a reliable interpretation can be made. From our own (42) studies in which the results of four consecutive analyses of 1199 men were compared, we concluded that, in normal circumstances and with comparable days of abstinence, the first sample can be regarded as representative of the other three samples. We concluded that in these circumstances one sample is sufficient.

Another factor that must be considered is the cost. The tendency is to keep the number of samples to a minimum. A good policy, therefore, is that in cases where the first sample is classified as normal according to the laboratory's standards, no repeat is needed. In cases where the analysis is abnormal, the patient should be reevaluated two or three times within 3 months so that a good semen profile can be obtained.

Physical Parameters

The physical parameters of the sample are classified by Freund (49) and Zaneveld (43) as volume, color, liquefaction, pH, and viscosity; coagulation and smell can also be included.

COAGULATION

This is an important aspect of the semen analysis which is ignored by many investigators, mainly because many samples are still produced at home instead of at the laboratory. Human semen is ejaculated in a liquefied state but is quickly transformed into a semisolid state or coagulum, probably under the influence of the enzyme proteinkinase (50) secreted by the seminal vesicles. Normally, nearly the whole sample is transformed into the coagulated state and only a very small part remains liquefied. When coagulation does not occur, it may be the result of a congenital absence of the vas deferens and the seminal vesicles and is then associated with the absence of fructose in seminal plasma.

LIQUEFACTION

In a normal sample, liquefaction occurs within 10 to 20 minutes of collection. This is caused by a proteolytic enzyme, fibrinolysin, secreted by the prostate (51), as well as two other proteolytic enzymes, fibrinogenase and aminopeptidase (52). If liquefaction takes more than 20 minutes or does not occur at all, it is a sign that the prostate is not functioning normally, usually as a result of previous prostatitis. In some cases, non-liquefaction may be a cause of infertility, as the spermatozoa are not released from the coagulum. Small coagulated particles may still be present after a period of time; however, this can be regarded as normal, and they will dissolve eventually.

VISCOSITY

In 1934, Cary (38) described the consistency of semen as slightly viscous, a parameter that could easily be determined by forcing the semen slowly through a pipette. Similar techniques have been described by other authors (18, 36, 41). Another method is determining the length of a semen thread that can be drawn with the aid of a small wooden rod (5, 32).

Portnoy (20) pointed out that the presence of an infection in the genital tract, prostate, or seminal vesicles can increase the viscosity, which in turn can have a deleterious influence on motility. An increase in viscosity, according to Amelar (29), is not a cause of infertility but can have an adverse effect on the determination of sperm concentration. To reduce viscosity, the semen can be drawn into a 5- or 10-ml pipette and forced out several times through a number 18 or 19 needle (51).

It is also important to distinguish between a delayed period of liquefaction and an increase in viscosity. An increased viscosity may be the result of abnormal prostate function or the use of an unsuitable type of plastic container.

VOLUME

Determinations of semen volume, according to Lode (14), were made in 1864 by Mantegazza, while Benedict in 1910 (53), Macomber in 1929 (54), and Belding in 1933 (55) and 1934 (31) also reported on different aspects of semen volume. Cary (38) stated in 1934 that a semen analysis must include a note on the semen volume and that the volume for a male under the age of 40 years should not be less than 3.5 ml. According to Hotchkiss (5), a volume of this magnitude is needed for good buffering of the seminal pool against the acid secretions of the vagina.

Volumes have been determined by means of glass syringes (32), graduated glass cylinders (39), or weighing (36). The most commonly used method today is to measure the volume by a graduated centrifuge tube or cylinder to the nearest 0.1 ml.

If the volume is less than 1.0 ml, it is important to establish whether it was a complete sample. This is important because the first portion, containing the most sperm with the best motility, is often lost. A low volume may also result from an obstruction due to a previous infection of the genital tract or from a congenital absence of the seminal vesicles and vasa efferentia. This condition will be associated with the absence of fructose (43). A small volume may also be due to retrograde ejaculation, especially if the patient has had surgery of the prostate or the bladder neck. Retrograde ejaculation can be diagnosed by investigation of the urine after an ejaculation.

COLOR

Cary (38) described the color of semen as opaque and grayish, changing to yellowish with an increase in the days of abstinence. Hotchkiss (5) noticed that fresh blood will give semen a reddish color and old blood a brownish color, while samples with a low concentration and white blood cells will usually have a transparent and watery consistency. Schirren (1) found that certain types of medicines, such as antibiotics, can discolor the semen. The color can also indicate possible pathology.

ODOR

Although semen has a strong, distinctive odor, this parameter is seldom used. The odor has been compared to flowers of the chestnut or the St. John's bread tree. It is thought that the odor is caused by oxidation of the spermine secreted by the prostate. An absence of the odor can therefore be associated with abnormal prostate function due to an infection (43).

pH

One of the first articles to mention the pH of semen was that of Muschat (56) in 1926. Early studies on the pH were also done by Cary (38) and Messer (57). Both came to the conclusion that the pH was of little significance, although Messer found that the pH increased with time after ejaculation. Colorimetric methods (41) and glass electrodes (57, 58) have been used to determine the pH. Today both methods are still used (1), but the electronic method is more accurate (43).

Schirren (1) stressed the importance of pH measurements. In cases of acute prostatitis, vesiculitis, or bilateral epididymitis, the pH will always be more than 8.0. In cases of chronic infection of the aforementioned organs, the pH will always be below 7.2 and can be as low as 6.6. With an obstruction of the ejaculatory ducts, or in cases where only prostatic fluids are secreted, the pH will also be less than 7.0.

Quantitative and Qualitative Analysis

The parameters under this heading are those regarded by most laboratories as a standard, basic semen analysis. They include the estimation of quantitative and qualitative motility, the supravital staining procedure to determine sperm vitality, and the concentration and morphology of the spermatozoa.

DETERMINATION OF QUANTITATIVE (PERCENTAGE OF MOTILE SPERMATOZOA) AND QUALITATIVE (SPEED OF FORWARD PROGRESSION) MOTILITY

The importance of the presence of motile spermatozoa in the endocervical mucus (3, 59) and semen (15, 60, 61) has been stressed by many authors, and the development of motility evaluation has resulted in the establishment of three categories. These were identified in 1938 by Hotchkiss (41): (*a*) the type and aggressiveness of movement (speed of forward progression); (*b*) the percentage of inactive spermatozoa; and (*c*) the duration of motility (in vitro).

The estimation of motility duration and the relevance of this estimation are controversial. Hühner (15) claimed that this determination was of no relevance for a normal semen analysis, while Moench (60) thought it of great importance. MacLeod (21) pointed out that the seminal plasma is only a temporary transport medium and that it is not physiological to assess the duration of sperm motility in this way. However, it is known that motile spermatozoa can still be present in a semen sample after 24 hours at room temperature. Therefore, we believe that valuable information can be obtained by regular examination of a wet preparation. An estimation of the motile quality of the spermatozoa, the formation of spermine crystals and sperm agglutination, and the presence of microorganisms (42) can be obtained.

Grading the type of movement or aggressiveness and the speed of forward progression is usually done according to an arbitrary grading system on a scale of 0 to 4 (41, 62, 63), 1 to 5 (36), or 0 to 10 (39), 0 meaning no motility and no forward progression, and 4, 5, or 10 meaning excellent forward progression.

The motility is usually expressed as the percentage of motile spermatozoa to the nearest 5% or 10% (36, 39, 62, 63). MacLeod (64) introduced the so-called motility index, which is obtained by multiplying the motility by the forward progression. More elaborate methods (36) have also been described, including the use of a hemocytometer (32, 58, 63). Atherton (65) devoted a chapter to six newer methods, including the photographic sperm track technique of Janick (66) and the sperm velocity test developed by Barták (67).

Newer techniques used today are the light-scattering technique, where a laser beam and the Doppler effect are used (68), and the multiple-exposure photographic technique of Makler (69), which he has improved (70) by incorporating a computerized system. More recently, automated semen analyses have been introduced, with varying degrees of success (71).

Poor motility (asthenozoospermia) can have several etiologic factors, which can be divided into four categories: (*a*) artifacts, (*b*) morphological abnormalities, (*c*) inherent factors, and (*d*) other factors.

Artifacts can be caused by using an inadequate method of collection, such as a regular condom, which may be sperm-toxic and may allow the sample to be contaminated by vaginal secretions; by the use of lubricants (72); by collecting an incomplete sample; by a long delay in transferring the sample to the laboratory; or by exposure of the sample to extreme temperatures. Artifacts can also be caused by technical factors such as cold shock from cold laboratory containers, slides, and pipettes; by the use of unsuitable, contaminated, or wet containers; by the storage of the sample at adverse temperatures (73, 74), and by inadequate technique used for the wet preparation, resulting in wrong thickness (75).

Morphological abnormalities include structural aberrations of the head (round head cell syndrome), the midpiece, and the tail (Kartagener's and short-tail syndromes). Inherent factors are those caused by a fault during formation and maturation of the spermatozoa before they are released from the Sertoli cells (65, 76) or during transport through the ductal system, or through abnormal function of the prostate or seminal vesicles. Other factors that can cause poor motility are hematospermia, varicocele, chromosomal aberrations, bacterial infections with an abnormal pH (74, 77), and the presence of certain metals or metal ions (78) in non-physiologic concentrations.

SPERMATOZOA CONCENTRATION

According to Lode (14), Mantegazza was the first person who, in 1864, performed sperm counts on human samples. Lode (14), in 1891, reported the results he obtained in sperm counts that he performed with an erythrocyte-counting chamber after diluting the semen samples four to five times. The average count of 24 samples provided by four men was $60,876 \times 10^6$/ml. In 1929, the well-known article of Macomber (54) described a sperm-counting technique that is the basis for most of the techniques used today. A 1:20 dilution was made with a white blood cell pipette, and the count was performed on a hemocytometer. The diluting fluid consisted of a 5% $NaHCO_3$ solution, to which 1% formalin was added. Macomber concluded that the possibility of conception was small if the sperm count was less than 60×10^6/ml.

Several improvements on the original method of Macomber (54) have been described (17, 31, 49, 79). Hotchkiss (41) pointed out that it is important for the count to be performed within 3 hours after ejaculation to ensure accuracy. Instead of the white blood cell pipette, Eliasson (8) used micropipettes to make a 1:50, 1:100, or a 1:200 dilution. Van Zyl (26) introduced the use of a glass tuberculin syringe instead of the white blood cell pipette. With this method, it is possible to make a 1:10, 1:20, or 1:100 dilution.

In 1962, Segal (80) introduced the electronic counting method with the aid of the Coulter counter. This method requires thorough training, a high degree of skill, and much time devoted to the calibration of the apparatus. The preparation of the correct dilutions is important, and attention must be paid to the interference of background particles (81). High—and especially low—concentrations can cause problems, and special dilutions should be made in these cases (82).

Makler (83) introduced a special sperm-counting chamber in 1979 and improved it in 1980 (84). With this method, it is possible to do sperm counts directly on undiluted semen, after immobilization of the spermatozoa. In low sperm concentration the method has a high coefficient of variation, and several drops must be counted (83). Menkveld (85) demonstrated that the results of the tuberculin syringe (TS) method compared well with the results of the white blood cell pipette (WCP) method. We (86) also compared the TS method with the Makler chamber (MC) and WCP methods and found that in our hands the TS method had the best relative accuracy, followed by the MC and then the WCP method, with an error variability of 1.96, 31.05, and 147.05, respectively, for a series of 20 samples with a sperm concentration of more than 50×10^6/ml. Today counting spermatozoa with the aid of computerized equipment is gaining ground, but more work must be done on the standardization of the procedure (71).

Differences still exist as to what can be regarded as a normal sperm concentration, and many different so-called normal counts have been proposed: 60×10^6/ml by Macomber (54), 20×10^6/ml by Eliasson (23) and MacLeod (87), and 10×10^6/ml by van Zyl (26, 46, 88) and Santomauro (89), to name a few. In 1962, MacLeod, stated that he was still of the opinion that a count of 20×10^6/ml was a good cut-off point but that fertilization could still take place if the count was as low as 10×10^6/ml, on the condition that a good motility and forward progression were present (21). Although MacLeod made this concession, he was not prepared to go along with the statements by Nelson (90) and others (91–93) that there is a decline in the spermatozoa concentration as time passes (94). This is in agreement with our own findings (42, 95) in a study where we statistically compared the trends of the average yearly sperm counts of three ethnic groups over a 15-year period (1976 to 1982). Very small negative correlation coefficients of -0.0425, -0.0211, and -0.0547 were found, which were of no statistical significance.

MORPHOLOGICAL EVALUATION OF SPERMATOZOA

After van Leeuwenhoek's first letter to the Royal Society in London with detailed descriptions and drawings of the morphology of the human spermatozoon, little attention was paid to the morphology. Only after the late 19th and early 20th century did the morphological appearance of spermatozoa become a focus of interest, and it was accepted that normal and pathological forms could simultaneously appear in a semen sample (2, 5). Significant contributions have since been made by Cary (38, 96) Parkes (97), Moench (98), and Williams (16, 99, 100). These advances were made possible through the development of new staining techniques (16, 38, 44, 99, 100) and the introduction of systems to classify spermatozoa into groups according to the type of abnormality (38, 41, 98).

In 1937, Williams (100) made a major contribution to the classification system. He pointed out that since evaluation of morphology depends largely upon objective findings, comparable results may be anticipated by different observers provided a uniform method of examination is adopted. This is possible only if the spermatozoa are examined minutely and classified into a limited number of groups (no more than six), based on their morphological characteristics. This system was improved by Hotchkiss (41), MacLeod (101–103), Freund (7), Eliasson (8), and Menkveld (104).

Moench (17) stressed the importance of other cells, such as the germinal epithelium, spermiophages, leukocytes, and unknown cells, that could be associated with infertility. Contributions in this regard were also made by Frank (105), Hartmann (106), and MacLeod (102).

However, sperm morphology remains one of the most controversial semen parameters in terms of its role in male fertility potential (31, 40, 63) as a prognostic parameter for fertilization in normal in vivo fertilization, IVF, the hamster test (107), artificial insemination by husband (AIH), and gamete intrafallopian transfer (GIFT) (108–110). This controversy can mainly be ascribed to the fact that there are still no clear and standardized criteria for a normal spermatozoon. The consequence is that diverse results are found in different laboratories and even within the same laboratory, as has been shown by the classic work of Freund (7) and more recently by Fredricsson (111) and Jequier (112). Freund (7) and Eliasson (8) proposed criteria for standardization. In our laboratory, we laid down even more stringent criteria (104). With this method (42, 104), we were able to obtain a high degree of relative accuracy among four observers with an error variability of 2.89 to 19.67. High Spearman's correlation coefficients of 0.8675 to 0.6537 ($P<0.001$) were also obtained among the four observers, in comparison with the correlation coefficients of 0.633 to 0.389 reported by Ayodeji (113) in a similar study. Our results (42, 104) can only be obtained if the following guidelines are strictly followed: (*a*) morphology smears of high quality must be prepared, and set rules must be followed with the evaluation of the spermatozoa; and (*b*) for the identification of a normal spermatozoon, a reference population of normal spermatozoa must be available. The definition of a normal spermatozoon based on this population must allow as little variation as possible.

Although the following principles are basic, they are often neglected: The slides must be thoroughly cleaned before use. Very thin smears must be prepared, so that the spermatozoa are in one focus level, each sperm can be visualized separately, and there are no more than five to 10 sperm per visual field. This can be done by altering the size of the semen drop and by adjusting the angle and speed of the slide used to make the smear (5). The slides are left to air-dry and are fixed in alcohol before staining. For routine work, a staining method such as the Papanicolaou procedure (114) is preferred; it gives a good staining of both the spermatozoa and other cells, such as the precursors or germinal epithelium cells and white blood cells (25). Other possible staining methods are described by Aitken (9). For special circumstances, rapid staining methods such as the Diff-Quik (115), Test Simplets (116), and toluidine blue-pyronine (117) can be used.

At least 100, but preferably 200, spermatozoa should be evaluated. They should be measured when there is any doubt about the classification of the sperm as too small, too large, or possibly elongated. Spermatozoa should never be evaluated in only one area but in several areas. Experience has shown that unrepresentative evaluations can be obtained if this is not done. The highest possible magnification should always be used; if this is not done, only the grossest abnormalities will be noted.

The second important aspect is the normal reference population. We (42, 104) used spermatozoa found in good periovulatory cervical mucus drawn from the upper endocervical canal after coitus (Fig. 4.1). Based on this, we define a normal spermatozoon as one having an oval form with a smooth contour and an acrosome comprising 40% to 70% of the distal part of the head; no abnormalities of the neck, midpiece, or tail; and no cytoplasmic droplets of more than half the sperm head, as described by Eliasson (8). We also use the dimensions described by Eliasson. The normal dimensions may differ according to the staining method used. The dimensions for head length and width given by Kruger (118) for the Diff-Quik method are larger than those given by Eliasson (5 to 6 μm $\times$ 2.5 to 3.5 μm vs. 3 to 5 μm $\times$ 2 to 3 μm, respectively).

Our system takes the whole sperm into consideration; borderline normal is taken as abnormal. The rationale for this is that the stricter the criteria and the less variation allowed, the more repeatable the results will be between and within observers.

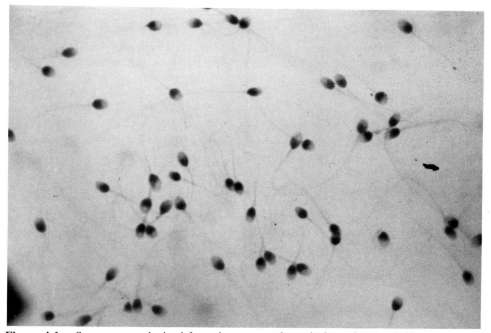

Figure 4.1. Spermatozoa obtained from the upper endocervical canal and suitable for use as a normal reference population for the evaluation of sperm morphology. A few slightly amorphous (borderline normal) spermatozoa are present.

The value of this method as a prognostic tool has been shown in an analysis of our IVF results (119). When the percentage of normal spermatozoa was 14% or less, there was a drastic drop in the fertilization rate, and no pregnancies were recorded. A further modification was introduced by Kruger (118), who found that in the group of men with 14% or less normal spermatozoa, two subgroups could be distinguished: those with a good prognosis (G pattern) and those with a poor prognosis (P pattern). Kruger included an extra class comprising slightly amorphous forms. Men with a combination of 30% or more slightly amorphous and normal forms were those with a good prognosis.

The morphological phenotype of spermatozoa is genetically determined (120); under normal circumstances and standardized conditions, it stays relatively constant with respect to the type of abnormalities and the percentage of normal forms (102, 106, 121). However, morphology must be regarded as a very sensitive parameter. Any stress caused by abnormal physical conditions (42, 103, 122), environmental influences of certain occupations (42, 123)—as seen in men working at lead (124) and DBCP (125) plants and drivers of vehicles (126)—and other factors such as the frequency of ejaculation (42, 127) will be reflected in the reduced percentage of normal forms (42, 128, 129). It is thought that abnormal morphology can be caused by two mechanisms. One is thought to be inherent or local, with abnormalities originating at the spermatogonia/spermatocyte I level and caused by abnormal biochemical functions of the Leydig cells, lamina propia, or Sertoli cells. This type is manifested especially in abnormalities of the acrosome and is irreversible. The second type is caused by environmental factors or stress acting on the Sertoli cells in the early stages of spermatogenesis. It is manifested by simple elongation, which is thought to be reversible, followed by more severe elongation, which is thought to be irreversible (130).

The question now arises whether it is time for a more clinically oriented approach to the evaluation and classification of sperm morphology. Based on our principles (42, 104, 119) and the work of Hofmann (130) and Kruger (118), classifications such as round heads, large heads, duplication, etc., should be disregarded. More attention should be given to acrosomal abnormalities, elongation, and slightly amorphous (borderline normal) forms. The latter are especially important in making a better diagnosis of male fertility potential in cases with a low percentage of normal forms and in establishing a better prognosis for possible treatments using such procedures as IVF, AIH, and GIFT.

SUPRAVITAL STAINING TECHNIQUE

Supravital staining for determining the percentage of live spermatozoa was performed in 1930 by Moench (61), but he found that this method added no more information than he could obtain with the direct evaluation of motility. MacLeod (131) used a similar method and also found the results unsatisfactory. The method most often used today is based on the eosin-nigrosin method described by Blom (132) in 1950 and modified by Dougherty (133) in 1975. Eliasson (134), who described his own technique, together with Treichl (135), modified the method of Dougherty by reducing the eosin concentration from 5% to 1%.

The performance of a supravital technique is important to distinguish between live and dead spermatozoa, since spermatozoa can be alive but immotile due to cold shock, etc., as discussed above. The results of supravital staining should always be some percentage points higher than the estimated motility. A diagnosis of necrozoospermia (all spermatozoa dead) cannot be made unless supravital staining has been performed.

Standards for Normal Semen Parameters

Minimum standards or values for normal semen based on the parameters of volume, motility, speed of forward progression, and morphology have been proposed. These were mostly obtained through studies on fertile populations (9). Some of these values (1, 8, 21, 38, 40, 41, 46, 58, 136–140) are shown in Table 4.1.

From Table 4.1, it can been seen that the threshold values have been lowered as time passed. In 1950, Falk (141) stated that the values published up to that time were too high in regard to the chances for conception and that it was not necessary for all semen parameters to conform to normal values. A few good parameters could compensate for abnormal ones, with the most important parameter being a high percentage of normal forms.

In 1976, we (46) called attention to the fact that patients seen at an infertility clinic do not constitute a normal population. Therefore, it is more important to establish whether or not they have a chance of fertilizing their wives—if normal—than to measure their potential fertilizing abilities according to fertile male standards. It is of utmost importance to define minimum standards or thresholds, above or below which clear differences in the pregnancy rates can be observed. Table 4.2 shows these values, together with currently accepted international standards based on the lower values obtained from Table 4.1.

Table 4.1.
Normal Semen Values Used by Different Authors

Author (date; ref. no.)	Volume (ml)	Motility (% motile)	Forward Progression	Concentration ($\times 10^6$/ml)	Morphology (% normal)
Cary 1934 (38)	3.5	75	—	70.0	?
Hotchkiss 1938 (41)	3.0	60–65	—	60.0	80–90
Pollak 1939 (136)	3.0–5.0	80	—	60.0–120.0	80
Davis 1943 (137)	4.0	80–95	—	60.0	80–95
Harvey 1945 (58)	—	45	—	50.0	65
Williams 1946 (138)	—	70–100	—	40.0	80
MacLeod 1965 (21)	2.0–5.0	40	2.5	20.0	60
Freund 1968 (40)	1.0–5.0	50	5[a]	20.0	60
Eliasson 1971 (8)	1.0	60	4[b]	60.0	60
Schirren 1972 (1)	2.0–6.0	70	—	40.0	60
Bustos-Obregón 1981 (139)	1.5–6.0	40	—	20.0	50
Eliasson 1981 (140)	2.0–6.0	50	Good	20.0	40
van Zyl 1976 (46)	—	30	2.0	10.0	20

[a] On a scale of 1 to 10.
[b] On a scale of 1 to 5.

With the aid of our own parameters and the international values, we calculated the percentage of patients who could be classified as normal or fertile in a series of 1285 men (including 233 pregnancies) in 1976 (46) and in a series of 2266 men in 1987 (42). The

Table 4.2.
Summary of Lower International Normal Parameters and Normal Values Used at Tygerberg Hospital

	International Values	Tygerberg Hospital Values (42, 46)
Volume (ml)	2–6	1–6
Count ($\times 10^6$/ml)	≥20.0	≥10.0
Motility (% motile)	≥40	≥30
Forward progression[a]	≥3.0	≥2.0
Morphology (% normal)	≥40 (60)[b]	≥20

[a] On a scale of 1 to 4.
[b] For the 1976 series (46), 60% was used as the normal international value.

Table 4.3.
Percentage of Men Classified as Fertile or Normal in Two Tygerberg Series (42, 46) According to Internationally Used Normal Values and Normal Values Used at Tygerberg

	First Series, 1976 (46)	Second Series, 1987 (42)
International values	18.8 (21.0)[a]	20.5
Tygerberg values	68.4 (87.6)[a]	64.5

[a] Percentage of 233 pregnancies which occurred in the fertile group. The rest occurred in the group of men classified as subfertile or infertile.

results, including the percentage of pregnancies in the first series, are shown in Table 4.3. If the current international standards are used, only 18.8% and 20.5% of our male patients can be regarded as normal or fertile, and only 21% of the total 233 pregnancies occurred in the fertile group. However, with our own normal values, 68.4% and 64.5% of men are classified as normal or fertile, and 87.6% of the pregnancies occurred in the fertile group. There seems to be a good chance that a pregnancy can occur in vivo with semen parameters well below the international standards (140, 142, 143) and even below our values. This is even more true for IVF, AIH, and GIFT. Minimum standards should be established according to each laboratory's own experience and results.

Performing semen analyses that include only the basic parameters is not sufficient; more extensive tests or procedures should be requested. A semen analysis now must include a screening test for antisperm antibodies. If the parameters are normal, further functional tests are indicated, especially in cases of unexplained infertility.

References

1. Schirren C: Practical Andrology. Berlin: Verlag Brüder Hartman, 1972, p 10
2. Joël CA: Historical survey of research on spermatozoa from antiquity to the present. In Joël CA (ed): Fertility Disturbances in Men and Women. Basel: Karger, 1971, p 3
3. Sims JM: On the microscope as an aid in the diagnosis and treatment of sterility. NY Med Bull 8:393, 1869
4. Ross LS: Diagnosis and treatment of infertile men: a clinical perspective. J Urol 130:847, 1983
5. Hotchkiss RS: Fertility in Men. London: William Heinemann, 1945
6. Abarbanel AR, Brown WE, Greulich WW, Pommerenke WT, Simmons FA, Sturgis S: Evaluation of the barren marriage: minimal procedures. Fertil Steril 2:1, 1951
7. Freund M: Standards for the rating of human sperm morphology: a cooperative study. Int J Fertil 11:97, 1966
8. Eliasson R: Standards for investigation of human semen. Andrologia 3:49, 1971
9. Aitken RJ, Comhaire FH, Eliasson R, Jager S, Kremer J, Jones WR, de Kretser DM, Nieschlag E, Paulsen CA, Wang C, Waites GMH: WHO Laboratory Manual for the Examination of Human Semen and Semen-Cervical Mucus Interaction, 2d ed. Cambridge, England: Cambridge University Press, 1987
10. Yanagimachi, R, Yanagimachi H, Rogers BJ: The use of zona-free hamster ova as a test-system for the assessment of the fertilizing capacity of human spermatozoa. Biol Reprod 15:471, 1976
11. Talbot P, Chacon R: A triple stain technique for evaluating normal acrosome reaction of human sperm. J Exp Zool 215:201, 1981
12. Schill W-B, Feifel M: Low acrosin activity in polyzoospermia. Andrologia 16:589, 1984
13. Mortimer D: The male factor in infertility. II Sperm function testing. Curr Probl Obstet Gynecol Fertil 8:4, 1985
14. Lode A: Untersuchungen über die zahlen- und regenerationsverhältnisse der spermatozoiden bei hund und mensch. Archiv Gesammte Physiol 50:278, 1891
15. Hühner M: Methods of examining for spermatozoa in the diagnosis and treatment of sterility. Int J Surg 34:91, 1921
16. Williams WW, McGugan A, Carpenter HD: The staining and morphology of the human spermatozoon. J Urol 32:201, 1934
17. Moench GL: Relation of certain seminal findings to fertility with special reference to sperm concentration and the significance of testicular epithelium cells in semen. Arm J Surg 47:586, 1940
18. Hotchkiss RS: Factors in stability and variability of semen specimens: observations on 640 successive samples from 23 men. J Urol 45:875, 1941
19. MacLeod J, Hotchkiss RS: Semen analysis in 1500 cases of sterile marriages. Am J Obstet Gynecol 52:34, 1946
20. Portnoy L: The diagnosis and prognosis of male infertility: a study of 44 cases with special reference to sperm morphology. J Urol 48:735, 1946
21. MacLeod J: The semen examination. Clin. Obstet Gynecol 8:115, 1965
22. Moench GL: A technique for accurate determination of sperm motility. Urol Cutan Rev 53:406, 1949

23. Eliasson R: Analysis of semen. In Behrman SJ, Kistner RW (eds): Progress in Infertility, 2d ed. Boston: Little, Brown & Co, 1975, p 691

24. Hendry WF: Male infertility. Br J Hosp Med 22:47, 1979

25. Mortimer D: The male factor in infertility. I Semen analysis. Curr Probl Obstet Gynecol Fertil 8:4, 1985

26. van Zyl JA: A review of the male factor in 231 infertile couples. S Afr Obstet Gynecol 10:17, 1972

27. Pryor JP: Seminal analysis. Clin Obstet Gynecol 8:571, 1981

28. Alexander NJ: Male evaluation and semen analysis. Clin Obstet Gynecol 25:463, 1982

29. Amelar RD: Infertility in Men. Philadelphia: FA Davis, 1966, p 13

30. Mehan DJ, Chehval MJ: A clinical evaluation of a new silastic seminal fluid collection device. Fertil Steril 28:689, 1977

31. Belding DL: Fertility in the male. II. Technique of the spermatozoa count. Am J Obstet Gynecol 27:25, 1934

32. Farris EJ: An improved method for semen analysis. J Urol 58:85, 1947

33. MacLeod J, Gold RZ: The male factor in fertility and infertility. V. Effect of continence on semen quality. Fertil Steril 3:297, 1952

34. Freund M: Effect of frequency of emission on semen output and an estimate of daily sperm production in man. J Reprod Fertil 6:269, 1963

35. Mortimer D, Templeton AA, Lenton EA, Coleman RA: Influence of abstinence and ejaculation-to-analysis delay on semen analysis parameters of suspected infertile men. Arch Androl 8:251, 1982

36. Freund M, Peterson RN: Semen evaluation and fertility. In Hafez E (ed): Human Semen and Fertility Regulation in Men. St. Louis: CV Mosby, 1976, p 344

37. Cary WH: Sterility diagnosis: the study of sperm cell migration in female secretion and interpretation of findings. NY State J Med 30:131, 1930

38. Cary WH, Hotchkiss RS: Semen appraisal: differential stain that advances the study of cell morphology. JAMA 102:587, 1934

39. Freund M: Interrelationships among the characteristics of human semen and factors affecting semen specimen quality. J Reprod Fertil 4:143, 1962

40. Freund M: Performance and interpretation of the semen analysis. In Rolands M (ed): Management of the Infertile Couple. Springfield, IL: Charles C Thomas, 1968, p 48

41. Hotchkiss RS, Brunner EK, Grenley P: Semen analysis of two hundred fertile men. Am J Med Sci 196:362, 1938

42. Menkveld R: Ondersoek na omgewingsinvloede op spermatogenese en semenparameters (Ph.D. Proefskrif). Universiteit van Stellenbosch, 1987

43. Zaneveld LJD, Polakoski KL: Collection and the physical examination of the ejaculate. In Hafez E (ed): Techniques of Human Andrology. Amsterdam: Elsevier/North-Holland Biomedical Press, 1977, p 147

44. Amelar RD, Dubin L, Schoenfeld C: Semen analysis: an office technique. Urology 2:605, 1973

45. Taylor PJ, Martin RH: Semen analysis in the investigation of infertility. Can Fam Phys 27:113, 1981

46. van Zyl JA, Menkveld R, Kotze TJvW, Van Niekerk WA: The importance of spermiograms that meet the requirements of international standards and the most important factors that influence semen parameters. In: Proceedings of the 17th Congress of the International Urological Society (Paris) 2:263, 1976

47. Sherins RJ, Brightwell D, Sternthal PM: Longitudinal analysis of semen of fertile and infertile men. In Troen P, Nankin HR (eds): The Testis in Normal and Infertile Men. NY: Raven Press, 1977, p 473

48. Poland ML, Moghissi KS, Giblin PT, Ager JW, Olson JM: Variation of semen measure within normal men. Fertil Steril 44:396, 1985

49. Freund M: Semen analysis. In Behrman SJ, Kistner RW (eds): Progress in Infertility. Boston: Little, Brown & Co, 1968, p 593

50. Mandal A, Bhattacharyya AK: Studies on the coagulational characteristics of human ejaculates. Andrologia 17:80, 1985

51. Amelar RD: Coagulation, liquefaction and viscosity of human semen. J Urol 87:187, 1962

52. Mann T: Biochemical appraisal of human semen. In Joël CA (ed): Fertility Disturbances in Men and Women. Basel: Karger, 1971, p 146

53. Benedict AL: Enumeration of spermatozoids. NY Med J 91:1169, 1910

54. Macomber D, Sanders MB: The spermatozoa count: its value in the diagnosis, prognosis and treatment of sterility. N Engl J Med 200:981, 1929

55. Belding DL: Fertility in the male. I. Technical problems in establishing standards of fertility. Am J Obstet Gynecol 26:868, 1933

56. Muschat M: The chemical reaction of the prostatic secretion and semen: a hydrogen-ion study. J Urol 15:593, 1926
57. Messer FC, Almquest BR: The hydrogen ion concentration of seminal fluid from sterile men. J Urol 37:319, 1937
58. Harvey C, Jackson MH: Assessment of male fertility by semen analysis: an attempt to standardise methods. Lancet 2:99, 134, 1945
59. Hühner M: The practical scientific diagnosis and treatment of sterility in the male and female. Med Rec 85:840, 1914
60. Moench GL: A consideration of some of the aspects of sterility. Am J Obstet Gynecol 13:334, 1927
61. Moench GL: Evaluation of the motility of spermatozoa. JAMA 94:478, 1930
62. MacLeod J, Heim LM: Characteristics and variation in semen specimens in 100 normal young men. J Urol 54:474, 1945
63. Farris EJ: The number of motile spermatozoa as an index of fertility in man: a study of 406 semen specimens. J Urol 61:1099, 1949
64. MacLeod J: Seminal cytology in the presence of varicocele. Fertil Steril 16:735, 1965
65. Atherton RW: Evaluation of sperm motility. In Hafez E (ed): Techniques of Human Andrology. Amsterdam: Elsevier/North-Holland Biomedical Press, 1977, p 173
66. Janick J, MacLeod J: Measurement of human spermatozoa motility. Fertil Steril 21:140, 1970
67. Barták V: Sperm velocity test in clinical practice. Int J Fertil 16:107, 1971
68. Jouannet P, Volochine B, Deguent P, Serres C, David G: Light scattering determination of various characteristic parameters of spermatozoa motility in a series of human sperm. Andrologia 9:36, 1977
69. Makler A: A new multiple exposure photography method for objective human spermatozoal motility determination. Fertil Steril 30:192, 1978
70. Makler A, Tatcher M, Mohilever J: Sperm semi-autoanalysis by a combination of multiple exposure photography (MEP) and computer techniques. Int J Fertil 25:62, 1980
71. Knuth UA, Yeung C-H, Nieschlag E: Computerized semen analysis: objective measurement of semen characteristics is biased by subjective parameter setting. Fertil Steril 48:118, 1987
72. Goldenberg RL, White R: The effect of vaginal lubricants on sperm motility in vitro. Fertil Steril 26:872, 1975
73. Carruthers GB: Assessment of semen. In Philipp EE, Carruthers GB (eds): Infertility. London: William Heinemann, 1981, p 195
74. Appell RA, Evans PR: The effect of temperature on sperm motility and viability. Fertil Steril 28:1329, 1977
75. Makler A: The thickness of microscopically examined seminal samples and its relationship to sperm motility estimation. Int J Androl 1:213, 1978
76. MacLeod J, Pazianos A, Ray BS: Restoration of human spermatogenesis by menopausal gonadotrophins. Lancet 1:1196, 1964
77. Bar-Sagie D, Mayevsky A, Bartoov B: A fluorometric technique for simultaneous measurement of pH and motility in ram semen. Arch Androl 7:27, 1981
78. Kesserü E, León F: Effect of different solid metals and metallic pairs on human sperm motility. Int J Fertil 19:81, 1974
79. Freund M, Carol B: Factors affecting hemocytometer counts of sperm concentration in human semen. J Reprod Fertil 8:149, 1964
80. Segal SJ, Lawrence KA: Automatic analysis of particulate matter in human semen. Ann NY Acad Sci 99:271, 1962
81. Brotherton J, Barnard G: Estimation of number, mean size and size distribution of human spermatozoa in oligospermia using a Coulter counter. J Reprod Fertil 40:341, 1974
82. Gordon DL, Herrigel JE, Moore DJ, Paulsen CA: Efficacy of Coulter counter in determining low sperm concentrations. Am J Clin Pathol 47:226, 1967
83. Makler A: A new chamber for rapid sperm count and motility estimation. Fertil Steril 30:313, 1978
84. Makler A: The improved ten-micrometer chamber for rapid sperm count and motility evaluation. Fertil Steril 33:337, 1980
85. Menkveld R, van Zyl JA, Stander FSH, Conradie E, Kopper K: Vergelykende studie tussen die witselpipet- en Makler-telkamermetodes vir die tel spermatozoa. S Afr Med J 58:536, 1980
86. Menkveld R, van Zyl JA, Kotze TJvW: A statistical comparison of three methods for the counting of human spermatozoa. Andrologia 16:554, 1984

87. MacLeod J, Gold RZ: The male factor in fertility and infertility. II. Spermatozoa counts in 1000 men of known fertility and in 1000 cases of infertile marriage. J Urol 66:436, 1951
88. van Zyl JA, Menkveld R, Kotze TJvW, Retief AE, Van Niekerk WA: Oligozoospermia: a seven-year survey of the incidence, chromosomal aberrations, treatment and pregnancy rate. Int J Fertil 20:129, 1975
89. Santomauro AG, Sciarra JJ, Varma AD: A clinical investigation of the role of the semen analysis and postcoital test in the evaluation of male infertility. Fertil Steril 23:245, 1972
90. Nelson CMK, Bunge RG: Semen analysis: evidence for changing parameters of male fertility potential. Fertil Steril 25:503, 1974
91. James WH: Secular trend in reported sperm counts. Andrologia 12:381, 1980
92. Leto S, Frensilli FJ: Changing parameters of donor semen. Fertil Steril 36:766, 1981
93. Osegbe DN, Amaku EO, Nnatu SN: Are changing semen parameters a universal phenomenon? Eur Urol 12:164, 1986
94. MacLeod J, Wang Y: Male fertility potential in terms of semen quality: a review of the past, a study of the present. Fertil Steril 31:103, 1979
95. Menkveld R, van Zyl JA, Kotze TJvW, Joubert G: Possible changes in male fertility over a 15-year period. Arch Androl 17:143, 1986
96. Cary HW: Examination of semen with reference to gynecological aspects. Am J Obstet Dis Women Child 74:615, 1916
97. Parkes AS: Head length dimorphism of mammalian spermatozoa. J Micr Sci 67:617, 1923
98. Moench GL, Holt H: Sperm morphology in relation to fertililty. Am J Obstet Gynecol 22:199, 1931
99. Williams WW, Savage A: Observations on the seminal micropathology of bulls. Cornell Vet 15: 353, 1925
100. Williams WW: Spermatic abnormalities. N Engl J Med 217:946, 1937
101. MacLeod J, Gold RZ: The male factor in fertility and infertility. IV. Sperm morphology in fertile and infertile marriage. Fertil Steril 2:394, 1951
102. MacLeod J: Human seminal cytology as a sensitive indicator of the germinal epithelium. Int J Fertil 9:281, 1964
103. MacLeod J: The clinical implications of deviations in human spermatogenesis as evidenced in seminal cytology and experimental production of these deviations. Excerpta Medica International Congress Series No. 133. Proceedings of the Fifth Congress on Fertility and Sterility, Stockholm, 1966, p 563
104. Menkveld R, Stander FSH, Kotze TJvW, Joubert G, Conradie E, Smith K, De Villiers A, Kruger TF, van Zyl JA: The evaluation of morphological characteristics of human spermatozoa. Clin Reprod Fertil (submitted for publication)
105. Frank IN, Benjamin JA, Segerson JE: Cytologic examination of semen. Fertil Steril 5:217, 1954
106. Hartmann GG, Schoenfeld C, Copeland E: Individualism in the seminal picture of infertile men. Fertil Steril 15:231, 1964
107. Rogers BJ, Bentwood BJ, Van Campen H, Helmbrecht G, Soderdahl D, Hale RW: Sperm morphology assessment as an indicator of human fertilizing capacity. J Androl 4:119, 1983
108. de Kretser DM, Yates C, Kovacs GT: The use of IVF in the management of male infertility. Clin Obstet Gynecol 12:767, 1985
109. Mahadevan MM, Trounson AO: The influence of seminal characteristics on the success rate of human in vitro fertilization. Fertil Steril 42:400, 1984
110. Yovich JL, Stanger JD: The limitations of in vitro fertilization from males with severe oligospermia and abnormal sperm morphology. J In Vitro Fertil Embryo Trans 1:172, 1984
111. Fredricsson B: Morphologic evaluation of spermatozoa in different laboratories. Andrologia 11:57, 1979
112. Jequier AM, Ukombe EB: Errors inherent in the performance of a routine semen analysis. Br J Urol 55:434, 1983
113. Ayodeji O, Baker HWG: Is there a specific abnormality of sperm morphology in men with varicoceles? Fertil Steril 45:839, 1986
114. Papanicolaou GN: A new procedure for staining vaginal smears. Science 95:438, 1942
115. Kruger TF, Ackerman SB, Simmons KF, Swanson RJ, Brugo SS, Acosta AA: A quick, reliable staining technique for human sperm morphology. Arch Androl 18:275, 1987
116. Schirren C, Eckhardt U, Jachczik R, Carstensen CA: Morphological differentiation of human spermatozoa with Testsimplets slides. Andrologia 9:191, 1977
117. Schütte B: Human spermatozoa stained with toluidine blue-pyronine: a rapid method for differentiation. Andrologia 18:567, 1986

118. Kruger TF, Acosta AA, Simmons KF, Swanson RJ, Matta JR, Oehninger S: Predictive value of abnormal sperm morphology in in vitro fertilization. Fertil Steril 49:112, 1988

119. Kruger TF, Menkveld R, Stander FSH, Lombard CJ, Van der Merwe JP, van Zyl JA, Smith K: Sperm morphologic features as a prognostic factor in in vitro fertilization. Fertil Steril 46:1118, 1986

120. Wyrobek AJ, Bruce WR: Induction of sperm-shape abnormalities in mice and humans. In Hollander A, deSerres FJ (eds): Chemical Mutagens, vol 5. NY: Plenum, 1978, p 257

121. MacLeod J, Gold RZ: The male factor in fertility and infertility. VIII. A study of variation in semen quality. Fertil Steril 7:387, 1956

122. MacLeod J: Effect of chickenpox and of pneumonia on semen quality. Fertil Steril 2:523, 1951

123. Steeno OP, Pangkahila A: Occupational influences on male fertility and sexuality. Andrologia 16:5, 1983

124. Lancranjan I, Popescu HI, Gavanescu O, Klepsch I, Serbanescu M: Reproductive ability of workmen occupationally exposed to lead. Arch Environ Health 30:396, 1975

125. Whorton MD, Meyer CR: Sperm count results from 861 American chemical/agricultural workers from 14 separate studies. Fertil Steril 42:82, 1984

126. Sas M, Szöllösi J: Impaired spermiogenesis as a common finding among professional drivers. Arch Androl 3:57, 1979

127. Baker HWG, Burger HG, de Kretser DM, Lording DW, McGowan P, Rennie GC: Factors affecting the variability of semen analysis results in infertile men. Int J Androl 4:609, 1981

128. MacLeod J: A possible factor in etiology of human male infertility. Fertil Steril 13:29, 1962

129. Fredricsson B: On the development of different morphologic abnormalities of human spermatozoa. Andrologia 10:43, 1978

130. Hofmann N, Haider SG: Neue ergenbnisse morphologischer diagnostik der spermatogenesestörungen. Gynäkologie 18:70, 1985

131. MacLeod J: An analysis in human semen of a staining method for differentiating live and dead spermatozoa. Anat Rec 83:573, 1942

132. Blom EB: A one-minute live-dead stain by means of eosin-nigrosin. Fertil Steril 1:176, 1950

133. Dougherty KA, Emilson LBV, Cockett ATK, Urry RL: A comparison of subjective measurements of human sperm motility and viability with two live-dead staining techniques. Fertil Steril 26:700, 1975

134. Eliasson R: Supravital staining of human spermatozoa. Fertil Steril 28:1257, 1977

135. Eliasson R, Treichl L: Supravital staining of human spermatozoa. Fertil Steril 22:134, 1971

136. Pollak OJ, Joël CA: Sperm examination according to the present state of research. JAMA 113:395, 1939

137. Davis CD, Pullen RL, Madden JHM, Hamblen EC: Therapy of seminal inadequacy. I. Use of pituitary, chorionic and equine gonadotropins. J Clin Endocrinol 3:268, 1943

138. Williams WW: Routine semen examinations and their interpretation. Trans Am Soc Stud Steril 139, 1946

139. Bustos-Obregón E, Guadarrama A, Thumann A, Zegers F, Barros C: Normal semen values and sperm fertilizing ability. In Franjese G, Hafez E, Conti C, Fabbrini A (eds); Oligozoospermia: Recent Progress in Andrology. NY: Raven Press, 1981, p 21

140. Eliasson R: Analysis of semen. In Burger H, deKretser D (eds): The Testis. NY: Raven Press, 1981, p 381

141. Falk HC, Kaufman SA: What constitutes a normal semen? Fertil Steril 1:489, 1950

142. Abyholm T: An andrological study of 51 fertile men. Int J Androl 4:646, 1981

143. Homonnai ZT, Paz G, Weiss JN, David MP: Quality of semen obtained from 627 fertile men. Int J Androl 3:217, 1980

Section B:

SPERMATOZOA SEPARATION

MARIE-LENA WINDT, M.S., ROELOF MENKVELD, PH.D., AND THINUS F. KRUGER, M.D.

Indications

In normal coitus, sperm are separated from seminal plasma by a filtration process as the sperm progress through the cervical mucus. For assisted reproductive procedures, sperm separation is essential for two reasons. The first is to remove the seminal plasma, because substances in the plasma can cause severe cramps when used for intrauterine insemination; also it is believed that long exposure to seminal plasma can decrease sperm fertilizing potential. The second reason is to obtain a higher proportion of motile and morphologically normal sperm.

Different sperm separation methods to obtain these objectives have been reported for assisted reproductive procedures such as artificial insemination with husband's semen (AIH) (1–4), in vitro fertilization (IVF) (5), and gamete intrafallopian transfer (GIFT) (5), as well as for patients with retrograde ejaculation (6, 7) or with antisperm antibodies (8, 9).

Techniques

SPERM WASHING AND SWIM-UP

Glass (4) used a method wherein equal volumes of semen and Tyrode's medium are mixed and then centrifuged once at 2800 to 3200 rpm for 10 minutes. The pellet is resuspended in Tyrode's to obtain a sperm count of 20 to 80 $\times$ 10^6/ml. Of this suspension, 0.5 ml is layered on top of a liquid human serum albumin (HSA) column (10% HSA). After 1 hour, the sperm suspension and top tenth of the column are removed and discarded. The most active and motile sperm are in the bottom part of the column; they are again washed with an equal volume of Tyrode's. The resultant pellet is resuspended in 0.25 ml of Tyrode's and used for insemination. This method, according to the author, results in sperm fractions with improved motility, numbers adequate for conception, a more nearly uniform morphology, and freedom from seminal debris.

Leong (3) used a similar method but resuspended the final sperm pellet in 0.5 ml of fasting serum, so that the sperm were further activated.

In Wiltbank's method (1), semen samples were diluted to 10 ml with sterile Biggers, Whitten, and Whittingham's medium (BWW). The mixture was centrifuged at 500 $\times$ g for 5 minutes. The resultant pellet was washed two more times in 10 ml of BWW. The final pellet was resuspended in 0.3 to 0.5 ml of BWW + 1% HSA and used for insemination. Washing of semen resulted in good motile sperm recovery, elimination of foreign debris, and, for the woman, no side effects, no infection, and minimal cramping.

Wiltbank (1) also described a modified method in which the sperm pellet from the first centrifugation was resuspended in a small volume (0.3 ml) of medium and layered with 10 ml of the same medium. After 1 hour of incubation, motile sperm that had migrated into the upper layer were aspirated, centrifuged, and resuspended in 0.5 ml of medium for insemination.

Toffle (2) used a single wash with an equal volume of phosphate-buffered saline (PBS). The mixture was centrifuged for 15 minutes at 300 $\times$ g. The pellet was resuspended in 0.5 ml of PBS for insemination.

The main advantage of a wash and swim-up method is that high percentages of motile sperm (80% to 100%) can be recovered. However, the recovery rate of total motile sperm is low, especially if the initial motility is low.

LAYERING AND SWIM-UP

To obtain motile and seminal plasma-free sperm, Berger (10) and Harris (11) used a layering and swim-up procedure in which centrifugation was excluded. Liquefied semen samples were layered beneath a volume of culture medium in culture tubes. After 60 minutes, the upper interface was aspirated, either washed through centrifugation or used as it was. An increase in motile sperm was obtained, and samples were free of seminal plasma and debris (11). The recovery rate was not very good, however, and in attempts to improve this, some non-motile sperm were also aspirated (10).

ALBUMIN GRADIENT SEPARATION

The principle of this method involves the layering of washed sperm over serum albumin (HSA or bovine serum albumin (BSA)) in a vertical column, allowing the progressively motile sperm to swim into two or more discontinuous albumin gradients. The albumin medium acts as a filter, and after a period of time, debris-free and seminal plasma-free sperm can be obtained from the albumin gradients (12–14). Sperm in the gradients are then washed free of the albumin medium and resuspended in insemination medium. This separation method has pronounced advantages. The motility of the treated sample is significantly increased (12–14). An improvement of forward progression is found (14), and the percentage of abnormal forms is significantly decreased (13, 14). Albumin gradient-separated sperm are also free of debris, seminal plasma, and foreign cells (12–14). The only disadvantage of the separation method is the decrease of total sperm count (14).

GLASS WOOL SEPARATION

In this method (15), a Pasteur pipette is filled with glass wool; semen samples are placed on top of the glass wool column to remove most of the debris and dead sperm. A sample with improved motility and better fertilization potential is obtained. Cervical mucus penetration is also increased. Although samples with high viscosity can be improved, glass wool separation does not remove all the seminal plasma (15). Retention of glass fiber material in the sample and ultrastructural damage to the membrane and acrosome of the sperm can also be a problem (16).

GLASS BEAD COLUMN SEPARATION

The use of small glass beads packed in a column to separate motile sperm from dead sperm and other debris was performed with success by Daya (16, 17). Since dead sperm stick to glass, the glass bead column is an efficient way of filtering out dead sperm. Diluted semen samples are placed on top of the packed glass bead column. The separation yields a semen sample of enhanced quality, with a significantly higher percentage of viable and progressively motile sperm. These sperm also have a better fertilizing capacity (16). The total number of sperm recovered, however, is less than that added to the column (16).

PERCOLL GRADIENT SEPARATION

In this method, human sperm are separated on the basis of their motility in a discontinuous or continuous Percoll gradient made up in tissue culture medium (18, 19). Motile sperm cells penetrate into the denser regions of the gradient when gently centrifuged (19). The sperm-containing layers are washed again to remove the Percoll, and pelleted sperm are resuspended in insemination medium. The Percoll separation method ensures the concentration of sperm into a small volume (20). It is also effective for isolating sperm of higher motility and viability, and for increasing fertilization capability (21). Separated samples are free of seminal plasma and other debris and leukocytes (21). The Percoll method is useful especially in cases of asthenozoospermia and oligozoospermia, where normal wash and swim-up procedures are unsuccessful (20). Some articles indicate that this method can damage the sperm membrane (22). We (23) have an average recovery rate of 81.3% motile sperm. However, we have found that there is a decrease in the median percentage of morphologically normal sperm from 10.0% to 8.0%. If the median percentage of normal forms is brought into the calculation, a median recovery rate of 62% is obtained for the total number of motile normal sperm.

Special Procedures

SPERM WASH FOR RETROGRADE EJACULATION

Retrograde ejaculation is caused by dysfunction of or damage to the internal urethral sphincter (6, 7). The diagnosis is made from sperm in the urine after masturbation in patients who are usually aspermic (7). One method of treatment is insemination with washed sperm retrieved from the urine (6, 7).

Because sperm are sensitive to fluctuations in pH and osmolarity, washing procedures should change the environment for better sperm survival. Urine can be made alkaline by giving the patient sodium bicarbonate. The osmolarity can be maintained within the normal range with an increased intake of fluid at breakfast (6).

Debris in the urine can also be a problem. An effort should be made to remove significant amounts of debris and cells. Braude (6) proposed two methods. Sedimentation by gravity of bigger cells and debris is possible when sperm suspensions are allowed to stand for 30 to 45 minutes. The supernatant can be aspirated from the sedimented debris and further prepared. A 60% Percoll gradient can also be used, leaving debris and cells in the uppermost layers of the gradient and motile sperm in the lower layers of denser gradients. The sperm-Percoll preparation is then washed before use for insemination.

Glezerman (7) used the following method of sperm preparation: The patient was asked to urinate before masturbation and 15 minutes after masturbation. The urine collected was added to 15 ml of Eagle's solution and centrifuged at 1500 rpm for 10 minutes. The pellet was washed and resuspended in medium for insemination.

Braude (6) used a similar method. Post-ejaculatory urine was centrifuged for 5 minutes at 300 $\times$ g. The pellet was diluted with 10 ml of warmed phosphate-buffered medium (PB1) containing 1.5% BSA, penicillin, and gentamicin, and centrifuged for 10 minutes at 300 × g. This was repeated once. The final pellet was resuspended in 0.5 to 1.0 ml of the supernatant and used for intracervical insemination. BSA was added to the wash medium to provide a buffering effect against pH fluctuations.

In our laboratory, we follow similar procedures. Urine pH is made alkaline by morning intake of sodium bicarbonate. Post-ejaculatory urine is centrifuged for 10 minutes at 1500 rpm. Pellets are washed once with 2 ml of Ham's F-10 + 10% human serum by centrifugation at 1500 rpm for 10 minutes. The final pellet is resuspended in 0.5 ml of Ham's F-10 + 10% serum and used for insemination.

We have found that when a sufficient number of sperm with good motility are present, a swim-up procedure can be performed, as described for AIH.

SPERM WASH FOR SEMEN WITH ANTISPERM ANTIBODIES

Sperm washing with a specified medium followed by a swim-up procedure into this medium is one of the treatments proposed for antisperm antibodies (24). The washed sperm samples are used in AIH, IVF, and GIFT. The aim of the process is to remove seminal plasma and possibly antibodies from the sperm membrane. Although most literature states that sperm-bound antibodies cannot be washed off (25), a study of Adeghe (26) showed that immediate sperm washing can rescue sperm from some extent of immunoglobulin G (IgG) antibody coating. He could not demonstrate the same effect on sperm immunoglobulin A (IgA) binding.

Boettcher (8) and Harrison (9) used a modified washing method, collecting semen into a volume of warm medium followed by a normal wash process. They postulated that, because antibody secretion is distal to the vas, antibodies attach to sperm antigens after ejaculation or liquefaction. Collection of the ejaculate directly into a large volume of medium and immediate washing should minimize the capacity of antibodies to attach to the sperm. Boettcher (8) recorded a weaker reaction for IgA in sperm thus treated. This observation was not confirmed in work performed in our unit (27). Although antibodies bound to the sperm were not reduced, semen parameters (motility and morphology) were significantly improved.

References

1. Wiltbank MC, Kosasa S, Rogers B: Treatment of infertile patients by intrauterine insemination of washed spermatozoa. Andrologia 17:22, 1985
2. Toffle RC, Nagel TC, Tagatz GE, Phansey SA, Okagaki T, Wavrin CA: Intrauterine insemination: the University of Minnesota experience. Fertil Steril 43:743, 1985
3. Leong J, Haddad Y, Osborn RA: An improved method for preparation of semen for artificial insemination by husband. Med J Aust 2:474, 1982
4. Glass RH, Ericsson RJ: Intrauterine insemination of isolated motile sperm. Fertil Steril 29:53, 1978
5. Kruger TF, Van der Merwe JP, Stander FSH, Menkveld R, Van den Heever AD, Kopper K, Odendaal HF, van Zyl JA, De Villiers JN: Results of the in vitro fertilization programme at Tygerberg Hospital, phases II and III. S Afr Med J 69:297, 1986
6. Braude PR, Ross LD, Bolton VN, Ockenden K: Retrograde ejaculation: a systematic approach to non-invasive recovery of spermatozoa from post-ejaculatory urine for artificial insemination. Br J Obstet Gynaecol 94:76, 1987
7. Glezerman M, Lunenfeld B, Potashnik G, Oelsner G, Beer R: Retrograde ejaculation: pathophysiologic aspects and report of two successfully treated cases. Fertil Steril 27:796, 1976
8. Boettcher B, Kay DJ, Fitchett SB: Successful treatment of male infertility caused by antispermatozoal antibodies. Med J Aust 2:471, 1982

9. Harrison KL, Hennessey JF: Treatment of male sperm autoimmunity by in-vitro fertilization with washed spermatozoa. Med J Aust 141:498, 1984

10. Berger T, Marrs RP, Moyer DL: Comparison of techniques for selection of motile spermatozoa. Fertil Steril 43:268, 1985

11. Harris SJ, Milligan MP, Masson GM, Dennis KJ: Improved separation of motile sperm in asthenospermia and its application to artificial insemination homologous (AIH). Fertil Steril 36:219, 1981

12. Broer KH, Dauber U: A filtering method for cleaning up spermatozoa in cases of asthenospermia. Int J Fertil 23:234, 1978

13. Ericsson RJ: Isolation and storage of progressive motile human sperm. Andrologia 9:111, 1977

14. Dmowski WP, Gaynor L, Lawrence M, Rao R, Scommegna A: Artificial insemination homologous with oligospermic semen separated on albumin columns. Fertil Steril 31:58, 1979

15. Paulson JD, Polakoski K, Leto S: Further characterization of glass wool column filtration of human semen. Fertil Steril 32:125, 1979

16. Daya S, Gwatkin RBL: Improvement in semen quality using glass bead column. Arch Androl 18:241, 1987

17. Daya S, Gwatkin RBL, Bissessar H: Separation of motile human spermatozoa by means of a glass bead column. Gamete Res 17:375, 1987

18. Pousette A, Akerlof E, Rosenborg L, Fredricsson B: Increase in progressive motility and improved morphology of human spermatozoa following their migration through Percoll gradients. Int J Androl 9:1, 1986

19. Gorus FK, Pipeleers DG: A rapid method for the fractionation of human spermatozoa according to their progressive motility. Fertil Steril 35:662, 1981

20. Iizuka R, Kaneko S, Kobanawa K, Kobayashi T: Washing and concentration of human semen by Percoll density gradients and its application to AIH. Arch Androl 20:117, 1988

21. Pardo M, Barri PN, Bancells N, Coroleu B, Buxederas C, Pomerol JM, Sabater J: Spermatozoa selection in discontinuous Percoll gradients for use in artificial insemination. Fertil Steril 49:505, 1988

22. Gellert ST, Clarke GN, Baker HWG, Hyne RV, Johnston WIJ: Evaluation of Nycodenz and Percoll density gradients for the selection of human motile spermatozoa. Fertil Steril 49:335, 1988

23. Menkveld R, Swanson RJ, Kotze JvW, Kruger TF: Comparison of a discontinuous Percoll gradient method versus a swim-up method: effects on sperm morphology and other semen parameters. (submitted for publication)

24. Rümke P: Autoimmunity against sperms in infertile men. Asian Pac J Allergy Immunol 2:329, 1984

25. Bronson RA, Cooper GW, Rosenfeld DL: Sperm antibodies: their role in infertility. Fertil Steril 42:171, 1984

26. Adeghe AJ-H: Effect of washing on sperm surface autoantibodies. Br J Urol 60:360, 1987

27. Windt M-L, Menkveld R, Kruger TF, Van der Merwe JP, Lombard JC: The effect of rapid dilution of semen on sperm-bound autoantibodies. Arch Androl (in press)

Section C:

BACTERIOLOGY AND LEUKOSPERMIA: DIAGNOSIS OF MALE ACCESSORY GLAND INFECTION

FRANK H. COMHAIRE, M.D., LUTGARDE VERMEULEN, INDUSTRIAL ENGINEER IN CHEMISTRY, GERDA VERSCHRAEGEN, M.D., AND GEERT CLAEYS, M.D.

Relevance of Clinical Data

Male accessory gland infection (MAGI) is diagnosed in 13% of men with abnormal semen quality (1). The diagnosis is based on a combination of criteria from history taking, clinical examination, and laboratory tests on prostatic fluid and ejaculate.

Symptoms of urinary tract infection (cystourethritis) are commonly detected in the history of men with silent MAGI. Men with such history have an increased prevalence of azoospermia or abnormal semen quality, more particularly with impairment of sperm morphology and motility.

Often a few periods of dysuria and/or increased frequency are mentioned, sometimes not even requiring medical treatment because they spontaneously disappear in a few days. A short treatment with either antibiotics or urinary antiseptics may have been taken. Such treatment will have cleared the infection out of the bladder and the urethra without penetrating into the accessory glands.

It should be stressed that every urinary tract infection in the male is, in principle, accompanied by infection of the glandular tissue of the prostate. After inadequate treatment, glandular infection will persist as a silent MAGI: "men's hidden infection" (2).

A more detailed analysis of urinary symptoms reveals that the finding of abnormal semen is not related to a particular type of symptom but occurs in men with a history of either dysuria, urethral discharge, hematuria, or increased frequency. About one-fourth of men with a history of urinary symptoms present either abnormalities in the expressed prostatic fluid or relevant abnormalities in the bacteriological, cytological, or biochemical makeup of the ejaculate.

In addition to symptoms of cystourethritis, the patient may report episodes of dull scrotal pain extending along the spermatic cord, which corresponds with attacks of vaso-epididymitis. Some patients mention symptoms related to prostatic inflammation, such as pain in the perineal or suprapubic region, or cramps at or immediately after ejaculation. Furthermore, changes may occur in the characteristics of ejaculation or the seminal fluid, such as decreased volume, abnormal appearance or smell, or a decreased feeling of orgasm. Hemospermia may occur, which alarms the patient, who will rapidly seek advice for this usually innocuous symptom.

The prevalence of abnormal semen quality is also significantly higher in men with a history of sexually transmitted disease. Such a history, even when occurring in repeated episodes, does not appear to depress sperm concentration but results in impairment of sperm motility related to functional disturbance of the epididymides.

Men with a history of inflammatory disease of the scrotal content, excluding orchitis associated with infectious parotitis (mumps), have a higher prevalence of azoospermia and abnormal semen quality. Orchidoepididymitis is associated with a reduction in sperm concentration, sperm motility, and morphology. The total testicular volume of those patients is usually decreased.

Clinical Findings

Upon scrotal palpation, the consistency and volume of the epididymides may be abnormal and the testicular volume may be decreased. Epididymal abnormalities are commonly situated at the head or tail, which may be enlarged, slightly indurated, perhaps granular or nodular, and often electively tender upon pressure. These alterations are usually found at both sides but not necessarily presenting as symmetrical lesions. Palpation of the vas deferens at the external inguinal ring may elicit pain extending into the scrotum or intra-abdominally, taking the direction of the urinary bladder.

Rectal palpation should be performed gently and following a systematic sequence. First, the palpating finger examines the cranial part of the right lobe; it is then pulled back while gently pressing the gland. This maneuver is repeated at the left lobe. Any zone of induration is recorded, and the patient is requested to mention painful sensations. In normal men, the seminal vesicles are not felt during rectal examination. If the vesicles are clearly palpable just above the prostate, this may indicate inflammation of these glands.

Nearly 40% of men with an abnormal prostate on palpation present an increased number of white blood cells (WBC) in semen.

VISUALIZATION OF THE ACCESSORY GLANDS

The plain x-ray film may disclose calcifications in the pelvic region, but ultrasonography gives much more detail. Particularly if ultrasonography is performed by means of a rectal probe, the structure of the gland is clearly visible, including the possible presence of pus collections or microcalcifications.

The seminal vesicles can also be depicted, so that dilatation or incomplete contraction after ejaculation can be documented. These suggest functional disturbances in case of chronic inflammation or infection.

Examination of the Expressed Prostatic Fluid

Prostatic and sometimes vesicular fluid obtained during gentle massage should be examined either as a wet preparation between slide and coverslip or as a stained dry smear. The wet preparation should be observed preferentially in phase contrast at ×400 magnification, high-power field (HPF).

Under these circumstances, the number of WBC normally does not exceed 15 per HPF. The presence of 15 to 40 WBC per HPF is suggestive, with more than 40 WBC per HPF strongly indicative of prostatic inflammation (3). Furthermore, the occurrence of mucous streaks and/or clusters of WBC, as well as of the degenerated prostatic or vesicular cells, strengthens the diagnosis. The same criteria prevail for the evaluation of dried Giemsa-stained smears.

It has also been suggested that the number of WBC in the expressed fluid be counted. This would permit a better differentiation between normal and pathological conditions (4).

Bacteriological examination of the expressed fluid can be performed as well. The uniform growth of urinary pathogens such as *Escherichia coli, Klebsiella* species, *Streptococcus faecalis*, or *Proteus* species indicates present infection.

If no prostatic fluid can be obtained, the patient is requested to pass urine after prostatic massage. The sediment of the first voided 10 ml is examined both for WBC and altered prostatic cells, and for quantitative bacteriological culture. The presence of 5 or more WBC per HPF in the urinary sediment suggests prostatic inflammation. As far as bacteriology is concerned, a count of 10 times more bacteria than in the pre-massage urine is accepted as evidence of prostatic infection (5).

About 50% of men with an increased number of WBC in urine or a positive urine culture have an increased number of WBC in semen.

Semen Analysis

STAINING TECHNIQUES FOR WBC

It is very difficult to distinguish between immature spermatogenic cells and neutrophil granulocytes on semen smears stained with the Giemsa or Papanicolaou methods. Some authors argue that Leishman staining permits better differentiation, but it is rather difficult to set up and is time-consuming (6).

A simple and reliable approach consists of peroxidase staining of the round cells in the fresh ejaculate. This can be done by the method suggested by the World Health Organization, which has been described by Nahoum (4).

Preparation of Working Solution

- Reagents:
   A. Saturated NH_4Cl solution (25 g/100 ml);
   B. Na_2 EDTA; 5% volume/volume (v/v) in phosphate buffer (pH 6.0);
   C. Ortho-toluidine, 0.025% (v/v);
   D. H_2O_2, 30% (v/v) in distilled water.
- The working solution:
   1 ml of reagent A;
   1 ml of reagent B;
   9 ml of reagent C;
   One drop of reagent D.
   This solution can be used for 24 hours after preparation.

Procedure

1. Mix 0.1 ml of semen with working solution to achieve a volume of 1 ml.
2. Shake for 2 minutes.
3. Leave for 20 to 30 minutes at room temperature.
4. Shake again.
5. Peroxidase-positive cells stain brown, while peroxidase-negative cells are unstained.
6. Count in a hemocytometer chamber for leukocytes, or estimate the percentage of peroxidase-positive and negative cells in a wet preparation.

In semen samples of all men, a few cells other than spermatozoa are present. If the number of round cells exceeds 1×10^6/ml, one of the above-mentioned staining methods must be used. If over 1×10^6/ml cells react positively, displaying peroxidase activity, this suggests inflammation of the accessory sex glands. An increased number of peroxidase-negative cells suggests alteration of the seminiferous tubules, resulting in premature release of immature spermatogenic cells. Lymphocytes usually are present in small numbers; their significance is still under investigation.

TECHNIQUES OF SEMEN CULTURE

Semen collection for culture should be performed in such a condition that interpretation of results is meaningful. Semen should be obtained by masturbation after at least 3 days of abstinence. The patient should pass urine and wash his hands and penis before ejaculation. The sample should be collected in a sterile container, which should reach the laboratory within 1 hour after emission.

Sperm culture for aerobic bacteria can be performed on a blood agar medium or on Dip slides. Since seminal plasma may exert bacteriostatic activity, it is preferable to dilute the semen sample 1:1 or 1:2 before inoculation. An aliquot of 1:20 or 1:40 ml of (diluted) semen is evenly spread on the blood agar or Dip slide by a wire loop. After 24 hours of incubation at 37°C or 3 days at room temperature (Dip slide), the number of colonies is counted and their aspect is evaluated. If the colonies are uniform and the calculated number of bacteria per milliliter exceeds 1000, identification of the bacterial strain is indicated. In all other circumstances, contamination is suspected.

Culture for anaerobic bacteria is probably not useful, since these bacteria are rarely found in semen, and their presence can usually not be confirmed upon control culture of a subsequent semen sample. Hence, anaerobic bacteria are unlikely to play any role in the pathogenesis of MAGI.

The same is true for *T. mycoplasma* and *Ureaplasma urealyticum*, which are commonly found in semen samples of fertile and infertile men. Culture for mycoplasmata, however, is indicated in couples who are scheduled to undergo IVF. For mycoplasma and ureaplasma, ureaplasma differential agar medium (A7) and SP4 agar medium are used.

A7 consists of ureaplasma basal agar medium (Gibco), prepared as described by the manufacturers, to which the following components are added, using sterile techniques: normal horse serum (unheated) 400 ml, CVA enrichment (Gibco) 1.0 ml, yeast extract solution (Gibco) 2.0 ml, urea solution (10%) 2.0 ml, 1-cysteine-HCl solution (4%) 0.5 ml; penicillin G potassium has been replaced by ampicillin to reach a final concentration of 1 g/liter. SP4 is constituted of mycoplasma broth base without crystal violet (Gibco), to which the following ingredients are added per 500 ml: tryptone (Difco) 5.0 g, peptone 2.65 g, glucose 2.5 g, agar 6 g. The ingredients are dissolved by boiling, and the pH is adjusted to 7.5. The solution is then autoclaved for 15 minutes at 120°C. Next, the following components are added per 500 ml, also using a sterile technique: CMRL 1066 ($10\times$ concentrated Gibco 154 with glutamine) 25 ml, α-ketoglutaric acid (0.4%) 25 ml, yeast extract 25% (Gibco) 17.5 ml, fetal bovine serum 85 ml, and ampicillin to reach a final concentration of 1 g/liter.

A loop or a drop of semen is placed on the agar plates, and an isolation culture is made. The plates are incubated in a jar in anaerobiosis or in an anaerobic chamber at 37°C for 4 days. From day 2 on, plates are daily inspected under the microscope with a low magnification ($\times 100$) for colony formation. On A7 agar, mycoplasma colonies have their typical "fried-egg" appearance, while ureaplasma colonies are small and black.

Chlamydia are rarely found in the semen of men consulting for infertility, even though chronic epididymitis is alleged to be caused by this pathogen in a considerable proportion of cases. Negative results are possibly due to inadequate culture or detection techniques. The exact role of chlamydia in male infertility needs further study.

BIOCHEMICAL MARKERS OF SECRETORY FUNCTION OF THE ACCESSORY SEX GLANDS

Seminal fluid is ejaculated in a well-defined sequence. First, a volume of approximately 0.2 ml of fluid from the glands of Cowper and the periurethral glands of Littré is passed. Afterwards the secretory fluid of the prostate (approximately 0.5 ml) is rhythmically expelled, together with the spermatozoa that are stored in the ejaculatory ampulla of the vas deferens and in the epididymis. Finally, the secretory fluid of the seminal vesicles is voided. The volume of the latter fraction varies from 1 to 5 ml, depending, among other factors, on the duration of sexual abstinence.

Each of these secretory products has a specific aspect and biochemical composition. If functional disturbance occurs as a result of present or previous infection, changes in the physical and biochemical make-up of the seminal plasma will occur.

Suggestive evidence of decreased function of the prostate are the following: alkaline pH (> 7.8); decreased concentration of citric acid, calcium, and zinc; and decreased activity of acid phosphatase and γ-glutamyltranspeptidase. Furthermore, the seminal plasma may fail to liquefy or may remain hyperviscous after liquefaction. Of all prostatic marker substances, the total output per ejaculate of citric acid was found to be most specifically related to infection (7). Assessment of the concentration of citric acid in seminal plasma can be performed by a simple colorimetric test.

Reagents

- Boehringer kit 139076 (ultraviolet method). One kit is sufficient for 30 determinations. The kit contains:
  a. Bottle 1 (mainly reduced nicotinamide adenine dinucleotide (NADH)): Reconstitute *solution A* by adding 12 ml of distilled water; store at $-20°C$ (stable for 4 weeks).
  b. Bottle 2 (citrate-lyase): Reconstitute *solution B* by adding 0.3 ml of distilled water at $-20°C$ (stable for 4 weeks).
- TRA buffer (pH 7.7):
  a. Dissolve 14.9 g of triethanolamine in 750 ml of distilled water. Adjust to pH 7.6 by adding HCl.
  b. Dissolve 0.027 g of $ZnCl_2$ in 250 ml of distilled water. Be sure that the $ZnCl_2$ is completely dissolved.
  c. Add the $ZnCl_2$ solution to the triethanolamine solution.
  d. Add 0.5 g of sodium azide.

Procedure

1. Preparation of seminal plasma: Centrifuge the ejaculate at 3000 $\times$ g for 15 minutes or 2000 $\times$ g for 20 minutes.
2. Extraction:
   a. Add 0.1 ml of seminal plasma to 4.95 ml of 15% (v/v) trichloroacetic acid (TCA).
   b. Add 0.72 ml of 6-M NaOH.
   c. The pH must exceed 7; if necessary; add NaOH to make alkaline.
   d. The extract must be clear.

3. Measurement:
   a. Add in a measuring cuvette:
      0.5 ml of solution A;
      2.3 ml of TRA buffer;
      0.2 ml of seminal plasma extract.
   b. Mix and measure absorption at 340 nm ⟶ extinction value *E1*.
   c. Add 20 μl of solution B.
   d. Mix and wait exactly 5 minutes. Measure absorption ⟶ extinction value *E2*.

Calculations

$$\text{Concentration of citric acid in g/liter} = (E1 - E2) \times 0.13 \text{ g}$$

Normal values are 52 μmol (10 mg) or more per ejaculate.

Significance of Biochemical Markers

Decreased secretion of the seminal vesicles will result in a decreased volume of the ejaculate, acid pH (<7.2), and a decreased total output per ejaculate of fructose and prostaglandins. However, the incidence of subnormal fructose output is only weakly correlated with other signs or symptoms of MAGI, and fructose measurement gives less information for the diagnosis of MAGI than measurement of the ejaculate volume.

Several substances have been measured as markers of epididymal function. These include glyceryl-phosphorylcholine, L-carnitine, and α-glucosidase activity. The latter seems to be the most accurate test, and its measurement is simple (8, 9). However, the usefulness of assessing the concentration of secretory products of the epididymis for the diagnosis of MAGI has not yet been evaluated.

Diagnostic Criteria

Since any of the described alterations in clinical investigation, expressed prostatic fluid, or semen analysis may occur in conditions other than present infection, the diagnosis of male accessory gland infection should only be accepted if one of the following combinations of alterations is found: (*a*) If clinical abnormalities are present, either a pathological prostatic fluid or at least one suggestive alteration of the ejaculate should be present. (*b*) If no history or clinical alterations are found, a combination of abnormal prostatic fluid with at least one alteration in the ejaculate should be present. Obviously bacteria found in the prostatic fluid and the ejaculate should be identical. (*c*) In the absence of clinical signs and of abnormalities in the prostatic fluid, the diagnosis should be based on the occurrence of at least two alterations in the ejaculate, which should be present in at least two semen samples.

References

1. World Health Organization: Towards more objectivity in the diagnosis and management of male infertility. Int J Androl Suppl 7, 1987
2. Drach GW: Prostatitis: man's hidden infection. Urol Clin N Am 2:499, 1975
3. Johannisson E, Eliasson R: Cytological studies of prostatic fluids from men with and without abnormal palpatory findings of the prostate. Int J Androl 1:201, 1978
4. Nahoum CRD, Cardozo D: Staining for volumetric count of leukocytes in semen and prostato-vesicular fluid. Fertil Steril 34:68, 1980
5. Meares EM, Stamey TA: The diagnosis and management of bacterial prostatitis. Br J Urol 44:175, 1972

6. World Health Organization: Laboratory Manual for the Examination of Human Semen and Semen-Cervical Mucus Interaction. Cambridge, England: Cambridge University Press, 1987, p 52
7. Comhaire F, Pieters O, Debrock M, Vermeulen L, Rowe P, Farley T: Importance of male accessory gland infection in fertility disorders. In Weidner W, Brunner H, Krause W, Rothauge CH (eds): Therapy of Prostatitis. Munich: W Zuckschwerdt Verlag, 1986, p 223
8. Guerin JF, Ben-Ali H, Rollet J, Souchier C, Czyba JC: Alpha-glucosidase as a specific epididymal enzyme marker: its validity for the etiologic diagnosis of azoospermia. J Androl 7:156, 1986
9. Casano R, Orlando C, Caldini AL, Barni T, Natali A, Serio M: Simultaneous measurement of seminal L-carnitine, alpha,1-4-glucosidase, and glycerylphosphorylcholine in azoospermic and oligozoospermic patients. Fertil Steril 47:324, 1987

Section D1:

TESTS OF SPERMATOZOA FUNCTION: ACROSIN

PATRICIA PLEBAN, PH.D., LOURENS J. D. ZANEVELD, D.V.M., PH.D., AND RAJASINGAM S. JEYENDRAN, D.V.M., PH.D.

Sperm cell acrosin (E.C. 3.4.21.10) is an acrosomal enzyme first identified in human semen more than 18 years ago (1, 2). It has been characterized as a serine proteinase which catalyzes the cleavage of peptide bonds containing either an arginine or lysine amino acid residue. Acrosin is believed to be the major sperm cell serine proteinase, although several others have been identified in spermatozoa (3, 4). It remains to be established that these other serine proteinases are not different forms of acrosin. The physiological functions which have been attributed to acrosin include facilitation of the acrosome reaction, and sperm binding to and penetration of the zona pellucida (5).

The enzyme is primarily present in the acrosomal cap in the inactive zymogen form, proacrosin, and is thought to be released in its active form, acrosin, during the acrosome reaction and sperm penetration through the zona pellucida (5). In vitro, proacrosin rapidly converts to acrosin at pH 8.0. In addition, acrosin is highly autoproteolytic at that pH. Therefore, the extracts of the enzyme are prepared and stored at pH 2.8 to 3.0 to prevent degradation. Serine proteinase inhibitors such as *p*-amino-benzamidine, benzamidine, and leupeptin inhibit acrosin activity (6). Natural acrosin inhibitors have been identified in seminal plasma (7) and on the acrosomal membrane (1, 8, 9).

Methods for the assay of acrosin have been described by a number of investigators (10) and include assay of esterase or amidase activity, active enzyme staining in electrophoretic gels, measurement of proteolytic activity using a gelatin film substrate, and immunochemical assay. All assays involve specimen collection, preparation, and measurement of acrosin activity or content.

Methodology

SPECIMEN COLLECTION

Specimens should be collected into glass, ceramic, or polypropylene tubes or cups by masturbation. Following liquefaction, the sperm pellet can be obtained by centrifugation at 1000 $\times$ g for 15 minutes and the supernatant seminal plasma discarded. More gentle and effective methods of separation involve Ficoll or sucrose centrifugation (see below). If the specimen cannot be assayed immediately, the ejaculate can be maintained at 2° to 5°C for 24 hours without loss of acrosin activity (see Chapter 5, part I, Biochemistry: Acrosin). Some procedures add 0.5-M benzamidine after liquefaction to give a final concentration of 0.05-M benzamidine to prevent conversion of proacrosin to acrosin during extraction (11). However, this is not necessary when one is determining total acrosin activity (free acrosin plus activated proacrosin). It should be noted that Elce and McIntyre (12) have reported losses of proacrosin even when 0.05-M benzamidine was used.

METHOD 1: EXTRACTION AND DETERMINATION OF ACTIVITY

The standard technique for estimating acrosin, proacrosin, and acrosin inhibitor of human spermatozoa involves benzamidine treatment of the spermatozoa, and extraction and measurement of the esterolytic activity before and after activation of proacrosin by adjusting the pH of the extract (11). However, for clinical purposes it is probably necessary to measure only the total acrosin activity that can be generated by the spermatozoa, i.e., the free acrosin plus the acrosin formed by conversion of proacrosin to acrosin. Therefore, this method was modified by Pleban as follows.

All steps are performed at 4°C. The sperm pellet obtained following collection is resuspended in 0.5 ml of 0.1-M phosphate buffer (pH 7.2 to 7.5) and layered onto 1 to 2 ml of 1-M sucrose solution. The mixture is centrifuged at 6000 $\times$ g for 30 minutes, followed by aspiration of the upper sucrose layer. The remaining pellet is resuspended in enough extraction medium containing 1% acetic acid and 5% glycerol (pH 2.8) to give a final sperm concentration of 10 to 40 10^6/ml of extracting fluid. Sperm concentrations in this range give the highest and most reproducible recovery. A 10-μl aliquot of the well-mixed suspension should be transferred immediately to a sperm-diluting solution to be counted. The acrosin extraction procedure is continued at 4°C for 4 hours (it may be left overnight) with constant stirring. The extraction suspension is then centrifuged at 27,000 $\times$ g for 20 minutes. Acrosin may be determined directly in the supernatant after the pH is adjusted to 8.0 to allow proacrosin activation to occur for 30 minutes; then the pH is readjusted to 3.0.

The classic assay for the determination of serine proteinase activity involves determination of the esterase or amidase activity. Either *N*-α-benzoyl-DL-arginine-*p*-nitroanilide (BAPNA, amidase activity) (10) or *N*-α-benzoyl-L-arginine ethyl ester (BAEE, esterase activity) (11) may be used as substrate. To obtain maximal enzyme activity and prevent adsorption of the enyzme to plastic, 0.01% Triton X-100 is sometimes used in the assay buffer. Enzyme activities are reported in mIU/10^7 sperm ((nmol of substrate hydrolyzed per minute per ml of extract)/(sperm count per ml of extract)). When microcuvets are used, the assay can measure the acrosin activity of as few as 0.5 $\times$ 10^6 sperm.

When BAPNA is used as the substrate, the product of the reaction, *p*-nitroanilide, may be measured at 410 nm, allowing the use of a less expensive spectrophotometer. However, BAPNA is sparingly soluble in water and must be dissolved in dimethyl sulfoxide (DMSO). Use of BAEE as an acrosin substrate avoids the solubility problem, but since the product, benzoyl arginine, absorbs at 253 nm, a spectrophotometer capable of measurement in the low ultraviolet area of the spectrum is required. Thioesterase activity, followed by fluorometric assay of the released thiol using 4,4′-dithiodipyridine, provides a more sensitive assay for serine proteinases (13). This methodology, using synthetic peptide thioesters, has been used to map the active sites of many of the serine proteinases involved in coagulation (14), but this has not been applied to the determination of acrosin.

The proacrosin-acrosin system has been studied by separating the components using gel electrophoresis (polyacrylamide or agarose gel) or isoelectric focusing followed by visualization using a BAPNA substrate overlay technique (10). This technique is semiquantitative but allows the visualization of all forms of acrosin.

Proteolytic activity in gelatin-containing sodium dodecyl sulfate-polyacrylamide electrophoretic (SDS-PAGE) gels has also been used to study the proacrosin-acrosin activity of the extracts (15). Following separation on SDS-PAGE slab gels at 4°C, the gels were incubated at pH 8.0 at 37°C for 2 to 3 hours. The gels were then fixed, stained with amido black, and the areas cleared of gelatin were observed. Using this technique, Siegel and Polakaski (15) were able to observe clearing by acrosin in extracts from as few as 30,000 spermatozoa.

Radioimmunoassay is the most specific assay for the determination of acrosin content (but not activity). Several laboratories have developed antisera to acrosin and used them to measure the acrosin extracted from human spermatozoa (16, 17). However, development of a radioimmunoassay requires production of in-house antiserum, since this item is not commercially available. Also, the total acrosin content is probably less useful as a fertility marker than the total acrosin activity. It is conceivable in some cases that proacrosin conversion to acrosin cannot take place, which would not alter the total acrosin content but would greatly decrease the amount of active acrosin available to spermatozoa for function.

Elce and McIntyre (12) have described a Western blot technique for the determination of proacrosin and acrosin in SDS-PAGE gels. The technique is quite specific for acrosin and proacrosin but is semiquantitative.

METHOD 2: CLINICAL ACROSIN ASSAY

A simple clinical method has been developed in the laboratory of Zaneveld and Jeyendran to measure the total acrosin activity of human spermatozoa (18). This technique is performed entirely at room temperature and combines several of the methods described above into a single procedure.

The assay consists of three steps. First, the spermatozoa are washed free of seminal plasma by centrifugation over Ficoll to remove the soluble proteinase inhibitors in human semen which can interfere with acrosin activity. The sperm pellet is subsequently suspended in buffer which has (*a*) a detergent which facilitates disruption of the acrosomes and releases the acrosomal enzymes; (*b*) a basic pH which allows activation of proacrosin into enzymatically active acrosin; and (*c*) a synthetic arginine amide substrate which, when hydrolyzed, releases a chromophoric product. Finally, the total amount of color developed after a 3-hour incubation period is measured spectrophotometrically.

Reagents

Benzamidine hydrochloride, Ficoll (type 400), BAPNA, DMSO, HEPES (*N*-2-hydroxyethylpiperazine-*N'*-2-ethanesulfonic acid), and Triton X-100 are obtained from Sigma Chemical Company (St. Louis, Mo.).

Solutions

A. *Ficoll:* 11% Ficoll in 0.12 M NaCl, 0.025 M HEPES buffer, at pH 7.4 to 7.6. The solution is prepared by dissolving 0.70 g of NaCl, 0.60 g of HEPES, and 11.0 g of Ficoll in approximately 90 ml of distilled, deionized water. The solution is adjusted to pH 7.4 to 7.6 (with HCl or NaOH, as required) and is then adjusted with water to a final volume of 100 ml. The Ficoll solution is stable for only 3 days in the refrigerator unless sodium azide (0.1% or 100 mg added to 100 ml of solution) is added as a preservative.
B. *Detergent Buffer:* 0.01% Triton X-100 in 0.055-M HEPES, 0.055-M NaCl, at pH 8.0. The solution is prepared by dissolving 1.31 g of HEPES, 0.32 g of NaCl, and 1 ml of 1% Triton X-100 stock solution (1 ml Triton in 99 ml of water) in 95 ml of distilled, deionized water. The solution is adjusted to pH 8.0 (with 1-M NaOH, as required) and then adjusted to a final volume of 100 ml with distilled, deionized water. The detergent buffer is stable for 3 days but can be stored for extended periods in the refrigerator after addition of sodium azide (0.1% or 100 mg added to 100 ml) as a preservative.
C. *Benzamidine:* 500 mM in water. The solution is prepared by dissolving 87.3 g of benzamidine-HCl in 1 liter of distilled, deionized water. The solution can be stored in the refrigerator without any additives for at least 2 weeks.
D. *Substrate:* 23-mM BAPNA in DMSO. The solution is prepared by dissolving 25 mg of BAPNA in 2.5 ml of DMSO. The solution should be prepared fresh on the day of the assay. Complete dissolution of BAPNA in DMSO requires 5 to 10 minutes.
E. *Substrate-Detergent Mixture:* 22.5 ml of the detergent buffer (solution B) is mixed thoroughly with 2.5 ml of the BAPNA-DMSO substrate (solution D) in a 50-ml Erlenmeyer flask. This solution should be prepared while Ficoll centrifugation is taking place (see step 4 of the assay procedure, below). Cloudy precipitates will appear if the solution is allowed to stand for several hours or if it is chilled. The solution should not be used if such precipitates are formed.

Assay Procedure

1. The ejaculate is allowed to liquefy completely, and the sperm concentration is measured.
2. For each ejaculate, the volume is calculated that will contain 2 to 10×10^6 spermatozoa. Optimally, no more than 250 μl are layered over the Ficoll (see step 3) except as required in cases of severe oligozoospermia.
3. One control and several tests are preferably run simultaneously for each ejaculate. Aliquots (0.5 ml) of Ficoll (solution A) are pipetted into 5-ml plastic, conical centrifuge tubes (Fisher, Itasca, Ill.). The ejaculate is thoroughly mixed, and the calculated volume of the ejaculate (see step 2) is layered over the Ficoll in each tube (including the control tube), preferably with a pipettor (Pipetman, Rainin Instrument Co., Woburn, Mass.). The semen should float on the Ficoll and should not be mixed within that layer.
4. The tubes are centrifuged at $1000 \times$ g for 30 minutes at room temperature.
5. After centrifugation, the seminal plasma and Ficoll supernatant are removed, preferably by suction through a thin-stemmed (Pasteur) pipette. Care should be taken that the sperm pellet is not disturbed. As close to 0.1 ml as possible of the sperm pellet and Ficoll should be left in the tube.
6. One hundred microliters of the benzamidine solution (solution C) is immediately added to the control tube, and the contents of the tube are thoroughly mixed, e.g., by vortexing.
7. To each tube (including the control tube), 1 ml of the substrate-detergent mixture (solution E) is added, and the contents of the tube are thoroughly mixed. At least 1 ml of solution E should be saved for step 11.

8. The tubes are incubated at 22° to 24°C for exactly 3 hours after the addition of the assay solution. It is optimal to mix the contents of the tubes once every hour during the incubation period, e.g., by vortexing.
9. After 3 hours of incubation, 100 μl of the benzamidine solution (solution C) is added to all tubes except the control tube.
10. All the tubes are centrifuged at 1000 × g for 30 minutes, and the supernatant solutions are collected separately.
11. A spectrophotometer capable of holding 1-ml cuvettes is adjusted so that the substrate-detergent mixture (solution E) has an absorbance reading of 0.0 at 410 nm. Subsequently, the absorbance of each supernatant solution is recorded at 410 nm. The control solution should show no or almost no absorption. If significant absorption occurs in the control, the centrifugation (step 10) was probably inadequate, or the benzamidine solution was incorrectly prepared or was old. Although it is recommended that the spectrophotometric analysis of the supernatant solutions be performed immediately, the solutions can be stored for up to 3 days in the refrigerator or at room temperature. Changes in absorbance may occur over time, but these are nullified by subtracting the control from the test absorbance readings (see Calculations, below).
12. Trypsin (bovine pancreatic trypsin, type 1; Sigma Chemical Co., St. Louis, Mo.) can be used as a positive control. A solution of 0.50 μg/ml is prepared, and 100 μl are used in the assay system described in steps 7 through 11. In our hands, the absorbance of one lot of trypsin control was 0.435 ± 0.014 (mean ± SEM).

Calculations

One IU of acrosin activity is defined as the amount of enzyme that hydrolyzes 1 μmol of BAPNA per minute at 23°C. The acrosin activity is expressed in $\mu IU/10^6$ spermatozoa to obtain whole numbers. The activity is calculated as the difference in optical density (OD) at 410 nm between the mean of the test assays and the control, multiplied by 1 million (10^6) and divided by the product of 9.9 $mM^{-1} \cdot cm^{-1} \times 180$ minutes × the number of sperm in millions added to each tube divided by the total volume (1.2 ml). A change in absorbance of 9.9 corresponds to the hydrolysis of 1.0 μmol of BAPNA. For simplicity, the following formula can be applied:

$$\mu IU \text{ acrosin}/10^6 \text{ sperm} = \frac{[(\text{mean } OD_{test}) - OD_{control}] \times 10^6}{1485 \times \text{number of sperm (in millions layered over the Ficoll)}}$$

METHOD 3: PROTEOLYTIC ACTIVITY OF SPERM CELLS

The proteolytic activity of spermatozoa may be estimated directly by incubating sperm cells on ultrathin gelatin layers (1.5 μm) (10, 19, 20). During the procedure the acrosome is disrupted, and acrosin is released into the surrounding gelatin, resulting in a visible clearing. Semi-quantitative measurement of acrosin may be made by evaluating the diameter of the cleared halo around the sperm head using light microscopy.

References

1. Zaneveld LJD, Dragoje RM, Schumacher GFB: Acrosomal proteinase and proteinase inhibitor of human spermatozoa. Science 177:702, 1972
2. Fritz H, Schiessler H, Schleuning WD: Proteinases and proteinase inhibitors in the fertilization process: new concepts of control. Adv Biosci 10:271, 1972
3. Johnson RA, Jakobs KH, Schultz G: Extraction of adenylate cyclase activating factor of bovine sperm and its identification as a trypsin-like protease. J Biol Chem 260:114, 1985
4. Siegel MS, Bechtold DS, Willand J, Polakoski KL: Partial purification and characterization of human sperminogen. Biol Reprod 36:1063, 1987

5. Rogers BJ, Bentwood JB: Capacitation, acrosome reaction and fertilization. In Zaneveld LJD, Chatterton TR (eds): Biochemistry of Mammalian Reproduction. New York: John Wiley & Sons, 1982, p 203
6. Ishii S, Kasai K: Affinity methods using argininal derivatives. Methods Enzymol 80:842, 1981
7. Zaneveld LJD, Polakoski KL, Schumacher GFB: The proteolytic enzyme systems of mammalian genital tract secretions and spermatozoa. In Reich R, Rifkin DB, Shaw E (eds): Proteases and Biological Control, vol 2. Cold Spring Harbor, NY: Cold Spring Harbor Laboratory, 1975, p 683
8. Florke-Gerloff S, Topfer-Peterson E, Schill WB, Engel W: Evolution and development of the outer acrosomal membrane (OAM) and evidence that acrosin inhibitors are proteins of the OAM. Andrologia 19:121, 1987
9. Tschesche H, Wittig B, Decker G, Muller-Esterl W, Fritz H: A new acrosin inhibitor from boar spermatozoa. Eur J Biochem 126:99, 1982
10. Muller-Esterl W, Fritz H: Sperm acrosin. Methods Enzymol 80:621, 1981
11. Goodpasture J, Polakoski KL, Zaneveld LJD: Acrosin, proacrosin, and acrosin inhibitor of human spermatozoa: extraction, quantitation, and stability. J Androl 1:16, 1980
12. Elce JS, McIntyre EJ: Acrosin: immunochemical demonstration of multiple forms generated from bovine and human proacrosin. Can J Biochem Cell Biol 61:989, 1982
13. Tanaka T, McRae BJ, Cho K, Cook R, Frack JE, Johnson DA, Powers JC: Mammalian tissue trypsin-like enzymes. J Biol Chem 258:13552, 1983
14. McRae B, Kurachi K, Heimark RL, Fujikawa K, Davie EW, Powers JC: Mapping the active sites of bovine thrombin, factor IXa, factor Xa, factor XIa, factor XIIa, plasma kallikrein, and trypsin with amino acid and peptide thioesters. Biochemistry 20:7196, 1981
15. Siegel MS, Polakaski KL: Evaluation of the human sperm proacrosin-acrosin system using gelatin dodecylsulfate-polyacrylamide gel electrophoresis. Biol Reprod 32:713, 1985
16. Mohensian M, Syner FN, Moghissi K: A study of sperm acrosin in patients with unexplained infertility. Fertil Steril 37:223, 1982
17. Calamera JC, Quiros MC, Brugo S, Nicholson RF, Vilar O: Adenosine triphosphate (ATP) concentrations and acrosin activity in human spermatozoa: their relationship with the sperm penetration assay. Andrologia 18:574, 1986
18. Kennedy WP, Kaminski JM, VanderVen H, Jeyendran RS, Reid DS, Blackwell J, Bielfeld P, Zaneveld LJD: Simple clinical assay to evaluate acrosin assay in human spermatozoa. J Androl 10:221, 1989
19. Gaddum P, Blandau RJ: Proteolytic reaction of mammalian sperm on gelatin membranes. Science 170:749, 1970
20. Ficsor G, Binsberg LC, Oldford GM, Snokes RE, Becker RW: Gelatin substrate film technique for the detection of acrosin in single mammalian sperm. Fertil Steril 39:548, 1983

Section D2:

TESTS OF SPERMATOZOA FUNCTION: ATP

FRANK H. COMHAIRE, M.D., LUTGARDE VERMEULEN, INDUSTRIAL ENGINEER IN CHEMISTRY, AND BLAYSE FAGLA, B.S.

Progressive motility is the most important functional characteristic of fertile spermatozoa. The energy needed for motility is produced in the mitochondria of the midpiece of the sperm. Approximately 90% of the energy needed for motility is produced as adenosine triphosphate (ATP) and transported to the flagellum. This energy is necessary for maintenance of osmotic balance of the cell.

In the flagellum, ATP is hydroxylated into adenosine diphosphate (ADP) and adenosine monophosphate (AMP) by the ATPase enzyme, which is present in the contractile protein of the dynein arms located in contact with the microtubular doublets. A decreased ATP content or production will result in insufficient energy and poor sperm motility.

Method

The modern methods for assessment of ATP in human semen are based on bioluminescence. In the presence of ATP, the luciferine-luciferase complex is activated, resulting in the production of light (Fig. 4.2). The amount of light which is produced is proportional to the concentration of ATP.

The following method for ATP determination is recommended by the World Health Organization (1):

REAGENTS

- TRIS-EDTA buffer:

TRIS	12.10 g;
$Na_2EDTA \cdot H_2O$	0.37 g;
Sodium azide	0.50 g.

  1. Dissolve in 900 ml of distilled water.
  2. Adjust pH to 7.75 with sulphuric acid.
  3. Add distilled water to 1000 ml.
  4. Before use, a sample of the buffer is first filtered through a disposable millipore filter (0.22 μm).
- ATP monitoring reagent:
  1. Add 10 ml of sterile water to the freeze-dried ATP to reconstitute the reagent from a kit (e.g., 1243-102 LKB).
  2. Divide into samples of 0.5 ml (use cryotubes with stoppers).
  3. Store at $-20°C$.
- ATP standard (10^{-5} mol/liter):
  1. Add 10 ml of sterile distilled water to the freeze-dried ATP to reconstitute the standard.
  2. Divide into samples of 0.5 ml (use cryotubes with stoppers).
  3. Store at $-20°C$.

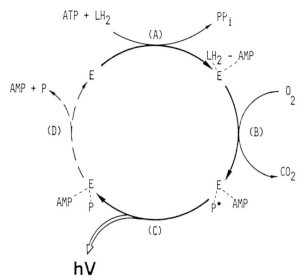

Figure 4.2. Mechanism of the luciferine-luciferase reaction. (Letters *A–E* refer to reagents defined in text.)

Additional ATP standard can be prepared by dissolving 6.052 mg of ATP in 10 ml of TRIS-EDTA buffer. Of the latter solution, 0.1 ml should be diluted in 10 ml of TRIS-EDTA buffer to obtain the standard with 10^{-5} mol/liter.

PROCEDURE

Preparation of Semen Extract

1. Add to a plastic cryotube with screw stopper:
   400 μl (0.4 ml) of TRIS-EDTA buffer;
   100 μl (0.1 ml) of liquefied fresh semen.
2. Place cryotube upright in a boiling waterbath for 15 minutes.
3. Either proceed immediately or store at $-20°C$ until determination.

Adjustment of the Luminometer with ATP Standard

1. Add in a disposable measuring (polystyrene) cuvette:
   1900 μl (1.9 ml) of TRIS-EDTA buffer;
   100 μl (0.1 ml) of monitoring reagent.
2. Place the cuvette into the luminometer and adjust background.
3. Add 50 μl (0.05 ml) of ATP-standard to the TRIS-EDTA buffer with monitoring reagent that is already present in the cuvette.
4. Read maximal luminescence in relative light units (RLU).

The reading for ATP-standard should be roughly comparable to previous readings with the same monitoring reagent. Monitoring reagent of a different lot may yield a different reading. Adjustment of the luminometer should be performed before each series of determinations.

Determination of ATP in Semen Extract

1. Let the fresh extract cool down, or thaw the frozen extract at room temperature.
2. Pour the contents of the cryotube into a disposable polystyrene measuring cuvette.

2. Pour the contents of the cryotube into a disposable polystyrene measuring cuvette.
3. Rinse the cryotube with 1450 μl (1.45 ml) of TRIS-EDTA buffer and pour the latter into the measuring cuvette.
4. Add 100 μl (0.1 ml) of monitoring reagent.
5. Mix by two brisk shakings.
6. Place into the luminometer and read maximal luminescence (value A, in RLU).
7. Add 50 μl (0.05 ml) of ATP standard.
8. Read maximal luminescence (value B, in RLU).

The whole procedure should be accomplished in less than 30 seconds.

CALCULATIONS

$$A = \text{ATP in 100 μl of semen}$$
$$B = \text{ATP in 100 μl of semen} + \text{ATP in 50 μl of standard solution } (10^{-5} \text{ mol/liter})$$

Therefore:

$$\frac{A}{2(B-A)} = \text{ATP in semen (in } 10^{-5} \text{ mol/liter)}$$

Results are expressed in μmol/liter, hence:

$$\text{ATP in semen (in μmol/liter)} = 10 \times \frac{A}{2(B-A)}$$

Relation between Sperm Characteristics and ATP Content

There is a linear correlation between sperm concentration and ATP concentration per milliliter (Fig. 4.3). A similar correlation is found between the ATP concentration per milliliter and the concentration of motile sperm. The ATP content per 10^6 sperm presents an inverse and non-linear correlation with sperm concentration, which is significant in semen samples where <40% of spermatozoa display a rapid linear progressive (type *a*) motility (Fig. 4.4). There is also an inverse relation between the ATP content of sperm and the proportion of vital cells.

Furthermore, the ATP content per spermatozoon decreases with time after ejaculation, but this effect is different in spermatozoa with good or poor motility. In the former, ATP starts to decrease after >4 hours, whereas in the latter, some decrease occurs within 4 hours after ejaculation. These differences may reflect differences in the potential of different cell types to generate energy, possibly related to cell aging.

Measurement of ATP should be performed as soon as possible after ejaculation, and certainly within 4 hours. The ATP content per milliliter is related to the number of sperm with rapid progressive motility. Because the relation between ATP and the concentration of type *a* motile sperm is not linear, the ATP concentration per spermatozoon changes with the concentration of type *a* cells. Therefore, it is not recommended that the ATP: spermatozoon ratio be used for clinical purposes.

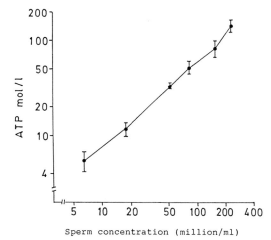

Figure 4.3. Relation between ATP concentration (mol/liter) and sperm concentration (10^6/ml).

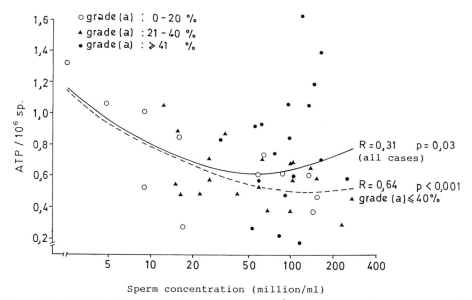

Figure 4.4. Relation between ATP concentration per 10^6 spermatozoa and sperm concentration.

Reference

1. World Health Organization: Laboratory Manual for the Examination of Human Semen and Semen-Cervical Mucus Interaction. Cambridge, England: Cambridge University Press, 1987, p 52

Section D3:

TESTS OF SPERMATOZOA FUNCTION: CERVICAL MUCUS PENETRATION

NANCY J. ALEXANDER, PH.D.

Although millions of sperm are deposited in the cervical mucus, only hundreds reach the fallopian tubes. A major factor in this reduction is the cervical mucus, which serves as a sperm filter, a mechanism for sperm selection. There is increasing evidence that more morphologically abnormal sperm are found in the vagina than at the internal cervical os. Cervical mucus serves to select morphologically normal sperm (1). This selection may occur because of an association between morphology and motility: sperm that are progressively more motile are more capable of penetrating the cervical mucus (2). The excluded spermatozoa are usually those with midpiece or tail defects, and are therefore those with impaired motility (3, 4).

In addition to providing a filter to separate sperm on the basis of morphology and motility, cervical mucus aids in the capacitation of sperm. This results from a direct interaction between sperm and mucus. Cervical mucus also plays an important role in allowing human sperm to reside for extended periods in the cervical canal and yet retain their fertilizing capacity (5).

If a careful test of sperm-mucus interaction reveals normal results, it probably indicates that there is no defect in sperm motility. Evaluation of cervical mucus and sperm penetration ability can be done in vitro or in vivo.

During the normal menstrual cycle, cervical mucus passes through an aqueous and a gel phase. During the low-viscosity aqueous phase, the mucus contains soluble proteins, inorganic ions, and low-molecular-weight organic compounds. In contrast, during the gel or cervical mucin phase, the mucin consists of high-molecular-weight glycoproteins with a polypeptide core. The extended entangled mucins are cross-linked molecules that are a framework for the mucus secretions.

Estrogens induce secretion of large amounts of a clear acellular mucus, whereas progestogens induce a mucus that is opaque and viscous. Consistency changes occur about 24 hours after the estrogen surge. The endocervical epithelial cells secrete approximately 600 mg of mucins in the preovulatory and ovulatory phases of the cycle. At midcycle, cervical mucus is about 98% water, whereas at other times the water content falls to 90%. During the luteal phase, the mucus acts as a mechanical barrier. The dense mucin network prevents spermatozoa and other organisms from reaching the uterus. It also prevents various sexually transmitted organisms from having access to the uterus. Progestational contraceptives, therefore, can prevent organism access.

Methodology

POSTCOITAL TEST

Although there is debate about the value of the postcoital test (PCT), it is still an important evaluation of fertility (6, 7). It is conducted 1 day before ovulation, when follicular estrogen is at its peak level and when the mucus shows good estrogenic features (transparency, spinnbarkheit, and ferning). Determination of the ovulatory cycle is usually made by a study of basal body temperature records, ultrasound monitoring, or daily examination of the cervical mucus. On the day of the test, some clinicians (8) instruct their patients to report to the clinic as soon as possible after coitus, whereas others (9) suggest that the patient be evaluated 4 to 5, or even 12, hours later.

Aliquots of mucus are collected from the internal os by means of a syringe. The mucus is assessed for ferning and the presence of a spinnbarkheit of ≥10 cm. The PCT involves placing a drop of cervical mucus on a slide, spreading and coverslipping it, then counting the number of motile sperm in 10 randomly chosen high-power fields ($\times 400$). A good PCT is defined as ≥10 sperm per field. Fewer sperm may indicate collection of non-midcycle mucus, poor mucus (sometimes called "hostile cervical factor"), mucus or sperm with antibodies on the surface, oligozoospermia, or sperm with poor motility.

Factors that contribute to poor-quality cervical mucus include infection, inadequate estrogen priming, deficient endocervical tissue (secondary to trauma), or previous surgery to the cervix. Scant viscous mucus at ovulation can be improved by increasing estrogen levels. In fact, some European clinics (W. Eggert-Kruse, personal communication) routinely provide oral estrogens (80 μg of ethinylestradiol per day for 7 days) before a PCT. Use of optimal mucus allows differentiation of sperm-cervical mucus problems from those of poor-quality mucus.

IN VITRO SPERM-CERVICAL MUCUS TESTING

Because of the problems of interpreting PCTs, many investigators use an in vitro test. Either a slide, or Kurzrok-Muller, test (a drop of semen and of cervical mucus are apposed under a coverslip) or a capillary tube, or Kremer, test (a capillary tube of mucus is placed in a reservoir of semen) is commonly used (10). The depth of penetration of the spermatozoa at particular time intervals is measured. As with in vivo testing, in vitro cervical mucus penetration depends upon collection of the cervical mucus in the periovulatory period. One of the advantages of an in vitro test is that, since the semen is produced by masturbation, a sample can also be used for semen analysis.

In the slide method, the spermatozoa appear to form phalanges, and a single spermatozoon appears to lead the penetration. In the presence of antisperm antibodies, these phalanges are not found. Because the size and shape of the semen-mucus interface vary, and because the coverslip exerts local forces, there are limits to the reproducibility and quantifiability of this test. When capillary tubes are used, the mucus is aspirated into a tube (10 cm $\times$ 3 mm $\times$ 0.3 mm flat capillary tube; Vitro Dynamics, Rockaway, N.J.) and sealed at one end. Although the couple is told to refrain from coitus for 3 days before collection, the mucus-filled capillary tube is checked before testing for the presence of spermatozoa. One open end of the tube is inserted into a small plastic vial containing 0.5 to 1.0 ml of semen. The mucus interface must be immersed in the semen. The tube and semen are incubated at 37°C for 60 minutes, after which the tube is removed and wiped gently to remove any residual semen, and the depth of sperm penetration is microscopically assessed (11). Some investigators evaluate the swimming speed and flagellar beat in addition to depth of penetration.

BOVINE CERVICAL MUCUS TEST

The advantage and disadvantage of the Kremer capillary approach is that both the wife's cervical mucus and the husband's spermatozoa are simultaneously evaluated. With repeated poor in vivo or in vitro tests, it is important for the clinician to determine whether the spermatozoa are the reason for poor penetration. One way to do this is to use donor mucus as well as the wife's mucus and donor sperm as well as the husband's sperm. The various combinations, called the cross-mucus test, can provide useful information (12). A standardized source of mucus makes access to donor mucus and sperm unnecessary and allows a more thorough evaluation of spermatozoa. Frequently, a homogeneous source of bovine cervical mucus can be used (Serono Diagnostics, Norwell, Mass.). Human and bovine mucus are rheologically similar: their glycoproteins are close in sugar and amino acid composition, as well as in electrophoretic mobility and sedimentation rate. When a drop of midcycle human cervical mucus is placed on a slide, crystallization occurs at right angles because of the presence of sodium and chloride. The ferning and viscous elastic patterns of bovine cervical mucus are similar at midcycle. Human sperm penetrate both bovine and human mucus in a similar unidirectional way with similar flagellar motions.

The procedure is straightforward. Two flat capillary tubes are taken from the freezer, allowed to warm briefly, and then are carefully tapped so that any air bubbles can float to one end of the tube. The tube is broken at the score mark and placed in a small aliquot containing semen. The sample is incubated at room temperature for 90 minutes (since sperm motility is temperature-dependent, shorter time periods at 37°C could be used) and, as in the Kremer test, is evaluated microscopically to determine the length of the progression of the vanguard sperm.

The literature indicates that the penetration is normal when it is >30 mm after 90 minutes. This method has been used to predict the outcome of the hamster sperm penetration test and the results of in vitro fertilization.

References

1. Pretorius E, Franken DR, DeWet J, Grobler S: Sperm selection capacity of cervical mucus. Arch Androl 12:5, 1984
2. Mortimer D, Pandya IJ, Sawers RS: Relationship between human sperm motility characteristics and sperm penetration into human cervical mucus in vitro. J Reprod Fertil 78:93, 1986
3. Gonzales J, Jezequel F: Influence of the quality of the cervical mucus on sperm penetration: comparison of the morphologic features of spermatozoa in 101 postcoital tests with those in the semen of the husband. Fertil Steril 44:796, 1985
4. Jeulin C, Soumah A, Jouannet P: Morphological factors influencing the penetration of human sperm into cervical mucus in vitro. Int J Androl 8:215, 1985
5. Lambert H, Overstreet JW, Morales P, Hanson FW, Yanagimachi R: Sperm capacitation in the human female reproductive tract. Fertil Steril 43:325, 1985
6. Moghissi KS: Significance and prognostic value of postcoital test. In Insler V, Bettendorf G (eds): The Uterine Cervix in Reproduction. Stuttgart: Georg Thieme, 1977, p 231
7. Collins JA, So Y, Wilson EH, Wrixon W, Casper RF: The postcoital test as a predictor of pregnancy among 355 infertile couples. Fertil Steril 41:703, 1984
8. Danezis J, Sujan S, Sobrero AJ: Evaluation of the postcoital test. Fertil Steril 13:559, 1962
9. Beck WW: The cervical factor. In Garcia C-R, Mastroianna L, Amelar RD, Dublin L (eds): Current Therapy of Infertility. Philadelphia: BC Decker, 1988, p 118
10. Kremer J: A simple sperm penetration test. Int J Fertil 10:209, 1965
11. Mortimer D: The male factor in infertility. Part II. Sperm function testing. In Leventhal JM (ed): Current Problems in Obstetrics, Gynecology and Fertility, vol. 8. Chicago: Year Book, 1985, p 1
12. Blasco L: Clinical approach to the evaluation of sperm-cervical mucus interactions. Fertil Steril 28:1133, 1977

Section D4:

TESTS OF SPERMATOZOA FUNCTION: HYPO-OSMOTIC SWELLING TEST

LOURENS J. D. ZANEVELD, D.V.M., PH.D., RAJASINGAM S. JEYENDRAN, D.V.M., PH.D., AND PATRICIA KRAJESKI, B.S.N.

In the diagnosis of male infertility, only limited attention has been devoted to assessing the functional integrity of the sperm membrane. Membrane integrity is not only important for sperm metabolism, but a correct change in the properties of the membrane is required for successful union of the male and female gametes: sperm capacitation, the acrosome reaction, and the binding to and penetration of the egg vestments. Therefore, assessment of membrane function may be a useful indicator of the fertilizing ability of spermatozoa.

Histological studies only show whether the membrane is morphologically intact. The same is true for the "live-dead" (supravital) stain, which measures the ability of eosin Y dye to permeate the membranes, a sign that they are either broken or morphologically altered by cell injury or death. These observations assess the functional status of the membrane.

A property of the cell membrane is its ability to selectively permit the transport of fluids and certain molecules. When exposed to hypo-osmotic conditions, fluid will enter the spermatozoon in an attempt to reach osmotic equilibrium. This inflow of fluid increases the sperm volume in order to maintain a more stable surface-to-volume ratio. As a result, the sperm membrane bulges or balloons, referred to as "swelling." Extra space is created in the sperm head and tail. Since the tail fibers are under tension, the excess space causes them to curl within the membrane (1); this is readily visible by phase contrast microscopy. The response of the sperm tail to hypo-osmotic conditions varies from a ballooning only at the tip of the tail to involvement of the entire tail. Therefore, curling of the tail fibers may occur to various degrees. It can be assumed that the ability of the human spermatozoon to swell under hypo-osmotic conditions is a sign that the transport of fluids across the membrane occurs normally, indicating membrane integrity and normal function.

Drevius and Eriksson (2) first reported the swelling phenomenon using bull spermatozoa. Since then, several studies (3–5) have confirmed the ability of bovine spermatozoa to swell in a hypo-osmotic medium and have shown that this phenomenon is correlated with fertility. In 1984, the swelling characteristic was developed into a test system (hypo-osmotic swelling test, or HOS) to evaluate the functional activity of the human sperm membrane (6). The HOS test was marginally correlated with sperm morphology, sperm motility, and the live-dead stain, but the correlation coefficients were too low to predict the outcome of the HOS test from the other sperm characteristics. The HOS test correlates highly ($r = 0.9$) with the outcome of the zona-free hamster penetration assay when normal ejaculates are used. A number of other observations have confirmed the clinical usefulness of the HOS test (Chapter 5). A distinct advantage of the test is that it is simple, cheap, and readily applicable clinically. Also, the spermatozoa can be fixed after being exposed to hypo-osmotic conditions and observed later. This is useful under field conditions or in a laboratory not fully equipped for microscopic observations.

Methodology

PREPARATION OF HYPO-OSMOTIC MEDIUM

1. Prepare:
   A. 2.7 g of fructose (M.W. 180.16) in 100 ml of distilled water;
   B. 1.46 g of sodium citrate · 2 H_2O (M.W. 294.11) in 100 ml of distilled water.
2. Add 100 ml of solution A to 100 ml of solution B and mix. This is the HOS solution (200 ml).
3. Pipette 1-ml aliquots of the HOS solution into separate test tubes. Cap and freeze at −20°C until use.

PROCEDURE FOR THE HYPO-OSMOTIC SWELLING TEST

1. Thaw a test tube of HOS solution by incubation at 37°C for 10 minutes.
2. Add 0.1 ml of well-mixed, fully liquefied semen to the solution and mix.
3. Incubate the mixture for at least 30 minutes but no longer than 3 to 4 hours (preferably 2 hours) at 37°C.
4. After incubation, place a drop of the well-mixed sample on a glass slide with a cover slip. Observe under a phase contrast microscope (×400) for curling of the sperm tail. (A bright-field microscope can be used but is less reliable.)
5. If desired, the treated spermatozoa can be fixed with formaldehyde (18.5%, 0.1 ml) for later evaluation (within 30 days).
6. Differentially count at least 100—preferably 200—spermatozoa per sample. Calculate the percentage of swollen sperm: (Number of swollen spermatozoa × 100%)/(Total number of spermatozoa counted).
7. Since some semen samples will have spermatozoa with curled tails before exposure to the HOS test, it is essential that the ejaculate is observed before exposure, especially when using a bright-field microscope. The percentage of spermatozoa with curled tails in the untreated sample should be subtracted from the percentage of spermatozoa that reacted in the HOS test.

Interpretation of Results

It is normal for an ejaculate to possess 60% or more swollen spermatozoa after being subjected to the HOS test. From 50% to 59% swollen spermatozoa represents a gray area in which no diagnosis can be reached. Less than 50% swollen spermatozoa is abnormal. Additional diagnostic information may be obtained by observing the type of swelling (tail curling) (see Chapter 5).

References

1. Schrader SM, Platek SF, Zaneveld LJD, Perez-Pelaez M, Jeyendran RS: Sperm viability: a comparison of analytical methods. Andrologia 18:530, 1986
2. Drevius LO, Eriksson L: Osmotic swelling of mammalian spermatozoa. Exp Cell Res 42:136, 1966
3. Bredderman PJ, Foote RH: Volume of stressed bull spermatozoa and protoplasmic droplets, and the relationship of cell size to motility and fertility. J Anim Sci 28:496, 1969
4. Foote RH, Bredderman PJ: Sizing of aging bull spermatozoa with an electronic counter. J Dairy Sci 52:117, 1969

5. Drevius LO: The permeability of bull spermatozoa to water, polyhydric alcohols and univalent unions upon the kinetic activity of spermatozoa and sperm models. J Androl Fertil 28:41, 1972
6. Jeyendran RS, Van der Ven HH, Perez-Pelaez M, Crabo BG, Zaneveld, LJD: Development of an assay to assess the functional integrity of the human sperm membrane and its relationship to other semen characteristics. J Reprod Fertil 70:219–228, 1984

Section E1:

EVALUATION OF THE ACROSOME: TRIPLE STAINING

KEVIN COETZEE, M.S., AND THINUS F. KRUGER, M.D.

Capacitated mammalian spermatozoa must first undergo the acrosome reaction to effect normal fertilization (1). The reaction is required for the penetration of the zona pellucida and the fusion with the egg plasma membrane. Numerous studies using zona-free and non-viable human ova have substantiated this prerequisite (2–4). The ability of spermatozoa to undergo a normal acrosome reaction and the rate of the reaction may thus be an important indicator of fertility. Nagae (5), in an electron microscopy study, showed that the acrosome reaction involves major alterations to the membrane system of spermatozoa. Changes result in the complete loss of the plasma and outer acrosomal membrane, exposing the inner acrosomal membrane. These changes should therefore allow for easy monitoring of the acrosome reaction.

The evaluation of the human acrosome reaction, however, is restricted by a practical limitation: the acrosome is too small to observe by light (phase contrast) microscopy. The best results were therefore initially observed by electron microscopy, which is time consuming and complex, discouraging routine use. The need thus arose for a relatively simple assay which could quantitate the acrosome reaction at the light microscope level. Another problem which had to be considered is that the human acrosome is relatively labile and may break down with sperm death (6). The assay must therefore be able to distinguish between normal and degenerative reactions. Several techniques have been proposed to differentiate intact acrosome from reacted spermatozoa. The following are important examples.

Methodology

TRIPLE STAINING TECHNIQUE

Although a number of techniques for staining the acrosomal contents of mammalian sperm have been reported (7, 8), these methods suffer from a common shortcoming: their inability to distinguish between normal and degenerative reactions. However, the triple stain technique permits direct assessment of viability and acrosome reaction in human sperm at the light microscope level (9, 10). Live and dead sperm are first differentiated by using the vital stain trypan blue. Next, the acrosomal and post-acrosomal regions are differentiated by using rose bengal and Bismarck brown, respectively. Rose bengal specifically stains the acrosome; loss of stain indicates loss of the acrosome observed by electron microscopy. Four staining patterns are thus obtained from this protocol: live, dead, acrosome-reacted, and non-reacted sperm.

The triple stain technique is laborious and subject to intra-assay and interassay variation. Most variations can be attributed to rose bengal, with batches varying in staining efficiency, and with stain intensity varying from patient to patient (10). A modified double stain technique, using only rose bengal and Bismarck brown, saves time but cannot distinguish between normal and degenerate reactions (11) or eliminate the variancy of rose bengal.

FLUORESCEIN-CONJUGATED LECTINS

Lectins are plant proteins with a high affinity for specific sugar residues. Numerous glycoproteins and glycolipids are present in cell membranes, many forming the receptor systems of the cell, which may bind lectins (12). Fluorescein-conjugated lectins bind to the acrosomal membranes and/or contents (soybean agglutinin, concanavalin A and *Pisum sativum* agglutinin, and *Ricinus communis* agglutinin 60, or RCA) due to the high concentration of glycoconjugates in the acrosomal region (13, 14).

Talbot and Chacon (13) found that RCA specifically labeled the acrosome region. Electron microscopy showed that a correlation exists between acrosome loss and loss of label. But this method has two major disadvantages: it cannot distinguish between normal and degenerate reactions, and RCA is highly toxic. A supravital stain (Hoechst 33258) and *Pisum sativum*, a non-toxic lectin, were used by Cross (14) to overcome the disadvantages encountered by Talbot and Chacon (13). Nevertheless, the use of lectins is restricted; they cannot be used in the presence of cervical mucus or zona pellucida, both of which are also rich in glycoconjugates.

INDIRECT IMMUNOFLUORESCENCE ASSAY

A fact generally accepted is that the sperm surface may alter during maturation, capacitation, and the acrosome reaction. Specific proteins may be incorporated, and/or integral membrane proteins may become unmasked or modified (15). Antibodies generated against spermatozoa can therefore be used to follow these developments by indirect immunofluorescence (16–18). Polyclonal and monoclonal antibodies can be raised against any species of spermatozoa in a host animal and cultured in vitro. Polyclonal antisera cannot, however, be purified to recognize specific antigens or be restricted to specific regions (15). Monoclonal antibodies, however, are highly specific immunoglobulins, recognizing specific antigens restricted to certain regions. The binding of the antibody is made visible under a fluorescent microscope when bound by fluorescein isothiocyanate—goat anti-mouse IgG, for example.

Wolf (16) identified two monoclonal antibodies specific for antigens in the acrosomal cap region: HS-19 and HS-21. Uniform and bright fluorescence over the whole acrosome in 87 (8.5%) of the sperm was seen using HS-21. A monoclonal antibody, generated against hamster epididymal spermatozoa and recognizing an acrosomal antigen, was used by Moore (18) to study capacitation and the acrosome reaction in live/motile as well as fixed spermatozoa. In this study, an intermediate stage, detected as "spotty fluorescence," was observed in unfixed sperm. This may represent initial acrosomal changes or late capacitation reactions. An important prerequisite is the ability to distinguish between degenerate and physiological reactions. Cross (14) included a supravital stain (Hoechst 33258) for viability differentiation. An alternative would be to use live/motile (unfixed) spermatozoa so that the motility and the acrosomal status of each sperm could be assessed simultaneously.

CHLORTETRACYCLINE FLUORESCENCE ASSAY

The chlortetracycline (CTC) fluorescent assay works on the principle that a complex of CTC and calcium bound to membranes shows highly enhanced fluorescence (19). Binding is to the surface and is affected by the changes in the plasma membrane surface. Initially used to follow the acrosome reaction in mouse spermatozoa (20), this assay is rapid and simple, allowing a sample to be processed within 5 minutes and presenting a finer resolution of the time-related progress of capacitation and acrosome reaction (19).

Discussion

To institute an assay for routine clinical use, it must comply with certain logistical requirements. The assay must be rapid and simple to perform, with no prolonged fixation, permeabilization, or extensive washing; it must use standard laboratory equipment and commercially available reagents. The assay must also be experimentally accurate, restricting ambiguous fixation and staining artifacts, and intraassay and interassay variances should be within acceptable limits. The ability to distinguish between physiological (normal) and degenerate reactions is also important. An assay able to differentiate between capacitation and the acrosome reaction, and the different stages of each, would be of critical importance. The availability of a monitor for the time course of capacitation and the acrosome reaction would provide valuable information. The percentage of reactions and/or the reaction rate might predict male fertility. The concordance with the fertility potential might be enhanced when used in combination with other semen parameters. The optimal capacitation time allowing maximal acrosome reaction could be calculated. In vitro fertilization and artificial insemination could be performed at the correct times. Conditions, environment, and media for the best capacitation rate could be optimized.

An interesting observation made by several investigators (9, 16, 19) is that the percentage of acrosome reaction never exceeds 50% and always averages about 30%. Therefore, not all capacitated sperm become acrosome-reacted. Is this an in vitro artifact, or can only 30% of a human ejaculate truly undergo a physiological acrosome reaction? Further studies may reveal the answer to this interesting question.

References

1. Yanagimachi R: Mechanisms of fertilization in mammals. In Mastroianni L, Biggers JD (eds): Fertilization and Embryonic Development in Vitro. New York: Academic Press, 1981, p 81
2. Rogers BJ: The sperm penetration assay: its usefulness reevaluated. Fertil Steril 43:821, 1985
3. Yanagimachi R: Zona-free hamster eggs: their use in assessing fertilizing capacity and examining chromosomes of human spermatozoa. Gamete Res 10:187, 1985
4. Overstreet JW, Yanagimachi R, Katz DF, Hayashi K, Hanson FW: Penetration of human spermatozoa into the human zona pellucida and the zona-free hamster egg; a study of fertile donors and infertile patients. Fertil Steril 33:534, 1980
5. Nagae T, Yanagimachi R, Srivastava P, Yanagimachi H: Acrosome reaction in human spermatozoa. Fertil Steril 45:701, 1986

6. Talbot P, Chacon RS: Observations on the acrosome reaction of human sperm in vitro. Am J Primatol 1:211, 1981
7. Wells ME, Awa OA: New technique for assessing acrosomal characteristics of spermatozoa. J Dairy Sci 53:227, 1970
8. Talbot P, Chacon RS: A new technique for rapidly scoring acrosome reactions of human sperm. J Cell Biol 83:2089, 1979
9. Talbot P, Chacon RS: A triple-stain technique for evaluating normal acrosome reactions of human spermatozoa. J Exp Zool 215:201, 1981
10. Talbot P, Dudenhausen E: Factors affecting triple staining of human sperm. Stain Technol 56:307, 1981
11. De Jonge C, Rawlins RG, Zaneveld LJD: Induction of the human sperm acrosome reaction by human oocytes. J Androl 9:39, 1988
12. Ahuja KK: Carbohydrate determinants involved in mammalian fertilization. Am J Anat 174:207, 1985
13. Talbot P, Chacon R: A new procedure for rapidly scoring acrosome reactions of human sperm. Gamete Res 3:211, 1980
14. Cross NL, Morales P, Overstreet JW, Hanson FW: Two simple methods for detecting acrosome reacted human sperm. Gamete Res 15:213, 1986
15. Moore HDM, Hartman TD: Localization by monoclonal antibodies of various surface antigens of hamster spermatozoa and the effect of antibody on fertilization in vitro. J Reprod Fertil 70:175, 1984
16. Wolf DP, Boldt T, Byrd W, Bechtol KB: Acrosomal status evaluation in human ejaculated sperm with monoclonal antibodies. Biol Reprod 32:1157, 1985
17. Suarez SS, Wolf DP, Meizel S: Induction of the acrosome reaction in human spermatozoa by a fraction of human follicular fluid. Gamete Res 14:107, 1986
18. Moore HDM, Smith CA, Hartman TD, Bye AP: Visualization and characterization of the acrosome reaction of human spermatozoa by immunolocalization with monoclonal antibodies. Gamete Res 17:245, 1987
19. Lee MA, Trucco GS, Bechtol KB, Wummer N, Kopf GS, Blasco L, Storey BT: Capacitation and the acrosome reactions in human spermatozoa monitored by a chlortetracycline fluorescence assay. Fertil Steril 48:649, 1987
20. Ward CR, Storey BT: Determination of the time course of capacitation in mouse spermatozoa using a chlortetracycline fluorescence assay. Dev Biol 104:287, 1984

Section E2:

EVALUATION OF THE ACROSOME: IMMUNOLOGICAL METHODS

COSIMA BRUCKNER, M.D., AND NANCY J. ALEXANDER, PH.D.

The acrosome reaction is the ultimate step in a series of events rendering spermatozoa capable of fertilizing an egg. The membrane-bound, cap-like acrosome covers the anterior portion of the sperm nucleus. Since it contains a broad spectrum of hydrolytic enzymes (1, 2), it is considered to be a "specialized lysosome" (3). Although the acrosomal matrix contains a carbohydrate component (4, 5), hyaluronidase and acrosin (6, 7) have been the most extensively studied of the enzymes.

The acrosome reaction in vivo is initiated by the binding of capacitated sperm to a glycoprotein receptor in the zona pellucida, called ZP3 in mice (8). Following binding, progressive multiple fusions and vesiculations between the outer acrosomal membrane and the periacrosomal plasma membrane enable the acrosomal contents to escape through the fenestrated membranes (9). Eventually, the entire acrosomal cap is sloughed from the head of the spermatozoon. The acrosome reaction is accompanied by changes in the antigenicity of the sperm head as well as in its carbohydrate composition.

Since the human sperm is too small to allow detection of morphological changes in acrosome-intact and acrosome-reacted sperm by phase contrast light microscopy, there is a requirement for more sophisticated techniques of visualization. The tools for detecting acrosomal status consist of lectins, on the one hand, and monoclonal or polyclonal antibodies, on the other. Lectins are proteins which bind and cross-link specific carbohydrate determinants on the cell surface; they allow visualization of changes in carbohydrate moieties. Changes are found in the lectin-binding pattern of acrosome-reacted and unreacted sperm. Monoclonal antibodies or polyclonal antisera can be raised against specific epitopes on the sperm surface. Since acrosome-reacted sperm, as opposed to acrosome-intact sperm, lack certain antigens, antibodies raised against acrosome-intact sperm may not react with acrosome-reacted sperm. In any evaluation of the acrosome reaction, it is important to differentiate between live and dead sperm, since the acrosomes of dead sperm undergo degeneration, which can be mistaken for the acrosome reaction.

Methods

SUPRAVITAL STAINING

Since the commonly used supravital stains, eosin (10) and trypan blue (11), are unsuitable for use in combination with immunofluorescent assays, another stain, Hoechst 33258, has been introduced (12). This dye fluoresces an intense blue when bound to DNA. It has a limited permeability through intact cell membranes and will therefore stain only dead cells (13). Sperm are incubated at 37°C in 5% CO_2-95% air in Biggers, Whitten, and Whittingham's (BWW) medium (3 μg/ml of bovine serum albumin (BSA)) containing 1 μg/ml of Hoechst 33258 for 10 to 15 minutes. Samples are then inspected by fluorescence microscopy. Fluorescent nuclei indicate non-viable spermatozoa, whereas unlabeled sperm represent the vital population. A thin band of fluorescence that can be seen at the posterior margin of the nucleus of some motile sperm is considered non-specific.

LECTIN LABELING

Lectin receptors are located within the acrosomal contents; if sperm are permeabilized by exposure to ethanol before staining, these receptors become accessible. After supravital staining, sperm are washed free of unbound stain by centrifugation (900 × g for 5 min) through a solution of 2% weight/volume (w/v) polyvinylpyrrolidone-40 (PVP) in phosphate-buffered saline (PBS), pH 7.4. Centrifugation is done in a soft 0.4-ml polyethylene centrifuge tube. The supernatant containing Hoechst 33258 is discarded, and the sperm are resuspended in 95% volume/volume (v/v) ethanol and incubated for 30 minutes at 4°C (12).

Several lectins have been screened for their ability to bind to the acrosomal region of permeabilized sperm (12). Of these, *Pisum sativum* agglutinin (PSA), *Lens culinaris* agglutinin (LCA), concanavalin A (Con A), *Maclura pomifera* agglutinin (MPA), *Ricinus communis* agglutinin-I (RCA-I), and wheat germ agglutinin (WGA) uniformly label the anterior and equatorial head regions of most sperm.

For labeling, permeabilized sperm are dried onto microscopic slides and covered with a droplet of FITC (fluorescein isothiocyanate)-conjugated lectin (Vector Laboratories, Inc., Burlingame, Calif.) at 100 μg/ml in PBS or distilled water for 5 to 10 minutes. The slides are rinsed with gentle agitation in distilled water and mounted in the medium of Johnson and Nogueira Araujo (14). Absence of acrosomal fluorescence indicates acrosome-reacted sperm, most likely due to the loss of acrosomal contents.

The use of FITC-conjugated PSA in combination with the supravital stain Hoechst 33258 has proven to be a rapid and safe method for detection of viable acrosome-reacted sperm (12). Talbot and Chacon (15) used FITC-conjugated *Ricinus communis* agglutinin-II (RCA-II), a lectin labeling the acrosomal region of the majority of sperm that had been fixed and permeabilized in ethanol, as a fast, simple, and widely available reagent; however, RCA-II is highly toxic. The disadvantage of lectin staining in general is that it cannot be used in the presence of other glycoconjugates, such as cervical mucus or zona pellucida components, since these also bind lectins and make the detection of a specific labeling pattern of the sperm unreliable.

Lectin labeling has been compared to labeling with polyclonal antisera. When 300 double-labeled sperm were inspected for their acrosomal status, only 5 (1.7%) scored differently with application of one technique or the other. In addition, when several sperm suspensions were assayed separately with the lectin or antisera method, the percentages of acrosome-reacted sperm determined by the two methods were very similar (12). The antisera method has also been used successfully to determine the acrosomal status of sperm attached to the zona pellucida of non-living oocytes (12).

LABELING WITH POLYCLONAL ANTISERA

The advantage of antisera over lectins is the possibility of evaluating the acrosomal status in the presence of glycoconjugates and other cellular material. Although polyclonal antisera usually do not detect one defined epitope, in conjunction with immunofluorescence they are suitable for demonstrating different staining patterns in acrosome-intact and acrosome-reacted sperm.

Ethanol-permeabilized sperm are dried on microscope slides and covered with a droplet of antisera (70 μg protein/ml in PBS containing 1 mg/ml BSA) for 15 minutes at room temperature, rinsed gently in PBS, incubated for 15 minutes with FITC-conjugated goat anti-rabbit immunoglobulin G (IgG), rinsed in PBS, and mounted in medium (14). This procedure can be combined conveniently with the Hoechst supravital stain.

LABELING WITH MONOCLONAL ANTIBODIES

The well-defined specificity of a monoclonal antibody and the possibility of producing it in virtually unlimited quantity without the sources of error inherent in the production of conventional antisera make it a valuable tool in the analysis of the biochemical alterations occurring during the acrosome reaction. To date, several monoclonals have been produced, mostly against whole, freshly ejaculated human sperm, that recognize different subcellular structures of human acrosome.

The monoclonal antibody C 11 H recognizes sperm acrosin (16, 17). The antigen recognized by C 11 H disappears during the acrosome reaction (18). Another monoclonal, 18.6, originally produced against hamster epididymal spermatozoa, also recognizes an antigen within the human acrosome (19).

To evaluate acrosomal status, Wolf (20) developed a rapid, reproducible assay using monoclonals HS-19 and HS-21, specific to antigens localized in the acrosomal cap region of the sperm head. In later work, another set of monoclonals was produced which recognize the intermediate filament proteins in human sperm heads. T15 is directed against vimentin, a cytoskeletal protein; T5 and T6 (Humagen, Charlottesville, Va.) recognize a keratin-like protein which may be unique to sperm cells (21). T15 characteristically binds to the equatorial segment in intact cells and gives uniform acrosomal cap binding in reacted cells; T5 and T6 reveal the reverse binding pattern.

For acrosomal status evaluation using monoclonal antibodies, sperm spreads are prepared in microwells defined by Mylar tape or glass spot slides (Robuz Surgical Instrument Co., Washington, D.C.). Drops of washed sperm are added to the wells, and sperm cells are allowed to settle and adhere to the slides for 5 to 10 minutes. The excess is removed, and the sperm are allowed to dry. Adherent sperm are then fixed for 5 minutes at 4°C in 1% paraformaldehyde in PBS, pH 7.4. The reaction is stopped with 0.2-M glycine, and the wells are washed with PBS. Sperm cells are exposed to the monoclonal antibody of choice for 1 hour, washed with PBS containing 1% BSA and 0.01% NP-40, then exposed to an FITC-conjugated affinity-purified goat anti-mouse IgG for 1 hour. After washing, slides are mounted in 10% PBS-90% glycerol containing 2% *n*-propylgallate (22).

In the determination of acrosomal status by the use of monoclonal antibodies, a homogeneous pattern has been obtained for fresh semen from 10 donors. A high percentage (87% ± 8.5%; mean ± SD) of the sperm cells in the samples showed uniform and bright fluorescence over the acrosome, indicating acrosome-intact sperm. Sperm that were negative are thought to have had defective or absent acrosomes (20).

Another approach compared the evaluation of acrosomal status of sperm that had been exposed to calcium ionophore A 23187 (to induce the acrosome reaction) by use of monoconal HS-21 with evaluation by transmission electron microscopy. The correlation for sperm from three different donors was $r = 0.96$, indicating that HS-21 allows an accurate quantitation of acrosomal status (20).

Clearly, the most useful approach is one that allows examination of living cells so that acrosomal status and motility of an individual sperm can be assessed simultaneously. Nevertheless, the methods described allow a reasonable approximation of the state of a spermatozoon. To corroborate observations made by indirect immunofluorescence methods, transmission electron microscopy—although it is not suitable for routine use—can readily be applied.

References

1. Stambaugh R, Smith M: Tubulin and microtubule-like structures in mammalian acrosome. J Exp Zool 203:135, 1978
2. Srivastava PN, Farooqui AA, Gould KG: Studies on hydrolytic enzymes of chimpanzee sperm. Biol Reprod 25:363, 1981
3. Allison AC, Hartree EF: Lysosomal enzymes in the acrosome and their possible role in fertilization. J Reprod Fertil 21:501, 1970

4. Holt WV: Development and maturation of the mammalian acrosome: a cytochemical study using phosphotungstic acid staining. J Ultrastruct Res 68:58, 1979

5. Kopecny V, Flechon JE: Fate of acrosomal glycoproteins during the acrosome reaction and fertilization: a light and electron microscope autoradiographic study. Biol Reprod 24:201, 1981

6. McRorie RA, Williams WL: Biochemistry of fertilization. Ann Rev Biochem 42:777, 1974

7. Morton DB: Acrosomal enzymes: immunological localization of acrosin and hyaluronidase in ram spermatozoa. J Reprod Fertil 45:375, 1975

8. Wassarman PM: The biology and chemistry of fertilization. Science 235:553, 1987

9. Yanagimachi R: Mammalian fertilization. In Knobil E, Neill J (eds): The Physiology of Reproduction. New York: Raven Press, 1988, p 135

10. Eliasson R, Treichl L: Supravital staining of human spermatozoa. Fertil Steril 22:134, 1971

11. Talbot P, Chacon R: A triple-stain technique for evaluating normal acrosome reactions of human sperm. J Exp Zool 215:201, 1981

12. Cross NL, Morales P, Overstreet JW, Hanson FW: Two simple methods for detecting acrosome-reacted human sperm. Gamete Res 15:213, 1986

13. Visser JWM: Vital staining of hemopoietic cells with the fluorescent biobenzimazole derivatives Hoechst 33342 and 33258. Acta Pathol Microbiol Scand 274:86s, 1981

14. Johnson GD, Nogueira Araujo GMC: A simple method of reducing the fading of immunofluorescence during microscopy. J Immunol Methods 43:349, 1981

15. Talbot P, Chacon R: A new procedure for rapidly scoring acrosome reactions of human sperm. Gamete Res 3:211, 1980

16. Kallajoki M, Suominen J: An acrosomal antigen of human spermatozoa and spermatogenic cells characterized with monoclonal antibody. Int J Androl 7:283, 1984

17. Kallajoki M, Parvinen M, Suominen JJO: Expression of acrosin during mouse spermatogenesis: a biochemical and immnocytochemical analysis by a monoclonal antibody C11H. Biol Reprod 35:157, 1986

18. Kallajoki M, Virtanen I, Suominen JJO: The fate of acrosomal staining in acrosome reaction of human spermatozoa revealed by a monoclonal antibody and PNA-lectin. Int J Androl 9:181, 1986

19. Moore HDM, Smith CA, Hartman TD, Bye AP: Visualization and characterization of the acrosome reaction of human spermatozoa by immunolocalization with monoclonal antibody. Gamete Res 17:245, 1987

20. Wolf DP, Boldt J, Byrd W, Bechtol KB: Acrosomal status evaluation in human ejaculated sperm with monoclonal antibodies. Biol Reprod 32:1157, 1985

21. Ochs D, Wolf DP, Ochs RL: Intermediate filament proteins in human sperm heads. Exp Cell Res 167:495, 1986

22. Giloh H, Sedat JW: Fluorescence microscopy: reduced photobleaching of rhodamine and fluorescein protein conjugates by *n*-propyl gallate. Science 217:1252, 1982

Section F:

HAMSTER ZONA-FREE OOCYTE SPERMATOZOA PENETRATION ASSAY

KEVIN COETZEE, M.S., R. JAMES SWANSON, R.N., PH.D., AND THINUS F. KRUGER, M.D.

Male fertility depends on the quality of the ejaculated semen. Traditionally, this quality has been assessed according to the parameters of morphology, density, and motility, since in vivo conception was assumed to occur only if there was a certain critical number of morphologically normal, motile sperm in the ejaculate (1). However, there have been many reports of men with apparently normal semen who were clinically infertile. Therefore, an alternate test was sought, by which the fertilizing potential of sperm could be assessed more accurately.

An in vitro system using mature human ova and sperm would fulfill all of the requirements for such a test, but ethical and moral considerations preclude use of human gametes for this purpose. Surrogate ova would provide the alternative, but as a rule the sperm of one species cannot fertilize eggs of another. One site of species specificity in mammals is the zona pellucida (ZP), but most mammals retain strong species specificity even after the removal of the ZP.

The golden hamster is unique in that, on removal of the ZP, all species specificity is lost, allowing the hamster ovum to be penetrated by other species of sperm (2–4). Zona-free (ZPF) hamster eggs can therefore be used in determining the fertilizing capacity of human sperm. The test based on this fact is the hamster ZPF-human sperm penetration assay (SPA). The concept of the SPA was introduced by Yanagimachi in 1972 (2) and was modified for use in humans in 1976 (4).

A spermatozoon must undergo a series of poorly understood biophysical and biochemical changes before it can penetrate a ZPF hamster egg. These changes—capacitation and the acrosome reaction—can be induced under the appropriate culture conditions in vitro; in vivo, they are induced by the presence of mature oocytes (5). The SPA measures capacitation, the acrosome reaction, membrane fusion, incorporation of the sperm into the ooplasm, and the decondensation of the sperm chromatin. However, not all factors which may influence fertilization are measured, and that is its only disadvantage. Penetration of the ZP and normal embryonic development are not measured. Therefore, a positive SPA does not guarantee fertilization and embryonic development, and a negative SPA, which should correlate closely with fertilization failure in human in vitro fertilization (IVF), in reality is the exception rather than the rule (6).

Capacitation

Freshly ejaculated mammalian sperm are unable to fertilize eggs immediately, even in direct contact with them. Sperm acquire their fertilizing ability in vivo during their passage through the female genital tract. This phenomenon is called capacitation (5). The process is not yet fully understood but is known to involve major biochemical and biophysical changes in the membrane complex and the energy metabolism of the sperm. There is general agreement among andrologists that capacitation is a reversible event involving membrane surface-associated molecules which can be replaced on the plasma membrane of the capacitated spermatozoon to return it to its decapacitated state.

Capacitation is a hormone-dependent, estrogen-stimulated phenomenon, which usually occurs in the female tract. However, it can be induced in vitro in chemically defined media (7, 8). Capacitation is also a time-dependent process in which the time varies between men, between ejaculates of the same man, and between sperm of the same ejaculate. Van Kooij (9) highlighted the individuality of the process by finding that there is a more pronounced difference in the capacitation rate between men than between ejaculates of the same man.

Factors which inhibit capacitation (decapacitators) are incorporated into the membrane of sperm during maturation in the epididymis (10, 11). This state of decapacitation is maintained after ejaculation by the presence of inhibitory macromolecules in the seminal plasma (12) and lower reaches of the female reproductive tract. A glycoprotein has been identified (10) as the primary decapacitator, but other molecules such as cholesterol may also play an important role in the stabilization of the acrosome. The precise mechanism by which this is achieved is not yet completely understood. Epididymal maturation also induces a significant increase in the net negative charge by the incorporation of sialoglycoproteins, sulphoglyceralipids, and steroid sulfates into the outer acrosomal membrane (13).

Capacitation involves major restructuring and destabilizing of the sperm surface, increasing membrane fluidity and permeability (12). An elevation in the energy metabolism of the sperm also occurs (14). This new status is achieved as follows:

1. The modification, redistribution, and/or loss of the epididymal, seminal plasma, and cervical decapacitating factors—by exogenous or endogenous proteases (plasmin, kallikrein, and acrosin) (10, 11).
2. The net negative charge is decreased by endogenous hydrolases (sterol sulfatase) (13).
3. The fluidity is increased by the efflux of cholesterol, altering the cholesterol:phospholipid ratio and the influx of unsaturated fatty acids. These changes are serum albumin-mediated (13, 15, 16).

The altered permeability allows the increased uptake of calcium ions, glucose, and oxygen, resulting in an elevated energy state and inducing hyperactivated motility and the ability to acrosome react (14, 17).

Acrosome Reaction

Although capacitation is reversible and is essential for the occurrence of the acrosome reaction, there is no clear demarcation between the two reactions. Rather, capacitation and the acrosome reaction must be seen as a continuous process divided into different stages, preparing the sperm for fertilization. To allow for maximal control, there are specific and non-specific inducers that may act synergistically or as an intricate backup system (albumin, hydrolytic enzymes, glycosaminoglycans, zona components, steroids, calcium ions, and lysophospholipids) (11).

An endogenous calcium ion threshold concentration is the primary inducer of the acrosome reaction (7, 14, 18). Yanagimachi and Usui (7) showed that on the addition of calcium—but not magnesium—guinea pig sperm incubated for several hours in calcium-free medium underwent the acrosome reaction within 10 minutes. Since then, calcium has been implicated in many reactions leading to the complete loss of the acrosome and eventually of fertilization (18), the activation of many enzymes (acrosin, hyaluronidase, phospholipase A_2), enzyme systems (adenylate cyclase), neutralization of the net negative charge, and the induction of hyperactive motility (13).

However, the acrosome reaction is characterized by significant ultrastructural changes leading to the complete loss of the outer acrosomal cap. Nagae (19) proposed a unique morphological sequence for the acrosome reaction:

1. The anterior part of the acrosomal cap swells due to decondensing of the acrosomal matrix.
2. The outer acrosomal membrane—alone, or with the plasma membrane—invaginates to form vesicles.
3. There is fusion of the plasma and outer acrosomal membrane. Fusion in the acrosomal cap is rarely seen, but fusion is consistently seen at the anterior end of the equatorial segment. Visualization of fusion in the cap region may not yet be technically possible because dispersion of the fused membranes occurs rapidly and is difficult to fix.
4. The plasma and outer membranes of the acrosomal cap region disappear, leaving many vesicles on or near the inner acrosomal membranes.
5. These vesicles disperse, leaving the spermatozoon surrounded by the single, continuous inner acrosomal membrane.

In addition to these changes, the plasma membrane overlying the equatorial/post-acrosomal region of the sperm head, which is involved in the fusion of the sperm with the egg vitelline membrane, undergoes a conformational change in the membrane proteins, resulting in activation (5, 7, 13, 20). The loss of the membranes also releases or exposes activated lysins, assisting the sperm penetration of the cumulus matrix and the ZP (11).

Acrosin, a trypsin-like serine proteinase found in the acrosome, may not only enable the sperm to penetrate the ZP but also may be involved in triggering the acrosome reaction (11). Studies (21) using *p*-aminobenzamidine (PABA), an inhibitor of mouse sperm acrosin, have shown that acrosin is necessary for the dispersal of the acrosomal matrix, probably through activation of proacrosin, a process known as self-activation. In the presence of PABA, the membranes undergo normal vesiculation, but ZP penetration is inhibited. Thus, without acrosin, fertilization may be impossible.

There is still uncertainty concerning the precise time when the acrosome reaction is initiated. Three major proposals have been made (5, 13):

1. While the sperm are in the oviductal fluid of the ampulla;
2. While the sperm are in the cumulus matrix;
3. While the sperm are on the surface of the ZP.

The majority of sperm acrosome reaction studies have been performed on the cauda epididymal sperm of the golden hamster because of its relatively large acrosomal cap. The progress of the acrosome reaction can therefore be followed by phase contrast microscopy. Data from the oviductal fluid studies are equivocal. Cummings and Yanagimachi (22) recently studied the ampullary contents of female hamsters by phase contrast microscopy 4 to 10 hours after insemination with golden hamster caudal epididymal sperm and observed that 93 of 96 sperm swimming freely had modified and swollen acrosomal caps. In an earlier study, Yanagimachi and Phillips (23), also using phase contrast microscopy, found that only 4 of 14 free-swimming golden hamster sperm had modified acrosomal caps.

In looking at the cumulus matrix as the site of acrosomal reaction, Cummings and Yanagimachi (22) reported that all 25 motile golden hamster sperm detected in the cumuli from oviducts had undergone or were undergoing the acrosome reaction. Yanagimachi and Phillips (23) reported that 8 of 11 motile sperm within cumuli of golden hamster cumulus-intact complexes from the ampulla had modified acrosomes. In a videotaped study, Cherr (24) found that only 3% to 6% of sperm had actually *completed* the acrosome reaction within the cumulus matrix, which was comparable to the control levels of the acrosome reaction occuring in free-swimming sperm. Their study included both cumulus-intact and cumulus-free eggs, with a higher percentage of reacted sperm found in association with the ZP of cumulus-intact eggs than with the ZP of cumulus-free eggs.

In an in vitro system, depolymerization (softening) of the cumulus matrix may occur because of the high sperm concentrations used. This may allow sperm to reach the ZP with intact acrosomes. Cummings and Yanagimachi (22) studied the ability of hamster sperm to penetrate intact cumulus matrices at low (3:1) sperm:egg ratios. Uncapacitated sperm were unable to penetrate the cumuli; at least 2 hours of pre-incubation were required. Of the 628 in vitro capacitated sperm seen in and on the cumuli, 270 could penetrate, of which only 10 had intact, unmodified acrosomes. They concluded that penetration of the cumuli was limited to a phase in capacitation before the completion of the acrosome reaction, since sperm that had lost the acrosomal cap penetrated poorly and showed reduced viability.

Corselli and Talbot (25) also developed a system in which physiological sperm numbers (1 to 100) were used to challenge fresh hamster oocyte-cumulus complexes in capillary tubes. Their results showed that capacitated, acrosome-intact hamster sperm can penetrate the extracellular matrix between the cumulus cells and can ultimately bind to the ZP. The results obtained by these two groups are quite similar, yet different. Both found that uncapacitated sperm tend to adhere to the cumulus cells on the periphery but do not penetrate, and that sperm that have lost the acrosomal cap penetrate poorly. The only difference seems to be the ability to identify, by phase contrast microscopy, changes occurring between capacitation and the loss of the acrosomal cap.

The cumulus matrix may thus be a selection barrier, allowing only sperm that can undergo a normal acrosome reaction to penetrate to the ZP, or it contains a molecule(s) that increases the rate of the acrosome reaction.

In two independent experiments, Barros (26) and Singer (27), using golden hamster sperm and human sperm, respectively, found that sperm became infertile with prolonged incubation, as judged by their ability to bind and penetrate the ZP. The reason for this decline in penetration with increasing incubation was attributed to an increase in the percentage of acrosome-reacted sperm (28). In contrast, an increase in the penetration of ZPF hamster eggs was seen with increasing incubation time (increase in the acrosome-reacted population). Thus, "old" sperm are prevented from penetrating the ZP. These results indicate that a certain stage of the acrosome reaction must be completed on the surface of the ZP.

In vitro studies by Saling and Storey (29) using mouse sperm were the first to demonstrate a role for the ZP in the acrosome reaction. They incubated cumulus-free eggs with sperm suspensions in which >50% of the population had undergone the acrosome reaction. After gradient centrifugation, only acrosome-intact sperm were detected on the ZP. They concluded that the acrosome reaction of a fertilizing mouse sperm occurs on the ZP. Saling (30) and Bleil and Wassarman (31) maintained that, at least in the mouse, the acrosome reaction is induced by a ZP constituent, the glycoprotein ZP3. They proposed the following concept:

1. Attachment to the ZP;
2. Binding to the ZP;
3. Induction of the acrosome reaction.

Species differences may account for some disagreement, but the major causes of differences among researchers are probably the differing experimental conditions and the varied assessment criteria. In vitro conditions may have a dramatic effect on the normal biochemical (metabolic and acrosomal) reactions of sperm. Oocyte-cumulus complexes may contain unnaturally trapped stimulatory molecules; these complexes must therefore be thoroughly washed. Also, using light microscopy to evaluate the early stages of the acrosome reaction is questionable. These are factors which must be kept in mind when one compares data.

Capacitation and the acrosome reaction may be a continuous event, divided into phases without a clear demarcation, initiated by specific stimuli or reactions. Each small change which enables the sperm to accomplish a specific task produces an additive effect, culminating in the capacity to fuse with the egg vitelline membrane. Our proposed sequence of events is as follows:

1. Capacitation during the passage through the female reproductive tract to the oocyte-cumulus complex;
2. Initiation of the acrosome reaction near the periphery of, on, or in the cumulus matrix;
3. Penetration of the cumulus matrix, during which the acrosome reaction continues;
4. Attachment of the sperm to the ZP;
5. Loss of the acrosomal cap and binding to the ZP (remnants of the acrosome must be present);
6. Penetration of the ZP.

Penetration

Transmission and scanning electron microscopy have revealed that all sperm bound to the oolemma (egg plasma membrane) have undergone the acrosome reaction (32, 33). The acrosome reaction may render the sperm plasma membrane—more specifically, the plasma membrane over the equatorial/post-acrosomal segment—capable of fusing with the oolemma. This area has been shown to be the primary location of sperm-egg fusion (30, 33).

Initial attachment of the sperm to the oolemma has been found to occur at different angles, but always head-first (32). The oocyte surface is covered with numerous microvilli, which actively assist penetration (32). Initially these microvilli appear to grasp and immobilize the anterior tip of the sperm head, but as gamete interaction proceeds, the microvilli begin to overlay the post-acrosomal/equatorial segment (32). Membrane fusion occurs between the plasma membrane overlying the midsegment of the sperm and the oolemma. Incorporation of the whole sperm head onto the ooplasm then follows a process akin to phagocytosis (34).

Sperm Penetration Assay: Methodology

ABSTINENCE

The length of abstinence is an important variable, with >48 hours required for maximum results; abstinence of <48 hours significantly reduces the sperm penetration potential (35). This reduction may be due to the reduced number of mature sperm and/or to a depletion of functional seminal plasma (36).

LIQUEFACTION

Native seminal plasma is believed to contain macromolecules, or factors associated with macromolecules, which can inhibit capacitation and/or the acrosome reaction; vigorous motility is also inhibited (12, 37). Kinetic studies have shown that maximum penetration is obtained with exposure times of 30 minutes (35) or 30 to 90 minutes (38). Long exposure times (>90 minutes) may irreversibly inhibit fertilization. Therefore, before the SPA, sperm must be thoroughly washed to remove all inhibiting substances.

SEMEN PREPARATION

After allowing 30 to 90 minutes for full liquefaction, an initial count and a motility/forward progression estimation is made, and a morphology slide is made for later assessment. The ideal washing technique is still a matter of dispute, although the World Health Organization (39) has issued a standard protocol. The following methods are used:

1. Non-swim-up wash only (28, 35, 40): Sperm are washed three times by dilution with equal volumes of medium and centrifugation at $600 \times$ g for 5 minutes. The resultant pellet is resuspended in medium; the density is adjusted to 1×10^7 cells/ml. Centrifugation and washes may be reduced to two in cases where it is necessary to decrease centrifugation damage.
2. Pre-swim-up centrifugation method (36, 39, 41): Sperm are washed twice with equal volumes of medium by centrifugation at $600 \times$ g for 5 minutes. The resultant pellet is overlaid with 0.5 to 1.0 ml of medium and placed at a $20°$ angle in a 5% CO_2-in-air incubator at $37°C$ for 60 to 90 minutes. The supernatant is removed by pipette, and the density of the sample is adjusted to 1×10^7 cells/ml.
3. Post-swim-up centrifugation method (5, 28, 39): Semen is placed in a test tube, overlaid with medium (1 part semen to 2 parts medium), and incubated at a $20°$ angle in 5% CO_2 in air for 60 to 90 minutes at $37°C$. The supernatant above the seminal plasma is removed and centrifuged at $500 \times$ g for 5 minutes (centrifugation may be repeated once) to remove all traces of seminal plasma. The resultant pellet is resuspended and adjusted to a density of 1×10^7 cells/ml.

The argument in support of method 2 is that, under normal in vivo conditions, only the actively motile sperm ascend to the upper region of the female genital tract; they are thus the only sperm that participate in in vivo fertilization. In method 2, one must give particular care to oligospermic and asthenospermic samples, since it can be quite difficult to recover a reasonable number of motile sperm for the assay.

After recovering the supernatant from the swim-up or resuspending the pellet from the last centrifugation, the prepared tubes are placed, loosely capped, in a humidified atmosphere of 5% CO_2 in air at $37°C$ for 6 to 20 hours. The tubes are placed at a $20°$ angle to prevent pelleting of the sperm and to increase the surface area for gaseous exchange.

The duration of pre-incubation has also been a point of dispute. Times varying from 1 hour (42) to 20 hours (43) have been reported. To complicate matters, the composition of media (especially the protein source) and incubation environments differ among laboratories, making comparisons extremely difficult. The selected pre-incubation time seems to be a balance between convenience and results. The most important factor to consider is the variability of capacitation times (44). A long incubation period (18 to 24 hours) is preferred, since this allows most samples to attain maximum levels of capacitation and acrosome reaction (27, 36, 45). However, there are a significant number of men whose sperm can penetrate the hamster oolemma after 6 to 10 hours but not after 18 to 24 hours of incubation (5).

After incubation, one of the following manipulations is made:

1. Motility of the sample is measured, and two aliquots (100 μl each) of sperm adjusted to 1×10^7 motile cells/ml are placed in a petri dish and covered with mineral oil (43). Alternatively, 1 ml can be placed in the center of a multi-well dish, while the moat is filled with plain medium to maintain a constant environment.
2. The pre-incubated tubes are returned to a vertical position for 20 minutes to allow settlement of the immotile sperm to the bottom. The sperm are aspirated, and the density is fixed at 3.5×10^6 motile cells/ml (39). Sperm are then placed under mineral oil, as in the method above.

Sperm concentration, and percentage and quality of motility in the insemination medium can considerably affect the outcome of the SPA, especially the number of motile acrosome-reacted sperm. Penetration may be proportional to the number of collisions of acrosome-reacted sperm (the only ones that can penetrate) with each ovum. For maximal penetration rates, the insemination mixture should have a minimum of 4% to 6% motile sperm if the concentration is adjusted to 1×10^7 cells/ml (46). However, not all acrosome-reacted sperm can penetrate ova (47), which may be due to residual species specificity. That is why the ova are inseminated with such a high concentration of sperm. The penetrating sperm may be those which exhibit all the necessary qualities to be recognized and engulfed by the hamster ovum, an event which should quantitatively evaluate the proportion of sperm per ejaculate which reach that endpoint. The SPA may therefore measure the number of sperm in the ejaculate which have fertilizing ability.

Numerous new techniques proposed since the conception of the SPA in 1976 have all been in search of the absolute test. The mechanical stress of centrifugation as the separation method has always been a problem, which has now been alleviated by use of Percoll-gradient centrifugation (48, 49). Rousette (50) modified this technique, allowing sperm to be separated by means of their own motility in a discontinuous Percoll gradient. Using this method, sperm are not pelleted but collect as a band at their specific buoyant density. An increase in the progressive motility index and frequency of sperm with normal morphology was obtained by this group.

Another parameter which might improve the SPA if it were standardized is the variability of capacitation time among individuals. With the use of calcium ionophore a23187 (51) or low-temperature (4°C) storage of sperm in TES-TRIS egg yolk buffer (52, 53), several groups have demonstrated almost instantaneous synchronization of several physiological events. In both treatments, capacitation is completed and the acrosome reaction is synchronized and enhanced by facilitating the influx of calcium into the sperm. Increased penetration with marked polyspermy is obtained by either method. These techniques can be viewed as a second generation SPA that almost elminates false negatives but at the same time balloons the number of false positives to uselessness.

EGG RECRUITMENT

The hamster egg recruitment and processing is a portion of the procedure which has remained reasonably standardized. Oocytes can be obtained from immature hamsters injected at random or from mature hamsters injected on day 1 of their estrous cycle. Day 1 is characterized by viscous, stringy (5 to 20 cm), visible vaginal discharge (54). Pregnant mare serum gonadotropin (PMSG) and human chorionic gonadotropin (hCG) are given by intraperitoneal injection at a dose of 30 to 40 IU, 48 to 72 hours apart. The hCG injection is given 15 to 18 hours before sacrifice by cervical dislocation. The cumulus masses are removed from the dissected oviducts and treated with 0.1% hyaluronidase and 0.1% trypsin to remove the cumulus cells and the ZPs, respectively. After each enzyme treatment, the ova are washed at least twice. From 25 to 50 ZPF eggs can routinely be collected from each yielding hamster. Mammalian eggs have a limited viability in vitro at a temperature of 25°C (55). Therefore, the time between recovery and insemination must be as short as possible. Egg viability can be extended by storage at 4°C (55).

INSEMINATION

Approximately 30 ZPF ova are placed with a single semen sample, adjusted to 1×10^7 cells/ml or 3.5×10^6 motile cells/ml. Coincubation occurs under mineral oil or in a multi-well dish for 3 hours in humidified 5% CO_2 in air at 37°C.

EVALUATION

After a 3-hour coincubation, the level of penetration is assessed by carefully removing the ova from the insemination medium and washing them free of loosely attached sperm. The ova are then placed on a microscope slide in a droplet. The ova are compressed with a coverslip which has petroleum jelly/paraffin wax 15:1 supports on the corners and are examined by phase contrast microscopy. To allow for future examination, the oocytes can be fixed in 1% gluteraldehyde, stained with lacmoid or aceto-orcein (36, 56), and the edges sealed with fingernail polish. Penetration has occurred if a decondensed sperm head is seen within the cytoplasm of the ovum. A tail must be attached to or associated with the decondensed sperm head to be counted, as it could be the pronucleus of the ovum (Fig. 4.5). The percentage of ova penetrated and the mean number of spermatozoa per ovum is then calculated. A donor sample run simultaneously must penetrate a minimum of 20% of the ova for the test to be considered valid. The number of sperm remaining attached to the ova after washing may also be recorded.

MEDIA

The media used for SPA have mostly been limited to Tyrode's, Biggers, Whitten, and Whittingham's (BWW) (57), or modifications of the two. Variations have been developed in the quest for a medium that eliminates false-positive and false-negative results, thus obviating the need to repeat the test.

The protein source in the medium is one of the most important factors in the induction of sperm capacitation. No consensus has been achieved concerning the source of this protein supplement. Rogers (36) prefers human serum albumin (HSA), Gould (28) prefers bovine serum albumin (BSA), and Van Kooij (58) finds no advantage in HSA over BSA. The reason for these contradictions could be the considerable differences between batches of albumin in their ability to capacitate sperm. For this reason, the

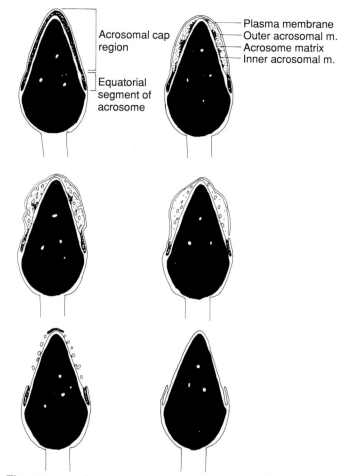

Figure 4.5. The sequence of events for the acrosome reaction of human spermatozoa (19).

World Health Organization (WHO) (39) decided that BSA should be the preferred protein source in its standardized protocol.

The concentration of the protein source has also been a variable, ranging from 0.3% to 3.5%. Barros (42) used 35 mg HSA/ml for a 1-hour capacitation period. Aitken (59) used 18 mg HSA/ml for a 6- to 7-hour incubation, while Rogers (43) used 3 mg/ml for a long capacitation period of 18 to 20 hours. An increased albumin concentration therefore seems to increase the capacitation rate or the ability to fuse with the oocyte plasma membrane (28, 60). This enhancement was not found by all investigators (61). In its protocol, the WHO (39) adopted the longer incubation period (18 to 24 hours) supplemented with 3.5 mg/ml of albumin.

Ions such as calcium, sodium, and potassium have been shown by several investigators (7, 14, 18, 62–64) to be essential for the natural progress of events leading to fertilization. Of these three ions, calcium is the most important, being essential for capacitation, induction of the acrosome reaction, hyperactivated motility, fusion of the sperm with the oocyte plasma membrane, and development of pronuclear oocytes into two-cell pre-embryos (8). These ions must be present in the medium at optimal concentrations to have a maximal effect (14). Mortimer (65) showed that calcium can be replaced by strontium without any loss in sperm motility. In a strontium/EGTA (ethylene glycol-bis-(β-amino ethylether)-$N_1N_1N^1N^1$) system for sperm capacitation, the penetration rate and polyspermy were significantly increased, although the mechanism of this action is unclear.

Spermatozoa pre-incubated for 10 to 20 hours before mixing with ZPF hamster ova in a glucose-free BWW medium penetrated a significantly lower percentage of ova (2% to 20%) than those handled in the normal manner (17% to 71%) (66). Also, the quality of motility deteriorated with time in the glucose-free medium. Murphy (14) found that precapacitated guinea pig sperm could undergo the acrosome reaction in the absence of any extracellular energy sources, although pyruvate was shown to be beneficial for the reaction. The energy needed for the acrosome reaction may thus be present within the sperm before they are capacitated. Additional energy sources in the medium may therefore be needed only to maintain motility and a maximal acrosome reaction rate, especially for long pre-incubations.

The standard medium used has an osmolarity of 305 mOsm/liter. Aitken (67) raised the osmolarity to 410 mOsm, which increased the rate of the acrosome reaction and the penetration rate of the sperm. A higher osmolarity increased the efficiency with which the decapacitating factors were removed (10). Murphy (14) found that precapacitated sperm could undergo the acrosome reaction in a medium with an osmolarity of 160 to 500 mOsm. However, the osmolarity range within which most sperm underwent the acrosome reaction, while retaining a degree of motility, was 220 to 380 mOsm. A medium of more physiological osmolarity should therefore be preferred for the test.

The pH of the medium may significantly influence the outcome of the test; a pH <7 may prevent or greatly retard sperm capacitation. The pH of the $NaHCO_3$-buffered BWW medium is 7.4 to 7.6 under humidified 5% CO_2 in air, but it is 8.1 to 8.3 under pure humidified air. Capacitation, the acrosome reaction, and penetration occur at a faster rate when exposed to a higher pH (5.65). However, prolonged exposure to this unphysiologically high pH may be stressful to the sperm. Some investigators (68) have included HEPES as an additional pH-buffering agent. A medium buffered with HEPES can maintain a constant pH in both 5% CO_2 and pure air. The WHO (39) decided that the medium should be within the physiological ranges of pH and osmolarity, and 20 mM of HEPES buffer should be included so that incubation could be carried out in pure air.

Results

CORRELATION OF THE SPA WITH CONVENTIONAL SEMEN PARAMETERS

The existence of a correlation between the SPA and the conventional semen parameters has been examined by numerous authors, but no consensus has been achieved, mainly because of the varied experimental conditions and assessment criteria of various laboratories (Table 4.4). Most earlier investigators (69–72) found no correlation between the SPA and any traditional semen parameters: sperm density, motility, and morphology. Cohen (73, 74) found low but significant correlations with the total motile sperm count and the percentage of morphologically normal sperm, with the former as the better predictor of the SPA. Rogers (75) also reported a correlation with motility and morphology but found the latter to be more important.

Table 4.4.
The Standard Semen Parameters Used by Different Authors

Author (year, ref. no.)	Density (10^6 cells/ml)	Motility (% motile sperm)	Morphology (% normal sperm)
van Zyl 1976(1)	>10	>30	>20
Overstreet 1980 (69)	>20	>40	>50
Tyler 1981 (72)	>20	>40	>60
Zausner-Guelman 1981 (71)	>20	>40	>60
Aitken 1982 (89)	>20	>40	>40
Margalioth 1983 (89)	>20	>40	>60
Cohen 1985 (74)	>10	>20	>20
Van Kooij 1985 (9)	>20	>60	>50
Albert 1986 (81)	>20	>40	>50
Hirsh 1986 (78)	>20	>60	>40
Van Duren 1987 (79)	>20	>50	>60

Aitken (59) conducted numerous studies in which the semen parameters and many characteristics of sperm motility were compared with the SPA. The characteristics of motility were analyzed by time-exposure photomicrography. In examining normally fertile men, he found that the only factors which correlated positively were the percentage of progressively motile sperm (>25 μm/sec) and the sperm exhibiting an amplitude of lateral head displacement >10 μm. In a group of patients with unexplained infertility (76), the majority of the semen parameters and characteristics of motility were depressed, compared to fertile donors; reduction in normal morphology was the most significant finding (76). Aitken (77), using seven post-capacitation characteristics of motility in a multivariate discriminant analysis, could correctly predict 91% of samples exhibiting normal penetration rates. However, only 60% of the samples with impaired penetration capacity were correctly identified. Defects not reflected in the motility patterns thus existed in 40% of this group. Aitken and Elton (46) confirmed this by comparing the penetration rates of normally fertile donors and patients with idiopathic asthenozoospermia using the Poisson model. They found that the reduced penetration rate of asthenozoospermia was not only due to the loss of motility but also was associated with defects which alter the normal sperm function related to fertilization.

More recent studies have also provided contradictory results. Van Kooij (9) found no correlations between semen parameters and SPA values, while others found correlations with motility and sperm density (78), amplitude of lateral head displacement and the percentage of abnormal acrosomes (41), and all semen parameters correlated with the SPA, especially motility (79).

The overall results so far indicate that of all the semen parameters, motility and morphology seem to be those most consistently correlated with the SPA. The percentage of motile sperm may not be as critical as the quality of motility, i.e., forward progression and lateral head displacement. Morphology may also be directly related to some biochemical/enzymatic factor not measured by other means.

In vivo, motility (forward progression) is of paramount importance in the fertilizing process, since only progressively motile sperm can pass through the cervical mucus and migrate to the ampulla. Logically, this characteristic is not needed in vitro. However, the in vitro concentration of motile sperm in the incubation medium is important because the more motile sperm present, the greater the number of collisions with the eggs and the level of penetration. This direct proportion between the percentage of motility and penetration has been shown with the SPA (59, 80, 81).

A parameter not measured by the SPA but one which must be kept in mind is the quality of motility needed for sperm to enter the cumulus cells and the ZP in human fertilization in vivo and in vitro, although immotile sperm can penetrate ZPF hamster ova (82, 83). There is also a difference between the penetrating potential of different fertile donors at a fixed motile concentration (74, 81). Under standardized conditions, the major reasons for this discordance would be the differences in (*a*) quality of motility; (*b*) biochemical status of the sperm; or (*c*) biochemical status of the ova. However, since this is a bioassay of biological events, the difficulty associated with interpretation of the results is multiplied.

The importance of morphology in predicting penetration and fertilization potential is greatly underestimated. Morphology may be the only factor related to the biochemical status of sperm which can be easily measured. However, morphology has been so poorly and inaccurately assessed in the past that its dismal predictive value is well deserved. In our laboratory, we use a modified classification system (1, 84, 85) based on an existing method (86). To be classified as normal, sperm must have a smooth, oval configuration (width of 2.5 to 3.5 μm; length of 4 to 5 or 5 to 6 μm, depending on the staining method), with a well-defined acrosome comprising 30% to 70% of the sperm head. Sperm with neck, midpiece, or tail defects, as well as ''borderline normal'' forms, are regarded as abnormal. With these criteria, morphology is an excellent predictor of penetration and fertilization potential (84, 87). Although the conventional semen parameters may not be linearly associated with the sperm fertilizing potential, these factors may reflect the underlying physiological status of the sperm.

CORRELATION BETWEEN THE SPA AND THE FERTILIZATION OF HUMAN OVA

Human IVF must be considered as the ultimate test for measuring the fertilization potential of sperm. A correlation between the SPA and IVF would thus stress the importance of the SPA as a screening test for male fertility. Before comparisons with IVF, Overstreet (69) inseminated non-living zona-intact human ova with the same semen sample used in the SPA. A positive correlation was seen in 85% ($n = 27$) of the inseminations with both hamster and human ova, whether penetrated or not. A false-positive result was obtained in 4 cases (15%). Sperm from 24 husbands participating in an IVF program were used in simultaneous inseminations by Wolf (88). In 89% (16 of 18) of the husbands whose sperm fertilized their wives' ova, a positive SPA ($>10\%$) was obtained. The two patients with false-negative assessments had limited penetration (6% and 7.7%, respectively). Margalioth (89) studied 20 men with normal spermiograms and found 100% correlation between a pathological SPA ($<10\%$) and IVF failure. Of the 13 patients with a normal SPA (20% to 100%), 10 (77%) fertilized at least one human ovum. Hall (90) also reported a high correlation (94%) between results of the SPA and human IVF, demonstrating a relationship between the percentage of hamster eggs penetrated and the ability to fertilize human ova in vitro.

More recent studies continue to report correlations. Rogers (36) indicated a correlation of 86% (25 of 29) between a positive SPA and IVF success. Ausmanas (91) found a good correlation between SPA and IVF outcome in 54 patients. An absolute lower limit of hamster egg penetration to define male infertility could not, however, be determined, since a poor SPA was not always indicative of the inability of the sperm to fertilize a human oocyte or produce a pregnancy. Margalioth (92) conducted a thorough investigation of 134 couples, divided into groups according to their indications for IVF (tubal disease, unexplained infertility, male factor, and male/female factors). The SPA was a good predictor of IVF success in 91 of 107. Of these four groups, tubal disease and unexplained infertility had the highest correlation with the SPA (94% and 76%, respectively). All of these authors supported the SPA as a pre-screening test for IVF, despite false-positive and false-negative results.

Two reports, however, did not support these results. Foreman (93) and Rudak (94) both found no evidence that the SPA had any usefulness in predicting IVF outcome. However, in both investigations the proportion of hamster eggs penetrated was significantly lower for men who could not fertilize their wives than for those who could. There was a discordance in false negatives between the two studies. Foreman reported that the occurrence of false negatives was rare, but Rudak reported a false-negative rate of 85.7%.

Most of these authors have found some level of correlation between the SPA and human IVF. Any discordance can be ascribed to the different techniques and conditions in which the SPA was performed. These discrepancies are compounded by the variables of patient classification, ovulation induction regimes, oocyte maturation criteria, and IVF laboratory techniques and conditions.

When comparing SPA and IVF, one must keep two other factors in mind. First, a man rarely ejaculates two identical samples; thus if the same sample is not used for comparison, it must be noted whether the samples were at least comparable in their semen parameters. For standarization, ejaculates should probably not be more than 4 weeks apart. Second, not all oocytes aspirated from a woman are of equal quality, especially at the molecular level, and therefore they are not equally susceptible to fertilization, even if only metaphase II ova are used. In contrast, large numbers of ZPF hamster ova can be obtained with relatively equivalent quality. For statistical accuracy, only preovulatory, mature metaphase II human ova with an extruded polar body should be used to compare IVF results with the SPA.

CAN THE SPA PREDICT FERTILITY OR INFERTILITY?

Can the SPA distinguish categorically between clinically infertile and fertile men? Is there a threshold above which all fertile men penetrate and below which all infertile men do not? (Table 4.5). With the arrival of human IVF, the two groups can now be compared more directly with regard to fertilization (pronuclei), embryo development (cleavage), and implantation. Most investigators (88, 90–92, 95) have shown a significant correlation between high hamster penetration and male fertility in human IVF. Yanagimachi (5) compared all published data and reported that sperm of men with proven fertility generally penetrated >10% of eggs, with an overall average of 57%. Many other investigators have observed that sperm of some fertile men penetrate 100% of eggs, while others penetrate <10%. This tendency has also been observed with infertile men. Sperm of clinically infertile men penetrated a significantly lower percentage of ova, with an overall average of 17%. Results must therefore be interpreted with caution because of the inherent overlap in penetrating ability. However, an absolute lower limit of penetration for defining infertility cannot be conclusively established (87, 91, 94). Aitken (47) followed 68 patients with unexplained infertility for 2 to 3 years; 24% (5 of 21) of these patients had scores of 1% to 10% but were successful in initiating a preg-

Table 4.5.
The Range and Mean Penetration Rates of Zona-Free Hamster Eggs by Spermatozoa of Men with Proven Fertility

Author (year, ref. no.)	Percentage Penetrated	Range (%)
Rogers 1979 (43)	56	14–100
Overstreet 1980 (69)	67	11–100
Hall 1981 (70)	66	20–100
Tyler 1981 (72)	60	24–89
Zausner-Guelman 1981 (71)	81	15–100
Aitken 1982 (59)	44	14–90
Cohen 1982 (73)	54	11–100
Martin and Taylor 1982 (68)	34	0–60
Margalioth 1983 (89)	—	20–100
Rogers 1985 (36)	40	0–100
Ausmanas 1985 (91)	37	0–100
Margalioth 1986 (92)	41	5–80

nancy. He therefore concluded that penetration scores below the normal fertile range ($<10\%$) are not incompatible with a pregnancy, although the fertility of such patients is significantly reduced.

The SPA thus seems to be subject to a high percentage of false-positive and false-negative results. There are many known factors directly responsible. Rogers (43) showed that improper sexual abstinence, an increased white blood cell count, and technical error might cause false-negative results. The species specificity of the ZPF hamster oocyte is not entirely abolished on the removal of the ZP with trypsin (96). A man may produce variable semen samples due to many factors; therefore, his penetration results may vary from test to test. This becomes especially important as the time between the SPA and IVF or pregnancy increases. Since the rates of capacitation and acrosome reaction differ, a man giving a negative result when his sperm are pre-capacitated for 20 hours may give a positive result when his sperm are capacitated for 5 to 8 hours, or vice versa. As fertile men may penetrate $<10\%$ of eggs, infertile men may penetrate $>10\%$ (0% to 100%), a false-positive result. In human IVF, sperm must be able to pass through the cumulus cells and the corona radiata, and to recognize and enter the ZP, whereas the barriers have been removed in the ZPF SPA. Sperm with a biophysical defect may thus be able to penetrate the ZPF eggs but be unable to fertilize human ova in vitro. Infertile men can be divided into two distinct groups: those with normal semen parameters and those with abnormal parameters. The average penetration rates for these two groups differ significantly: 24% and 10%, respectively (5). Thus it is advisable to consider the complete semen profile, i.e., the conventional semen parameters, the SPA, and any other biochemical tests, when one is evaluating a man's fertility. With the results of the semen analysis in mind, another group that may be worth further investigation is those men with normal semen parameters but with a repeatedly negative SPA.

Discussion

Most aspects of sperm function required for the normal fertilization of human oocytes are measured by the SPA: the ability of sperm to capacitate and acrosome react, to fuse with the vitelline membrane, to become incorporated into the ooplasm, and to undergo nuclear decondensation. Exceptions are the ability to penetrate the outer vestment of the oocyte—the cumulus cells, corona radiata, and ZP—as these barriers have been removed in the SPA. These factors alleviate the necessity for sperm motility, a major function required for the penetration of the outer vestments. Thus, some functions needed for normal fertilization are not reflected in the SPA, possibly giving a false-positive result.

Notwithstanding the inherent limitations of the SPA, it is a good measure of male fertility. Routine IVF has provided the yardstick for male infertility. Comparative studies have shown that the SPA can predict IVF success. The majority of men scoring within the normal range (>10%) have the potential to fertilize human ova, whereas men scoring below this level (<10%) may be incapable of fertilization. However, the SPA is unable to define an absolute lower limit for fertility, since fertile men may also penetrate <10% of eggs. We have discussed a number of reasons for this overlapping. Two important facts must be kept in mind. We are dealing with an in vitro heterologous system; all species specificity may not have been removed after the enzymatic treatment of the ova. Also, the mechanism of the biophysical and biochemical changes which the sperm undergo may be vastly different under in vitro and in vivo conditions. Further research is needed for the proper understanding of this heterologous gamete interaction to allow unequivocal interpretation of the results.

In view of the complexity of the test and the number of variables that may influence the results, it is essential that the results be reproducible and that the coefficient of interassay variation be as low as possible. Values reported for the SPA are encouraging in that a competent technician can obtain reasonably precise results in terms of interassay variation (35, 68, 73, 97). The SPA does not answer all questions about male infertility, but it comes the closest of any test to date, other than IVF itself, to evaluating the functional potential of sperm. In combination with sperm parameters, characteristics of motility, and other biochemical tests, a more precise overall definition of fertility may be determined.

References

1. van Zyl JA, Menkveld R, Kotze TJvW, Van Niekerk WA: The importance of spermiograms that meet the requirements of international standards and the most important factors influencing semen parameters. Proceedings of the 17th Congress of the International Society of Urology. Paris: Diffusion Doins, 1976, p 263
2. Yanagimachi R: Penetration of guinea-pig spermatozoa into hamster eggs in vitro. J Reprod Fertil 28:477, 1972
3. Hanada A, Chang ML: Penetration of the zona-free or intact eggs by foreign spermatozoa and the fertilization of deer mouse eggs in vitro. J Exp Zool 203:277, 1978
4. Yanagimachi R, Yanagimachi H, Rogers BJ: The use of zona-free animal ova as a test-system for the assessment of the fertilizing capacity of human spermatozoa. Biol Reprod 15:471, 1976
5. Yanagimachi R: Zona-free hamster eggs: their use in assessing fertilizing capacity and examining chromosomes of human spermatozoa. Gamete Res 10:187, 1984
6. Johnson AR, Lipshultz LI, Smith RG: Thermal shock (37°C) to spermatozoa stored at 4°C optimizes capacitation. J Urol 133:74, 1985
7. Yanagimachi R, Usui N: Calcium dependence of the acrosome reaction and activation of guinea pig spermatozoa. Exp Cell Res 89:161, 1974
8. Yanagimachi R: In vitro sperm capacitation and fertilization of golden hamster eggs in a chemically defined medium in in vitro fertilization and embryo transfer. In Hafez ESE, Semm K (eds): In Vitro Fertilization and Embryo Transfer New York: Alan Liss, 1982, p 65

9. Van Kooij RJ, Balerna M, Roatti A, Campana A: Oocyte penetration and acrosome reactions of human sperm. II. Correlation with other seminal parameters. Andrologia 18:503, 1985

10. Oliphant G, Reynolds ALB, Thomas TS: Sperm surface components involved in the control of the acrosome reaction. Am J Anat 174:269, 1985

11. Meizel S: Molecules that initiate or help stimulate the acrosome reaction by their interaction with mammalian sperm surface. Am J Anat 174:285, 1985

12. Kanwar KC, Yanagimachi R, Lopata A: Effects of human seminal plasma on fertilizing capacity of human spermatozoa. Fertil Steril 31:321, 1979

13. Langlais J, Roberts KD: A molecular membrane model of sperm capacitation and the acrosome reaction of mammalian spermatozoa. Gamete Res 12:183, 1985

14. Murphy SJ, Roldan ERS, Yanagimachi R: Effects of extracellular cations and energy substrates on the acrosome reaction of precapacitated guinea pig spermatozoa. Gamete Res 14:1, 1986

15. Fleming AD, Yanagimachi R: Effect of various lipids on the acrosome reaction and fertilizing capacity of guinea pig spermatozoa, with special reference to the possible involvement of lysophospholipids in the acrosome reaction. Gamete Res 4:253, 1981

16. Papahadjopoulos D, Vail WJ, Newton C, Nir S, Jacobsen KI, Poste G, Lazo R: Studies on membrane fusion. III. The role of calcium induced phase changes. Biochim Biophys Acta 465:579, 1977

17. Katz OF, Cherr GN, Lambert H: The evolution of hamster sperm motility during capacitation and interaction with the ovum vestments in vitro. Gamete Res 14:333, 1986

18. Yanagimachi R: Calcium requirements for sperm-egg fusion in mammals. Biol Reprod 19:949, 1978

19. Nagae T, Yanagimachi R, Drivastava PN, Yanagimachi H: Acrosome reaction in human spermatozoa. Fertil Steril 45:701, 1986

20. Yanagimachi R, Kamiguchi Y, Sugawara S, Mikamo K: Gametes and fertilization in the Chinese hamster. Gamete Res 8:97, 1983

21. Fraser LR: p-aminobenzamidine, an acrosin inhibitor, inhibits mouse sperm penetration of the zona pellucida but not the acrosome reaction. J Reprod Fertil 66:185, 1982

22. Cummings JM, Yanagimachi R: Development of the ability to penetrate the cumulus oophorus by hamster spermatozoa capacitated in vitro in relation to the timing of the acrosome reaction. Gamete Res 15:187, 1986

23. Yanagimachi R, Phillips DM: The status of acrosomal caps of hamster spermatozoa immediately before fertilization in vivo. Gamete Res 9:1, 1984

24. Cherr GN, Lambert H, Katz D: Completion of the hamster sperm acrosome reaction on the zona-pellucida in vivo. J Cell Biol 99:261, 1984

25. Corselli J, Talbot P: An in vitro technique to study penetration of hamster oocyte-cumulus complexes by using physiological numbers of sperm. Gamete Res 13:293, 1986

26. Barros C, Jedlicki A, Bize I, Aquirre E: Relationship between the length of sperm preincubation and zona penetration in the golden hamster: a scanning electron microscopy study. Gamete Res 9:31, 1984

27. Singer SL, Lambert H, Overstreet JW, Hanson FW, Yanagimachi R: The kinetics of human sperm binding to the human zona pellucida and zona-free hamster oocyte in vitro. Gamete Res 12:29, 1985

28. Gould JE, Overstreet JW, Yanagimachi H, Yanagimachi R, Katz DF, Hanson FW: What functions of the sperm cell are measured by in vitro fertilization of zona-free hamster eggs? Fertil Steril 40:344, 1983

29. Saling PM, Storey BT: Mouse gamete interactions during fertilization in vitro: chlortetracycline as a fluorescent probe for the mouse acrosome reaction. J Cell Biol 83:544, 1979

30. Saling PM, Irons G, Waibel R: Mouse sperm antigens that participate in fertilization. I. Inhibition of sperm fusion with the egg plasma membrane using monoclonal antibodies. Biol Reprod 33:515, 1985

31. Bleil DJ, Wassarman PM: Sperm-egg interactions in the mouse: sequence of events and induction of the acrosome reaction by a zona pellucida glycoprotein. Dev Biol 95:317, 1983

32. Tsuiki A, Hoshiai H, Takahashi K, Suzuki M, Hoshi K: sperm-egg interactions observed by scanning electron microscopy. Arch Androl 16:35, 1986

33. Sathananthan HA, Ng SC, Edivisinghe R, Ratnam SS, Wong PC: Human sperm-egg interaction in vitro. Gamete Res 15:317, 1986

34. Sathananthan HA, Chen C: Sperm-oocyte membrane fusion in the human during monospermic fertilization. Gamete Res 15:177, 1986

35. Rogers BJ, Perreault SD, Bentwood BJ, McCarville C, Hale RW, Soderdahl DW: Variability in the human-hamster in vitro assay for fertility evaluation. Fertil Steril 39:204, 1983

36. Rogers BJ: The sperm penetration assay: its usefulness reevaluated. Fertil Steril 43:821, 1985

37. Van der Ven H, Bhattacharyya AK, Binor Z, Leto S, Zaneveld LJD: Inhibition of human sperm capacitation by a high-molecular-weight factor from human seminal plasma. Fertil Steril 38:753, 1982

38. Wolf DP: The hamster egg bioassay in studies of sperm-egg interaction at fertilization. Int J Androl 6:49s, 1986

39. World Health Organization: WHO Protocol for the zona-free hamster oocyte penetration test. Int J Androl 6:197s, 1986

40. Martin RH, Taylor PJ: Effect of sperm concentration in the zona-free hamster ova penetration assay. Fertil Steril 39:379, 1983

41. Jeulin C, Feneux D, Serres C, Jouannet P, Guillet-Rosso F, Belaisch-Allart J, Frydman R, Testart J: Sperm factors related to failure of human in vitro fertilization. J Reprod Fertil 76:735, 1986

42. Barros L, Gonzalez J, Herrera E, Bustos-Obregon E: Human sperm penetration into zona-free hamster oocytes as a test to evaluate the sperm fertilizing ability. Andrologia 11:197, 1979

43. Rogers BJ, Van Compen H, Ueno M, Lambert H, Bronson R, Hale R: Analysis of human spermatozoal fertilizing ability using zona-free ova. Fertil Steril 32:664, 1979

44. Perreault SD, Rogers BJ: Capacitation pattern of human spermatozoa. Fertil Steril 38:258, 1982

45. Johnson JP, Alexander NJ: Hamster egg penetration: comparison of preincubation periods. Fertil Steril 41:599, 1984

46. Aitken RJ, Elton RA: Quantitative analysis of sperm-egg interaction in the zona-free hamster penetration test. Int J Androl 6:14s, 1986

47. Aitken J: The zona-free hamster egg penetration test. In Hargreave TB (ed): Male Infertility. Berlin: Springer-Verlag, 1983, p 75

48. Lessley BA, Garner DL: Isolation of motile spermatozoa by density gradient centrifugation in Percoll. Gamete Res 7:49, 1983

49. Forster MS, Smith WD, Lee WI, Berger RE, Karp LE, Stencher MA: Selection of human spermatozoa according to their relative motility and their interaction with zona-free hamster eggs. Fertil Steril 40:655, 1983

50. Rousette A, Akerlof E, Rosenburg L, Fredricsson B: Increase in progressive motility and improved morphology of human spermatozoa following their migration through Percoll gradients. Int J Androl 9:1, 1986

51. Aitken RJ, Ross A, Hargreave T, Richardson D, Best F: Analysis of human sperm function following exposure to ionophore A23187. J Androl 5:321, 1984

52. Bolanos JR, Overstreet JW, Katz DF: Human sperm penetration of zona-free hamster eggs after storage of the semen for 48 hours at 2°C to 5°C. Fertil Steril 39:536, 1983

53. Johnson AR, Syms AJ, Lipshultz LI, Smith RG: Conditions influencing human sperm capacitation and penetration of zona-free hamster ova. Fertil Steril 41:603, 1984

54. Mizoguchi H, Dukelow WR: Fertilizability of ova from young or old hamsters after spontaneous or induced ovulation. Fertil Steril 35:79, 1981

55. Syms AJ, Johnson AR, Lipshultz LI, Smith RG: Effect of aging and cold storage of hamster ova as assessed in the sperm penetration assay. Fertil Steril 43:766, 1985

56. Campana A, Gatti MY, Ruspa M, Van Kooij R, Buetti C, Eppenberger U, Balerna M: Relationship between fertility, semen analysis and human sperm penetration of zona-free hamster eggs. Acta Eur Fertil 14:331, 1983

57. Biggers JD, Whitten WK, Whittingham DG: The culture of mouse embryos in vitro. In Daniel JC (ed): Methods in Mammalian Embryology. San Francisco: Freeman, 1971, p 86

58. Van Kooij RJ, Balerna M, Roatti A, Campana A: Oocyte penetration and acrosome reactions of human spermatozoa. I. Influence of incubation time and medium composition. Andrologia 18:152, 1986

59. Aitken RJ, Best FSM, Richardson DW, Djahanbakhch O, Lees MM: The correlates of fertilizing capacity in normal fertile men. Fertil Steril 38:68, 1982

60. Wolf DP, Sokoloski JE. Characterisation of the sperm penetration bioassay. J Androl 3:445, 1982

61. Plachot M, Mandelboum J, Junca A-M: Acrosome reaction of human sperm used for in vitro fertilization. Fertil Steril 42:418, 1984

62. Hyne RV, Higginson RE, Kohlman D, Lopata A: Sodium requirement for capacitation and membrane fusion during the guinea-pig sperm acrosome reaction. J Reprod Fertil 70:83, 1984

63. Fraser LR: Potassium ions modulate expression of mouse sperm fertilizing ability, acrosome and hyperactivated motility in vitro. J Reprod Fertil 69:539, 1983

64. Mortimer D, Courtot AM, Giovangrandi Y, Jeulin C, David G: Human sperm motility after migration into, and incubation in, synthetic media. Gamete Res 9:131, 1984

65. Mortimer D, Curtis EF, Dravland JE: The use of strontium-substituted media for capacitating human spermatozoa: an improved sperm penetration method for the zona-free hamster egg penetration test. Fertil Steril 46:97, 1986

66. Perreault SD, Rogers BJ: Effects of various sugars on the course of human spermatozoal capacitation in vitro. J Androl 2:22, 1981

67. Aitken RJ, Wang YF, Liu J, Best F, Richardson DW: The influence of medium composition, osmolarity and albumin content on the acrosome reaction and fertilizing capacity of human spermatozoa: development of an improved zona-free hamster egg penetration test. Int J Androl 6:180, 1983

68. Martin RH, Taylor PJ: Reliability and accuracy of the zona-free hamster ova assay in the assessment of male fertility. Br J Obstet Gynaecol 89:951, 1982

69. Overstreet JW, Yanagimachi R, Katz DF, Hayashi K, Hanson FW: Penetration of human spermatozoa into the human zona pellucida and the zona-free hamster egg: a study of fertile donors and infertile patients. Fertil Steril 33:534, 1980

70. Hall JL: Relationship between semen quality and human sperm penetration of zona-free hamster ova. Fertil Steril 35:457, 1981

71. Zausner-Guelman B, Blasco L, Wolf DP: Zona-free hamster eggs and human sperm penetration capacity: a comparative study of proven fertile donors and infertility patients. Fertil Steril 36:771, 1981

72. Tyler JPP, Pryor JP, Collins WP: Heterologous ovum penetration by human spermatozoa. J Reprod Fertil 63:499, 1981

73. Cohen J, Weber RFA, Van Der Vijver JCM, Zeilmaker GH: In vitro fertilizing capacity of human spermatozoa with the use of zona-free hamster ova: interassay variation and prognostic value. Fertil Steril 37:565, 1982

74. Cohen J, Edwards R, Fehilly C, Fishel S, Hewitt J, Purdy J, Rowlands G, Steptoe P, Webster J: In vitro fertilization: a treatment for male infertility. Fertil Steril 43:422, 1985

75. Rogers BJ, Bentwood BJ, Van Campen H, Helmbrecht G, Soderdahl D, Hale RW: Sperm morphology assessment as an indicator of human fertilizing capacity. J Androl 4:119, 1983

76. Aitken RJ, Bet FSM, Richardson DW, Djahanbakhch O, Mortimer D, Templeton AA, Lees MM: An analysis of sperm function in cases of unexplained infertility: conventional criteria, movement characteristics, and fertilizing capacity. Fertil Steril 38:212, 1982

77. Aitken RJ, Warner P, Best FSM, Templeton AA, Djahanbakhch O, Mortimer D, Lees MM: The predictability of subnormal penetrating capacity of sperm in cases of unexplained infertility. Int J Androl 6:212, 1983

78. Hirsh I, Gibbons WE, Lipshultz LI, Rossavik KK, Young RL, Poindexter AN, Dobson M, Findley WE: In vitro fertilization in couples with male factor infertility. Fertil Steril 45:659, 1986

79. Van Duren DBPJ, Vemer HM, Bastiaans BLA, Doesburg WH, Willemsen WNP, Rolland R: Importance of sperm motility after capacitation in interpreting the hamster ovum sperm penetration assay. Fertil Steril 47:456, 1987

80. Binor Z, Sokoloski JE, Wolf DP: Penetration of the zona-free hamster egg by human sperm. Fertil Steril 33:321, 1980

81. Albert M, Bailly MA, Roussel L: Influence of the concentration of motile sperm inseminated on the ovum penetration assay results: towards a standardized method. Andrologia 18:161, 1986

82. Aitken RJ, Ross A, Lees M: Analysis of sperm function in Kartagener's syndrome. Fertil Steril 40:696, 1983

83. Williamson RA, Koehler JK, Smith WD, Karp LE: Entry of immotile spermatozoa into zona-free hamster ova. Gamete Res 10:319, 1984

84. Kruger TF, Menkveld R, Stander FSH, Lombard CJ, Van der Merwe JP, van Zyl J, Smith K: Sperm morphologic features as a prognostic factor in in vitro fertilization. Fertil Steril 46:1118, 1986

85. Menkveld R: An investigation of environmental influences on spermatogenesis and semen parameters (Ph.D. dissertation). University of Stellenbosch, Tygerberg, South Africa, 1987

86. Macleod J, Gold RZ: The male factor in fertility and infertility. II. Spermatozoon counts in 1000 men of known fertility and 1000 cases of infertile marriage. J Urol 66:436, 1951

87. Kruger TF, Swanson RJ, Hamilton M, Simmons KF, Acosta AA, Matta JF, Oehninger S, Morshedi M: Abnormal sperm morphology and other semen parameters related to the outcome of the hamster oocyte human sperm penetration assay. Int J Androl 11:107, 1988

88. Wolf DP, Sokoloski JE, Quigley MM: Correlation of human in vitro fertilization with the hamster egg bioassay. Fertil Steril 40:53, 1983

89. Margalioth EJ, Navot D, Laufer N, Yosef SM, Rabinowitz R, Yarkoni S, Schenker JG: Zona-free hamster ovum penetration assay as a screening procedure for in vitro fertilization. Fertil Steril 40:386, 1983

90. Hall JL, Engel D, Berger GS, Dingfelder JK, Marik J: Use of the hamster zona-free ovum test in human in vitro fertilization program. Fertil Steril 41:105, 1984

91. Ausmanas M, Tureik RW, Blasco L, Kopf GS, Ribas J, Mastroianni L: The zona-free hamster egg penetration assay as a prognostic indicator in a human in vitro fertilization program. Fertil Steril 43:433, 1985

92. Margalioth EJ, Navot D, Laufer N, Lewin A, Rabinowitz R, Schenker JG: Correlation between the zona-free hamster egg sperm penetration assay and human in vitro fertilization. Fertil Steril 45:665, 1986

93. Foreman R, Cohen J, Fehilly CB, Fishel SB, Edwards RB: The application of the zona-free hamster egg test for the prognosis of human in vitro fertilization. J In Vitro Fertil Embryo Trans 1:166, 1984

94. Rudak E, Dor J, Nebel L, Maschiach S, Goldman B: Assessment of the predictive ability of the zona-free hamster egg penetration test for the outcome of treatment by IVF-ET. Int J Androl 6:131s, 1986

95. Margalioth EJ, Laufer N, Navot D, Voss R, Schenker JG: Reduced fertilization ability of zona-free hamster ova by spermatozoa from male partners of normal infertile couples. Arch Androl 10:67, 1983

96. Overstreet JW: Human sperm function as assessed by fusion with zona-free hamster oocytes. Int J Androl 6:42s, 1986

97. Muller CH: Precision, reliability and biological variability in human sperm function measured by penetration of zona-free hamster oocytes. Int J Androl 6:31s, 1986

Part Two—Therapeutic Procedures

Section A:

MANIPULATION OF SEMEN
FOR SEX PRE-SELECTION

DAVID L. FULGHAM, B.A., AND NANCY J. ALEXANDER, PH.D.

To choose the sex of one's offspring has been a desire of couples since earliest times. Various schemes have been suggested and tried. With a 50% chance of success (boy or girl), some omens, douches, or potions have enjoyed an extended period of popularity even with no scientific basis (1, 2).

There is considerable evidence that certain conditions can result in a shift in the sex ratio. For example, more women who conceive by means of artificial insemination have male children than would be expected (2). Whether this phenomenon occurs because of insemination near the time of ovulation is not clear, but such hypotheses have resulted in timing inseminations depending on the sex desired in the offspring. Unfortunately, a statistical parameter that is predictive for a population is often not so for an individual.

Many sperm qualities have been attributed to gender: the mass is slightly lighter for Y-bearing sperm (3), the charge is more negative for Y-bearing sperm (4, 5), the swimming speed is higher for the Y-bearing sperm (6, 7, 8), and a male-specific antigen is preferentially expressed on Y-bearing sperm (9, 10). However, the only established difference between Y-bearing and X-bearing sperm is the DNA content: the Y-bearing sperm has about 3% less DNA.

We present the methods that seem to enhance a shift in favor of one gender over the other. The Y-bearing sperm enrichment technique is protected by patents in the United States and abroad. This method is used by more than 50 clinics; more than 500 babies have been born through its use. Selection for X-bearing sperm is a newer procedure; preliminary results look promising, although large numbers are not yet available.

With the advent of assisted reproduction, including in vitro fertilization and embryo transfer, it is no wonder that there is an increased interest in the possibilities of selecting the gender of one's progeny. Future effective possibilities do exist, for instance, sexing the embryo before transfer.

Enrichment of X-Bearing Sperm

This procedure, a modification of the protocol described by Quinlivan (11), involves preparation of a Sephadex G-50 column (1.0 × 12.0 cm), placing a sperm sample on the column bed, and collecting 1.0-ml fractions of sperm from the column. One might expect that sperm would completely pass through the column because of their size; however, they do not. This phenomenon may be due to interaction of the sperm surface with the sugar moieties of the Sephadex material. After the column void volume (usually the first 1.5 to 2.0 ml), the first fraction of sperm is collected and used for insemination. This fraction of sperm seems to be enriched for X-bearing sperm (i.e., there is a lower portion of Y-bearing sperm).

REAGENTS AND EQUIPMENT

- Sephadex G-50 (Pharmacia Fine Chemicals).
- Locke's solution:
    8.50 g of sodium chloride;
    0.42 g of potassium chloride;
    0.20 g of sodium bicarbonate;
    0.24 g of calcium dichloride.
    Combine the ingredients into 500 ml of tissue-grade distilled water. After the salts have gone into solution, bring the final volume to 1000 ml with more tissue-grade water; pH the solution to 7.2, and filter-sterilize it by passing it through a 22-μm filter. De-gas the solution for 2 hours under vacuum while stirring; store it in 100-ml aliquots at 4°C. (It can be stored for at least 4 months at 4°C.) Use a fresh aliquot each time.
- Human serum albumin solution (intravenous grade; 25% albumin, sterile).
- Disposable glass 10.0-ml graduated pipette.
- Glass beads (5 × 5 mm).
- Tygon tubing (3.2 ID × 0.81 wall thickness × 4.8 OD; in mm).
- Hemostat or other clamping device to turn the column on and off.
- Glass Pasteur pipette and glass test tubes.
- Calibrated swinging-bucket centrifuge.

METHOD

Two days before the procedure, the Sephadex G-50 must be swollen and degassed. Weigh out 10 g of dry Sephadex G-50 and place the gel into a 500-ml side-arm vacuum flask. Add 150 to 200 ml of Locke's solution and swirl the ingredients together. As the beads swell, more Locke's solution may be added. (Do not use a magnetic stir bar or any mechanical device to stir the ingredients because it can damage the Sephadex bead particles.) After 2 hours of swirling the mixture, de-gas it under vacuum for another 2 hours. Store at 4°C. For long-term storage, add sodium azide to a final concentration of 0.01%.) Two days before the gel is to be used, it should be checked by light microscopy for possible bacterial contamination. Bacteria can reside inside and outside the gel beads.

Using a diamond pencil or a triangle file, etch a 10-ml glass pipette below the mouthpiece and break the pipette at this mark; flame polish to remove any sharp edges. Attach the tubing to the end of the glass pipette, and place a glass bead inside. Gas-sterilize the column and let it de-gas for at least 2 weeks before using. (Alternatively, the column can be sterilized by washing the outside and inside with 70% ethanol in water.) With the glass bead seated in the pipette the flow rate from the column should be noted; very little flow retardation should occur.

The column is prepared on the day of use at least 2 hours before its possible need. Once it has been poured, care should be taken not to move it excessively to prevent shifting of the glass bead or Sephadex gel particles. Glass wool should not be used to support the G-50 gel matrix, since fiber particles may shed into the column eluate and contaminate the semen sample.

The column is mounted vertically in a ring stand and leveled. The G-50 gel and an aliquot of Locke's solution are allowed to come to room temperature; they are then de-gassed for 15 minutes. Approximately 10 ml of Locke's solution is added to the empty pipette column with the glass bead seated in the bottom. The tubing is clamped off after 8 ml of the solution has passed through the column, leaving 2 ml still in the column. (This allows a check to ascertain that the glass bead has not seated so well that flow is too restricted; if the flow is too slow, another column should be selected.) Washing the column with an aliquot of Locke's solution allows removal of any air bubbles from around the glass bead and provides a bed on which to add the G-50 slurry, which is made by swirling the gel gently in a minimum volume of Locke's solution. The column is filled with G-50 slurry, and the gel is allowed to settle for 10 minutes. The excess Locke's solution is removed from atop the gel, and another layer of G-50 slurry is poured on. This procedure is repeated until the column is filled. After the column has settled and no more than 1 to 2 cm of excess Locke's solution is at the top, the column is slowly opened and washed with Locke's solution. *The column must never run out of liquid; the gel bed would crack and require repacking!* The column is packed by running 20 ml of Locke's solution through it and removing any excess gel bed until there is a distance of 12 cm between the glass bead and the top of the gel bed. It is very important to wash the column with 60 ml of the solution if the gel was stored with sodium azide; otherwise, a total of 35 to 40 ml of Locke's solution is adequate for washing the gel before the procedure. Finally, 0.5 cm of liquid should remain over the bed, and the column is clamped off.

Collect a fresh human sperm sample and allow it to liquefy for 30 minutes at 37°C; dilute it two- to threefold with Locke's solution. Centrifuge at room temperature at 300 × g for 20 minutes: discard the supernatant. Resuspend the pellet to 1 ml in fresh Locke's solution.

Load onto the column the 1 ml of washed sperm. Allow the sperm solution to enter the bed of the column after the tubing is unclamped. Then load 1 ml of fresh Locke's solution, and collect 1-ml fractions off the column. Continue in this fashion until 5 ml (five 1-ml fractions) have been collected. Discard the first 2 ml (first two 1-ml fractions), but keep the next 1 to 2 ml. Pool these fractions together and centrifuge at 300 × g for 10 minutes. Discard the supernatant and resuspend the sperm pellet to 0.5 ml with 3.0% HSA and Locke's solution. Use this preparation for insemination.

The principle behind the enrichment of X-bearing sperm by G-50 chromatography is not understood. The gel matrix is not separating on the basis of size, since both the Y-bearing and X-bearing sperm are too large for the exclusion abilities of G-50. It would seem that the flow rate of the column would negate any differences in swimming velocities between the two populations of sperm. The only possibility is that Y-bearing sperm interact with the gel matrix more than do the X-bearing sperm, or that there is a subpopulation of X-bearing sperm that do not interact with the gel matrix as extensively as do the other sperm.

Enrichment for Y-Bearing Sperm

This method, a modification of the protocol described by Ericsson (7), has been patented and consists of exposing sperm to various albumin gradients. The end result is the collection of the sperm that exhibit a higher degree of linear swimming velocity.

The procedure is performed using discontinuous albumin gradients. The sperm that enter a 7.5% albumin solution are placed on a second gradient of 12.5% albumin solution overlaid on a 20% albumin solution. The sperm within the last gradient are used for insemination.

There is a significant loss of sperm by this procedure (as with the X-bearing sperm enrichment protocol); thus the initial quality of the semen sample must be taken into account.

REAGENTS AND EQUIPMENT

- Tyrode's solution, composed of the following stock-salt solutions ($10\times$) (prepared separately and combined in the order given):
    80 g of sodium chloride in 1000 ml of tissue culture-grade water;
    1.95 g of potassium chloride in 1000 ml of tissue culture-grade water;
    2.13 g of magnesium chloride ($MgCl_2 \cdot 6H_2O$) in 1000 ml of tissue culture-grade water;
    10.15 g of sodium bicarbonate in 1000 ml of tissue culture-grade water;
    1.554 g of calcium dichloride (anhydrous) in 1000 ml of tissue culture-grade water.
    On the day of the procedure, combine 20 ml of each of the stock-salt solutions; dissolve 0.2 g of glucose to bring the final volume to 200 ml with tissue culture-grade water.
- A 25% solution of liquid human serum albumin, salt poor.
- Glass Pasteur pipettes, 5¾ inch long

METHOD

The albumin gradients are prepared for the separation and loaded into Pasteur pipettes with the ends heat-sealed at the point of tapering. Alternatively, appropriate 8×75-mm glass tubes may be purchased from Arrow Glass Co. (South Vineland, N.J.).

Collect a fresh human semen sample and allow it to liquefy at 37°C for 30 minutes. Mix the semen sample 1:1 with Tyrode's solution and determine the volume. Prepare 7.5% albumin from the stock albumin solution using Tyrode's solution. For every milliliter of the diluted semen sample, prepare two 7.5%-albumin gradients. (If the diluted semen sample volume is 6 ml, prepare 12 7.5%-albumin gradient columns.)

For each milliliter of the diluted semen sample, place a glass tube vertically into a 37°C water bath. Place 1 ml of 7.5% albumin (0.3 ml of 25% stock albumin + 0.7 ml of Tyrode's solution) into each glass tube to be used. Gently overlay the albumin gradient with 0.5 ml of the diluted semen and incubate for 1 hour.

Gently remove the diluted semen sample from the albumin layer, taking a small amount of the albumin layer to ensure that the sperm used in the rest of the procedure are from the albumin layer and are not contaminated with sperm from the diluted semen layer. Discard the diluted semen layer. Pool the 7.5% albumin fractions and determine the sperm density. Centrifuge the albumin pool in 4-ml aliquots for 10 minutes at 300 $\times$ g. Discard the supernatants, and bring the sperm pellets to 60 $\times$ 10^6 sperm per milliliter with Tyrode's solution. In other words, if the sperm density in 10 ml of the 7.5% albumin pool were 12 $\times$ 10^6/ml, then the pellet would be resuspended in a total volume of 2 ml of Tyrode's solution.

For each milliliter of semen at the appropriate density, prepare two two-layer albumin gradient tubes, as described above. Each tube is filled at the bottom with 0.5 ml of 20% albumin (0.8 ml of 25% albumin + 0.2 ml of Tyrode's solution). Onto this layer, place 1 ml of 12.5% albumin (0.5 ml of 25% albumin + 0.5 ml of Tyrode's solution). Into each tube, place 0.5 ml of the appropriately diluted sperm.

Incubate the sample for 1 hour; carefully remove the 0.5-ml semen layer. Incubate the sample for an additional 0.5 hour. Remove the 12.5% gradient from the 20% gradient. Discard the 12.5% fractions and pool the 20% albumin fractions. Centrifuge the pool at 300 × g for 10 minutes; resuspend the pellet in 0.5 ml of Tyrode's solution. This sample is used for insemination.

As an alternative to overlayering the sample onto the portion of the gradients, one could underlay them. The only change in the protocol is the order of placement of the samples. For example, in the 7.5% columns, rather than 1 ml of the albumin solution being loaded first into the tubes, first the 0.5-ml diluted semen sample is placed into the tubes, following which the 1 ml of 7.5% albumin solution is delivered under the semen sample with a Pasteur pipette. Some technicians find this procedure easier for collecting sample fractions.

Histochemical Staining for the Y-Bearing Sperm

To determine the ratio of X- and Y-bearing sperm in a sample, an in vitro staining procedure can be used. The following is a modification of the quinacrine mustard dihydrochloride technique of Zech (12), later applied to sperm (13, 14).

The visualization of the Y body of the stained sperm requires fluorescent microscopy and analysis at 1000× magnification of at least 200 cells. The stained chromatin of the sperm will fluoresce with a mild yellow-green color. Normally the basal one-third of the sperm head will show a concentrated or denser spot of fluorescence when the Y chromosome is present. However, the spot may vary, and there may be two spots, possibly indicating the YY-bearing sperm. This pattern is often difficult to distinguish and is complicated by the fact that the fluorescence is quenched rather quickly. Usually 45 to 50% of the sperm in a normal sample are stained. Doing a sperm swim-up into buffer before staining the sperm does not alter this percentage.

REAGENTS AND EQUIPMENT

- Quinacrine mustard dihydrochloride (QMD; Sigma Chemical Co.): Store the reagent under desiccation and hold at 4°C.
- McIlvane's buffer (15): Prepare the following stock solutions:
  1. 0.1-M citric acid anhydrous: Start with 19.212 g of citric acid anhydrous. Bring to 1000 ml with tissue culture-grade water.
  2. 0.2-M disodium phosphate: Start with 28.396 g of disodium phosphate. Bring to 1000 ml with tissue culture-grade water.
  Prepare buffer:

Desired Volume (ml)	Citric Acid (ml)	Disodium PO$_4$ (ml)
20	3.53	16.47
100	17.65	82.47
500	88.25	411.75

All solutions should be at pH 7.0.
- Sucrose mounting solution:
  Dissolve 6 g of sucrose into 10 ml of tissue culture-grade water and heat gently until the sucrose goes into solution.
- Baker's buffer:
  0.2 g of sodium chloride;
  3 g of glucose;
  0.354 g of sodium phosphate, dibasic (anhydrous);

0.03 g of potassium phosphate, monobasic.

Bring all to 100 ml with tissue culture-grade water. The pH of the buffer will be 7.77; bring pH to 7.0 with sodium hydroxide.
- Methanol-acetic acid fixing solution:
  Mix 1 part absolute methanol with 1 part glacial acetic acid.
- Fluorescent microscope equipped with a mercury lamp and appropriate exciter barrier filters, a dark-field condenser, a 100 × objective.

METHOD

1. Dissolve 2.5 mg of QMD in 10 ml of tissue culture-grade water; further dilute with 40 ml of McIlvane's buffer. The final concentration of QMD will be 62.5 μg/ml. Protect the QMD solution from light *at all times*. Store the QMD solution in a dark, foil-wrapped bottle at 4°C for no more than 2 weeks. The fresher the QMD solution, the better the staining.
2. Wash the semen sample twice in Baker's buffer at 300 × g.
3. Prepare a sperm cell smear slide by dragging a film of sperm across a microscope slide, using a second slide edge. Let the slide air-dry.
4. Dip the sperm slide into methanol-acetic acid fixing solution for 5 minutes.
5. Air-dry the slide.
6. Wash the slide in McIlvane's buffer for 5 minutes.
7. While protecting the slide from exposure to light, stain it with QMD solution for 10 minutes (if the stain is fresh) or for 20 minutes (if the stain is about 2 weeks old).
8. While protecting the slide from exposure to light, wash it in two McIlvane's buffers for 5 minutes each.
9. Air-dry the slide.
10. Coverslip with sucrose mounting medium. Read the slide at a magnification of 1000 ×. Report the number of sperm seen with a fluorescent spot and the number seen without it.

Clinical Results

Since 1975, 45 centers in the United States and 9 centers abroad have performed the Y-bearing sperm pre-selection procedure. In 1983, 13 centers began a slightly modified version of the method by shortening the incubation time of the first layer.

There have been 509 births reported, with 380 males and 129 females. In addition, three centers have performed the procedure on sperm that were used in in vitro fertilization, with 11 males and 3 females resulting (16). The X-bearing sperm pre-selection method has been described more recently, and few centers have yet reported their results. Alexander (17) has reported that Corson had 30 females in 41 deliveries, while she has had 9 females and no males born in her series.

References

1. Parkes AS: Mythology of the human sex ratio. In Kiddy CA, Hafes HD (eds): Sex Ratio at Birth—Prospects for Control: A Symposium. University Park, PA: American Society of Animal Science, Pennsylvania State University, 1971, p 38
2. Corson SL, Batzer FR: Human gender selection. Semin Reprod Endocrinol 5:81, 1987
3. Sumner AT, Robinson TA: A difference in dry mass between heads of X- and Y-bearing human spermatozoa. J. Reprod Fertil 48:9, 1976
4. Shishito S, Shirai M, Matsuda S: Galvanic separation of X- and Y-bearing human sperm. Andrologia 6:17, 1974
5. Bhattacharya BC, Shome P, Gunther AH: Successful separation of X and Y spermatozoa in human and bull sperm. Int J Fertil 22:30, 1977
6. Rohde W, Portsmann T, Dorner G: Migration of Y-bearing human spermatozoa in cervical mucus. J Reprod Fert 33:167, 1973

7. Ericsson RJ, Langevin CN, Nishino M: Isolation of fractions rich in human Y sperm. Nature 246:421, 1973

8. Sarkar S: Motility, expression of surface antigen, and X and Y human sperm separation in in vitro fertilization medium. Fertil Steril 42:899, 1984

9. Goldberg EH, Boyse EA, Bennett D, Scheid M, Carswell MP: Serological demonstration of H-Y antigen (male) on mouse sperm. Nature 232:478, 1971

10. Koo GC, Stackpole CW, Boyse EA, Hamarling V, Dardis MP: Topographical location of H-Y antigen on mouse spermatozoa by immunoelectron-microscopy. Proc Natl Acad Sci USA 70:1502, 1973

11. Quinlivan WLG, Preciado K, Long TL, Sullivan H: Separation of human X and Y spermatozoa by albumin gradients and Sephadex chromatography. Fertil Steril 37:104, 1982

12. Zech L: Investigation of metaphase chromosomes with DNA-binding fluorochromes. Exp Cell Res 58:463, 1969

13. Barlow P, Vosa CG: The Y chromosome in human spermatozoa. Nature 226:961, 1970

14. Sumner AT, Robinson JA, Evans HJ: Distinguishing between X, Y, and YY-bearing human spermatozoa by fluorescence and DNA content. Nature New Biol 229:231, 1971

15. Humanson GL: Animal Tissue Techniques. San Francisco, WH Freeman, 1962, p 418

16. Beernink FJ, Alexander NJ, Corson SL, Dmowski WP, Ericsson RF: Male sex pre-selection through albumin separation of sperm (Abstract no. P 008). In: Program of the 44th Annual Meeting of the American Fertility Society (Atlanta, GA, 1988), p 547

17. Alexander NJ: Prenatal sex selection. In Garcia C-R, Mastroianni L Jr (eds): Current Therapy of Infertility. Philadelphia: BC Decker, 1988, p 157

Section B:

WASH AND SWIM-UP METHOD OF SPERMATOZOA PREPARATION AND SEX SELECTION

WELDI CLAASSENS, B.S., FRIK S. H. STANDER, M.T., THINUS F. KRUGER, M.D., ROELOF MENKVELD, PH.D., AND CARL J. LOMBARD, PH.D.

Due to the higher ratio of boys to girls (1.5:1) by in vitro fertilization (IVF) and gamete intrafallopian transfer (GIFT) at Tygerberg Hospital, the question arose whether the wash-up and swim-up method of semen preparation, used for our IVF procedure, plays a role in sex selection. Semen samples of 20 men were evaluated at different time intervals to determine the percentage of F body-positive sperm. We found that the swim-up time affects the relationship between Y- and X-bearing sperm, especially at intervals of 30 and 45 minutes, where an optimal percentage of Y-bearing sperm was found ($P = 0.0039$ and $P = 0.0092$, respectively). Sperm obtained at these intervals may influence the outcome of sex by IVF and GIFT in favor of males.

A successful sex selection technique is demanded by sociopsychological and genetic factors and, in veterinary medicine, by economic factors in animal breeding. Such a technique would play an important role in handling sex-linked defects such as hemophilia and muscular dystrophy. A sperm selection technique which provided a population of almost pure X-bearing sperm would offer the chance for healthy children to every woman heterozygous for harmful X chromosome-linked hereditary disorders (1). Research into the isolation of human X and Y sperm is now practical because of the fluorochrome quinacrine, which stains the Y chromosome (2–4).

Although the human sex ratio is generally 1.06:1 (boys:girls) (5), we found during the period 1984 to 1987 that, in the 113 births by IVF and GIFT at Tygerberg Hospital, a higher ratio (1.5:1) was attained. Because of this situation, the following question arose: Did the wash and swim-up method of semen preparation used for our IVF procedure play a role in sex selection? The effect of time and/or sperm motility may be inseparable from separation of X- and Y-bearing sperm.

Material and Methods

Semen samples of 20 men (14 donors) were used for a study in the Tygerberg Reproductive Biology Unit. An aliquot of 2 to 4 ml of donor sperm was divided into four equal parts and washed twice in Ham's F-10, supplemented with 10% heat-inactivated human serum. Washing was done by adding 2 ml of Ham's F-10 with serum to the sample and centrifuging for 10 minutes at 1000 rpm. The supernatant was discarded, and the pellet was resuspended in Ham's F-10 with serum. After the last wash, half the initial amount of medium was carefully layered onto the pellet. The test tubes were left at an angle for intervals of 15, 30, 45, and 60 minutes. A wet preparation was made of 1 drop of untreated semen to determine initial motility and forward progression. After each interval, half the overlaid medium was removed, and a wet preparation was used to determine sperm motility and concentration. An air-dried preparation for F body determination was also made. The control and the four preparations were fixed overnight (acetic acid:methanol = 1:3). The slides were stained with quinacrine mustard and were coded, after which the percentage of F body-positive sperm was determined blindly with a fluorescent microscope (Table 4.6).

Multivariate and univariate analyses of variance (MANOVA and ANOVA) were used to investigate the effect of time on the percentage of Y-bearing sperm.

Results

Wilks' criterion for the hypothesis of no time effect (MANOVA) indicates a probability value of 0.0499, which indicates that the swim-up time affects the relationship between the X- and Y-bearing sperm. ANOVA results of contrast variables represent the contrast between Y-bearing sperm at the five time levels and the control sample (Table 4.7). Significant differences are shown at time intervals 0 to 30 and 0 to 45 ($P = 0.0039$ and $P = 0.0092$, respectively). Figure 4.6 shows a non-linear swim-up time effect on the mean values. This is confirmed by a significant quadratic polynomial contrast for time ($P = 0.0202$).

Table 4.6.
The Effect of Time Lapse on the Percentage of Y-Bearing Spermatozoa

Patient	Swim-up Time (min)				
	0 Control	15	30	45	60
1	41.0	42.0	47.0	57.0	40.0
2	38.0	31.0	47.0	43.0	35.0
3	54.0	56.0	52.0	66.0	76.0
4	51.0	53.0	47.0	47.0	42.0
5	44.0	42.0	53.0	46.0	50.0
6	55.0	57.0	62.0	62.0	64.0
7	41.0	47.0	44.0	55.0	50.0
8	40.0	46.0	42.0	40.0	42.0
9	50.0	47.0	57.0	46.0	51.0
10	28.0	41.0	47.0	44.0	36.0
11	45.0	46.0	50.0	40.0	39.0
12	47.0	51.0	51.0	45.0	40.0
13	42.0	37.5	49.0	42.5	39.5
14	50.0	60.5	52.0	54.5	51.0
15	45.5	50.0	53.5	53.0	54.5
16	52.5	51.5	48.0	47.5	51.5
17	50.0	55.5	44.0	48.5	46.5
18	43.5	48.0	48.0	52.5	53.0
19	52.5	47.5	57.0	60.0	53.5
20	47.0	46.0	51.5	60.5	53.5
Mean	45.8	47.8	50.1	50.5	48.4
SD	6.5	7.0	4.9	7.7	9.9
CV[a]	14	15	10	15	20

[a] CV, coefficient of variation.

Discussion

The F body is the distal end of the long arm of the Y chromosome and shows up as a bright fluorescent spot (6, 7). The fluorochrome we used contains an alkylating terminal mustard group in the side chain; alkylating groups of the mustard variety have a well-known affinity for the N-7 atom of guanine (7, 8). Some investigations, however, doubt the reliability of the F body as a marker for the Y chromosome. Increases and decreases in the length of the Y chromosome directly reflect similar changes in fluorescent pattern. Therefore, normal males were described as possessing very short Y chromosomes which lacked an intensely fluorescent portion (9).

Since the direct analysis of human sperm chromosomes with the use of zona-free hamster ova was made possible (10, 11), a comparative study (10) was performed to assess the correlation of F body percentages with Y chromosomes in human sperm. Not all Y-bearing sperm were found to contain an F body, and some sperm with an F body were not true Y-bearing sperm. The number of sperm with two or more F bodies was also found to be inexplicably high (up to 5.6%).

Table 4.7.
ANOVA Results of Contrast Variables

Time (min)	Probability (P)
0–15	0.1101
0–30	0.0039
0–45	0.0092
0–60	0.1369

Another study compared the incidence of sperm with two F bodies with the manifestation of two Y chromosomes, as determined by chromosome analysis. The number of F bodies (0.6%) was more than 10 times the number of Y chromosomes (0.05%) (10). The counting of F bodies is also viewer-dependent.

However, our results indicate a good correlation between the percentage of F bodies and the birth ratio. An optimal number of Y-bearing sperm were found in the supernatant fluid at intervals of 30 and 45 minutes, which may influence the outcome of sex by IVF and GIFT in favor of males. The question remains to be answered whether this small and theoretical difference really can make a difference in practice.

References

1. Engelmann U, Krassnigg F, Schatz H: Separation of human X and Y spermatozoa by free-flow electrophoresis. Gamete Res 19:151, 1988
2. Caspersson T, Zech L, Modest EJ: Chemical differentiation with fluorescent alkylating agents in *Vicia Faba* metaphase chromosomes. Exp Cell Res 58:128, 1969

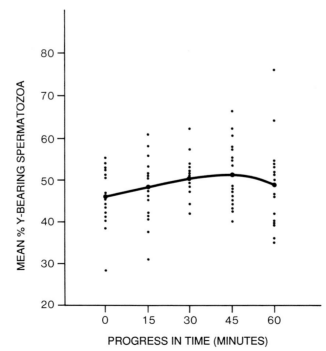

Figure 4.6.   The effect of time lapse on the percentage of Y-bearing spermatozoa.

3. Ueda K, Yanagimachi R: Sperm chromosome analysis as a new system to test human X- and Y-sperm separation. Gamete Res 17:221, 1987
4. Zech L: Investigation of metaphase chromosomes with DNA binding fluorochromes. Exp Cell Res 58:463, 1969
5. Chaudhuri JP, Schill WB: A possibility of unbiased sex preselection in humans by enrichment of X or Y chromosome bearing spermatozoa. Andrologia 19:157, 1987
6. Ericsson RJ, Langevin CN, Nishino M: Isolation of fractions rich in human Y sperm. Nature 246:421, 1973
7. Pearson P: The use of new staining techniques for human chromosome identification. J Med Genet 9:264, 1972
8. Brooks P: Reaction of alkylating agents with nucleic acids. In Plattner PA (ed): Chemotherapy of Cancer. Amsterdam: Elsevier/North Holland, 1964, p 32
9. Borgaonkar DS, Hollander DH: Quinacrine fluorescence of the human Y chromosome. Nature 230:52, 1971
10. Kamiguchi Y, Mikamo K: An improved, efficient method for analyzing human sperm chromosomes using zona-free hamster ova. Am J Hum Genet 38:724, 1986
11. Rudak E, Jacobs PA, Yanagimachi R: Direct analysis of the chromosome constitution of human spermatozoa. Nature 274:911, 1978

CHAPTER 5

Evaluation and Preparation of Spermatozoa for In Vitro Fertilization

Part One—Evaluation

Section A1:

BASIC SEMEN ANALYSIS: THE NORFOLK EXPERIENCE

R. JAMES SWANSON, R.N., PH.D., STEVEN B. ACKERMAN, PH.D., KATHRYN SIMMONS, M.S., ANIBAL A. ACOSTA, M.D., SERGIO OEHNINGER, M.D., AND MAHMOOD MORSHEDI, PH.D.

Collection Facility and Patient Information

In attempting to minimize the stress-producing factors facing couples undergoing infertility evaluation, a suitable facility for the collection of semen specimens is imperative. Although the necessary retention of the specimen for examination precludes production by completely natural means, a room with pleasant surroundings and comfortable accommodations for the couple, as well as provisions for use of a non-toxic condom as an alternative to masturbation, can help reduce the stress of the situation and may result in a more useful sample than might otherwise be obtained.

The layout of the Norfolk collection facility includes a bathroom for patient use, plus cabinets for the storage of containers, laboratory tissues, and toiletries. The room appointments have been chosen for comfort, durability, cleanability, and esthetics: a couch, chairs, end table, coffee table, lamps, wall hangings, draperies, and carpeting. Patients are free to use their own discretion in bringing whatever may be of assistance in the collection, although nothing of this nature is provided by the laboratory.

The routine collection method is masturbation into a laboratory-provided sterile container (Baxter, McGaw Park, Ill.). No lubricants are permitted because of their potential for contamination or spermicidal effects. If masturbation is not possible or is unacceptable to the patient, a seminal collection device (HDZ Corp., Mountain View, Calif.) with instructions is provided. This is a sterile, spermicide-free, non-lubricated, non-toxic silicone rubber condom, which is usually acceptable to the couple in these cases. If the patient is still unable to produce a specimen, he is referred to the physician for direction.

The containers provided to the patient are of sterile polypropylene or polystyrene construction with screw-on caps. The most frequently used container has a 110-ml capacity and a 6-cm opening diameter. Some patients prefer a 50-ml conical centrifuge tube, also of sterilized plastic. This container allows for inconspicuous delivery to the laboratory, but the opening diameter is only 3 cm, making spillage at the time of ejaculation more likely than when the larger container is used.

The Norfolk andrology laboratory operates by appointment. The husband or wife usually contacts the laboratory directly, although arrangements may be made through the clinic. When the appointment is made, instructions are given for the proper collection and transport of the semen. If any microbiological assays on the specimen have been requested, the patient is informed that he must empty his bladder before producing the ejaculate; this "flushing" helps to eliminate erroneously elevated microbial concentrations from semen culture. The patient is informed of the necessity for a 3- to 5-day abstinence before the appointment date, and he is given the option of collecting at the laboratory or elsewhere. If the collection is made elsewhere, he must obtain and use an appropriate container, and the transport of the specimen is critical. Maintenance of the semen at close to body temperature in transit is emphasized. This may be accomplished by placing the securely capped container in proximity to the body, as in a pocket, inside the waistband, or under an overcoat. Receipt of the specimen by the laboratory should be within 30 to 45 minutes after collection to evaluate liquefaction and to measure the sperm parameters at their peak.

In addition to the verbal explanation given when someone calls for an appointment, the laboratory provides a patient information/service request form (Fig. 5.1) with written instructions to the doctors' offices and the patients. The back of the form includes the written instructions, which patients are encouraged to read, along with maps and diagrams for locating the lab. The front of the sheet requests general information about patient and spouse, with a section pertinent to the semen specimen collected. Specifically requested is the time and location of the collection (if other than the laboratory facilities), whether the specimen is completely in the container or if spillage occurred, and if the latter, whether the loss was from the first or last portion of the ejaculate. To confirm the proper abstinence, the date of the last ejaculation before the appointment is also requested. Each patient must either present a completed form upon arrival or complete one at the laboratory. Also included on the front of this form is the service request section, ideally completed by the physician or an appropriate representative. If the doctor's office has not indicated the necessary assays, the laboratory personnel may complete this section based upon information obtained at the time the appointment was made. If any question remains as to which tests are to be performed, the doctor's office is called for clarification.

IMPORTANT: PLEASE READ INSTRUCTIONS ON BACK

PATIENT INFORMATION FORM
EVMS/ODU ANDROLOGY LABORATORY
Room A-8 Jones Institute Research Laboratories (JIRL)
P.O. Box 1980
Norfolk, Virginia 23501
(804) 446-5737

PATIENT TELEPHONE NUMBERS

Home: _____ Work: _____

Address: _____

_____

Specimen No. _____
(lab use only)

_____

Patient: _____ , _____ ; _____
last name   first name   spouse's name

Physician: _____

address to receive lab report

Appointment Date: _____ Appointment Time: _____

Husband's Birthdate: _____ Social Security No. : _____

Wife's Birthdate: _____ Social Security No. : _____

New patient or repeat patient (circle one)   Private or In Vitro patient (circle one)

Type of specimen: semen, cervical mucus, blood serum (circle one);

Other (explain): _____

Time specimen collected: _____ Time specimen arrived in lab: _____

Location of specimen collection: _____ Was specimen collection complete? _____
yes or no

If collection was incomplete, was loss from first or last part? (circle one)

Date of last ejaculation, intercourse, or emission: _____

SERVICE REQUEST

_____ 1. Basic Semen Analysis
_____ 2. Semen microbiology (Ureaplasma)
_____ 3. Cervical mucus microbiology (Ureaplasma)
_____ 4. Count only-semen
_____ 5. Morphology only-semen
_____ 6. Antisperm antibodies—male serum
_____ 7. Antisperm antibodies—female serum
_____ 8. Mar test for antibodies on sperm
_____ 9. Sperm/cervical mucus compatibility test
_____ 10. Sperm/cervical mucus penetration test
_____ 11. Combined sperm/cervical mucus compatibility and penetration tests
_____ 12. Biochemical evaluation of semen
    _____ a. total proteins
    _____ b. fructose
    _____ c. citric acid
    _____ d. acid phosphatase
    _____ e. glycerylphosphorylcholine
    _____ f. zinc
    _____ g. copper
    _____ h. acrosin
    _____ i. ATP

_____ 13. Hamster ova/human sperm penetration test
_____ 14. Electron microscopy of sperm
_____ 15. Indirect Mar test a. Male serum
    b. Female serum
    c. Follicular fluid
_____ 16. Preparation of specimen for AIH
_____ 17. Separation of motile sperm fraction
_____ 18. Evaluation of specimen from retrograde patient
_____ 19. Separation of motile sperm from antisperm autoimmune patient
_____ 20. Hypoosmotic Swelling Test (HOS)
_____ 21. Direct immunobead test for antibodies on sperm
_____ 22. Indirect immunobead test
    a. Male serum
    b. Female serum
    c. Follicular fluid

A

Figure 5.1.   Patient information form: directive for an andrology laboratory.

Routine Evaluation

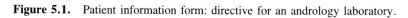

Once the semen specimen has been delivered to the laboratory, it is assigned a number and recorded in a daily log. A checklist is prepared (Table 5.1) based upon the information

BOOKING APPOINTMENTS AND SPECIMEN COLLECTION

1. It is necessary to call the Andrology Laboratory approximately one week in advance in order to make an appointment. Appointments are taken between   7:30 am-3:00 pm Monday-Friday. Exceptions may be possible in the event that special arrangements are necessary.

2. Cervical mucus specimens should be collected in the physician's office and transported by the patient to the Lab. Blood can be drawn in the physician's office or in the Lab. However, special collection and transportation procedures need to be followed for both mucus and blood, so prior arrangements with the Lab should be performed.

3. For assays involving semen we strongly recommend collection in our private facilities. Most of these assays necessitate the use of a fresh specimen to assure accurate determinations of sperm motility and viability. If it is impossible to collect the specimen in the Lab's facilities, then the sample must be collected in a **proper** collection container (provided by the Lab) and delivered to the Lab within 30-45 minutes after emission.

4. In order to ensure that the semen specimen is clinically useful, the following procedures should be employed:

    a. A period of sexual abstinence (no emission) of no more than 5 and no less than 3 days should be observed before collection of the ejaculate being tested.

    b. The specimen should be collected by manual masturbation, without the use of lubricants, condoms or oral sex. If masturbation is not possible, a SPECIAL SEMEN CONDOM will be provided by the Lab.

    c. The specimen should be collected in a container provided by the Lab or provided to the physician by the Lab.

    d. Avoid contamination of the inside of the collection container both before and after collection. (Note: the container is sterile until opened.)

    e. Collect the entire ejaculate and note on PATIENT INFORMATION form if any portion (first or last) of the ejaculate misses the container or if spillage occurs.

    f. During transport the specimen should not be subject to extreme heat or cold, nor to direct sunlight. We recommend that the container be carried in an inside pocket next to your body so that body temperature is maintained.

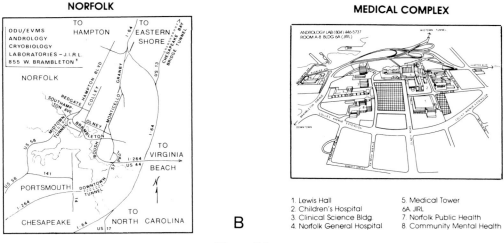

NORFOLK   MEDICAL COMPLEX

1. Lewis Hall   5. Medical Tower
2. Children's Hospital   6A JIRL
3. Clinical Science Bldg   7. Norfolk Public Health
4. Norfolk General Hospital   8. Community Mental Health

Figure 5.1.

included on the patient information/service request form. This checklist is further used for recording the data pertinent to the specimen as the requested tests are performed and for entering these data into a computer, ultimately to be reported to the physician.

VISUAL INSPECTION OF SEMEN

Before any analysis, the semen specimen must liquefy. Thirty minutes are routinely allowed for the liquefaction to occur, after which time an assessment is made of

Table 5.1.
Norfolk Andrology Laboratory Checklist

ANDROLOGY LABORATORY CHECKLIST

Logbook #: _____   Date: _____

Patient name: _____   SS#: _____

Spouse name: _____   SS#: _____

Physician: _____ Location: _____ Collection method: _____

Time collected: _____ Time at lab: _____ Last ejaculation: _____

Specimen complete: YES _____ NO _____   Portion lost: FIRST _____ LAST _____ NO _____

ORDERED	PREPARED	RESULTS	ENTERED
_____ Semen data	_____		_____
_____ Semen motility	_____		_____
_____ Morphology	_____		_____
_____ Microbiology	_____	_____	_____
_____ Acrosin	_____	_____	_____
_____ ATP[a]	_____	_____	_____
_____ ABs Male _____	_____	K: _____ I_o: _____ I_1 _____	_____
_____ ABs Female _____	_____	K: _____ I_o: _____ I_1 _____	_____
_____ SSM	_____		_____
_____ Chlamydia	_____	_____	_____
_____ Other:_____	_____	_____	_____

SEMEN DATA
Time analyzed: _____
Volume: _____
Viscosity: _____
Liquefaction complete: _____
Liquefaction time: _____
Agglutination: _____
pH: _____
COMMENTS:

OTHER ASSAYS
BIOCHEMICAL: _____
Fructose: _____
Citric acid: _____
Acid phosphatase _____
GPC: _____
Zinc: _____
Copper: _____
Total protein: _____

SPERM MOTILITY DATA
Sperm conc. _____ 10^6/ml
Percent motile: _____ %
Mean velocity: _____ μm/sec
Mean linearity: _____
Motile sperm/ejac.: _____ 10^6

MORPHOLOGY ANALYSIS DATA

# of sperm analyzed:	_____	
Normal sperm:	_____/_____	%
Small heads:	_____/_____	%
Large heads:	_____/_____	%
Amorphous heads:	_____/_____	%
Neck defects:	_____/_____	%
Cytoplasmic droplets:	_____/_____	%
Round heads:	_____/_____	%
Duplicate forms:	_____/_____	%
Tapered heads:	_____/_____	%

SPERM FUNCTION
SPERM/CM COMPATIBILITY
Husband/wife: _____
Husband/donor: _____
Donor/wife: _____
Donor/donor: _____
SPERM/BOVINE CM PENETRATION
Husband: _____
Donor: _____
COMMENTS:

IMMUNOLOGICAL
Direct: _____
Indirect male: _____
Indirect female: _____
COMMENTS:

Table 5.1.—*Continued*

Coiled tails:	_____/_____%
COMMENTS:	

ROUND CELL CYTOLOGY

Round cells counted: _____		Neutrophils: _____
Other round cells: _____		COMMENTS:

[a]Abbreviations: ATP, adenosine triphosophate, ABs antibodies; SSM, sperm swimup method; GPC, glycerylphosphorylcholine; CM, cervical mucus.

the completeness of the process. A completely liquefied specimen appears homogeneous when "rolled" against the sides of the container, with uniformity of color throughout. Occasionally a specimen will appear completely liquefied upon gross examination, yet will demonstrate incomplete liquefaction when observed microscopically, evidenced by "streaming" patterns among the cells and apparent droplets which disappear as the liquefaction process continues. If a specimen does not liquefy after 30 minutes, it is checked every 10 minutes by gross and/or microscopic observation until the process is complete, and the time required is recorded on the worksheet. In the infrequent event that the specimen does not liquefy after 90 minutes, an attempt is made to measure the necessary parameters regardless of the incomplete liquefaction, and this abnormality is noted on the worksheet.

Although homogeneity is the chief gross characteristic of a completely liquefied ejaculate, there are occasional exceptions. Macroscopic globules are present in some ejaculates, and their presence is sometimes confused with incomplete liquefaction. In most of these cases, a majority of the specimen volume consists of homogeneous liquid, with the globules interspersed. When the liquid portion is observed microscopically, it appears completely liquefied. When the globules are separately pipetted from the specimen and examined, they appear to be acellular masses with a gelatinous consistency. If left in the specimen, the globules usually disappear after several hours at room temperature, and the entire specimen appears uniform. In some instances the globules remain until disposal of the specimen. Again, this is not considered to be abnormal liquefaction but simply a variable characteristic among ejaculates, within the realm of normal features.

One final gross observation associated with the basic semen analysis is the assessment of color. The normal color for semen is grayish-white to slightly yellow. Other colorations are frequently associated with the presence of blood in the specimen, infection, or some additive from improper collection.

INITIAL DATA DETERMINATIONS

Evaluations of the specimen volume, pH, and viscosity are performed after complete liquefaction, or no longer than 90 minutes post-emission if liquefaction appears incomplete. Volume is determined by drawing the specimen from the container into a graduated 10-ml pipette using a bulb or Pi-pump for suction, noting the volume, redispensing the specimen into the container, and recording the measurement on the data worksheet. Subsequently the pH is determined by touching the tip of the pipette used to measure the volume to a piece of pH paper and comparing the color change with a chart on the side of the paper dispenser. The pH value on the chart corresponding to the color of the test strip is recorded as the appropriate measurement. A viscosity determination is made by observing the specimen while pipetting for the volume analysis. The degree of viscosity is noted as normal, slight, moderate, or excessive. *Normal* indicates free pipetting and redispensing of the specimen. *Slight* indicates a thickness to the specimen, yet relative ease of pipetting and redispensing. *Moderate* indicates a specimen which is difficult to pipette and redispense, with a stringy characteristic. *Excessive* viscosity indicates a specimen which is quite difficult or impossible to pipette and may require manipulation in some manner before further evaluation.

The first microscopic evaluation made on a specimen received for basic analysis is the viability. This requires the use of a 0.5% solution of eosin Y in distilled water. This stain may be prepared, aliquotted, and frozen in microcentrifuge tubes until needed. Once thawed for use, it may be left at room temperature indefinitely without adverse effects. The viability determination is performed by placing 15 µl of semen and 5 µl of eosin on a 24 × 75-mm slide, mixing them thoroughly with the pipette tip, and applying a 24 × 50-mm coverslip. The prepared slide is then scanned microscopically on high dry (400× or 450×). If cells are plentiful, the slide is evaluated using oil immersion (1000×). If cells are scarce, the high dry lens is used for the reading.

At least 10 fields uniformly distributed around the slide are observed. These fields display sperm which are motile and non-motile. Only the intact, non-motile sperm will be red (those which have absorbed the stain), and others will be colorless (those which have not absorbed the stain). The red-headed sperm are dead, and the rest of the non-motile sperm are alive though immobile. A tally is made of dead sperm and non-motile live sperm, and a percentage is calculated for each. The decimal form of the percentage of dead sperm is then multiplied by the percent form of the non-motile fraction obtained through the motility evaluation, and a percentage of dead sperm in the total specimen concentration is obtained.

COMPUTER-ASSISTED MICROSCOPIC EVALUATIONS

The Norfolk andrology laboratory employs the CellSoft computer-assisted semen analyser (CASA) (Labsoft Division of Cryo Resources, Ltd., New York, N.Y.) for motility and concentration determinations. The equipment includes an IBM computer with keyboard and terminal, a separate unit for CellSoft, an Okidata printer, an Olympus microscope with attached video camera, and two video screens. A VHS video cassette recorder is included with the setup, but it is not regularly used.

The program designed by CellSoft which is used for the specimen evaluations is referred to by the acronym *CSN*. This program is accessed by entering the acronym and following the menu information. The first step is to check the parameter settings to ensure that they are correct. Although these parameters are changed infrequently, they may be altered for particular types of evaluations. The parameters indicated are the values suggested by Cryo Resources as the most accurate when analyzing whole semen with a concentration of 20 to 200 × 10^6 sperm/per milliliter. Handling specimens with concentrations beyond these limits is considered later.

The second item which must be checked before evaluating concentration and motility is the threshold setting. This setting is important for telling the computer the size of the cells observed in the specimen. Since the CellSoft analyser uses a digitized image of a video projection to make its analysis, the optimal result is obtained when these two representations are essentially identical. The closer the digitized version of the cells resembles the video version, the more accurate the reading of the specimen characteristics by the computer. Adjusting the threshold allows the technician to simulate as closely as possible in the digitized image the cell sizes observed in the focused video image. The adjustment is performed using the "greater than" and "less than" keys on the computer keyboard. Increments of variation ("step changes") may be altered using the "up" and "down" (arrow) keys on the keyboard. The objective becomes clear as the changes in the digitization are noted with each adjustment, minimizing the background noise and sharpening the objects of focus.

For the Cellsoft CASA to perform a reliable concentration and motility analysis, the semen must be aliquotted into a specialized chamber. The Norfolk facility uses a Makler chamber (Sefi Medical Instruments, Haifa, Israel) for mounting the specimen. This chamber, when properly loaded, is designed to create a uniform distribution of the specimen over a planar surface, allowing a depth of 10 μm when the cover glass is properly placed on the chamber. This depth is adequate for liberal movement of the cells in the plane of the chamber surface without permitting excessive movement in other planes, although such movement is not impossible. Close observation of the cover glass reveals a grid in the center. This grid is calibrated into 100 squares, each measuring 0.1 × 0.1 ml, in place on the base of the chamber. The space bounded by the grid and the two planar surfaces is sufficient for a volume of exactly 0.00001 ml. The concentration of a specimen, in 10^6/ml, may be determined by counting the sperm cells in one row of 10 squares on the grid or by counting the sperm on the entire grid and dividing the total by 10. Although such a concentration determination technique is not required with the CASA, it is a valuable means of evaluating specimens with abnormalities such as oligozoospermia or excessive round cell concentration, as described later.

Before the Makler chamber is loaded for reading a specimen, the device must be clean and dry. Minimal wiping of the cover glass surface opposing the base is suggested to avoid scratching or marring the grid. Tissue or lens paper may be used to blot excess moisture from the base and cover glass, with forced air used to eliminate the final traces of dust and water. A 5-μl Eppendorf pipette is used to load the chamber. The aliquot of semen is placed in the center of the glass surface of the base, and the cover glass is placed over it. A properly loaded chamber will show prismatic effects on all four quartz-coated pillars upon which the cover glass rests. Slight movement of the glass may be necessary to achieve this condition, which is required for proper reading with the computer. If any bubbles are noted on the loaded chamber after the cover glass is applied, the chamber should be cleaned and the process repeated until a successfully loaded chamber is ready for reading. Cleaning of the chamber base and cover is attained by removing the cover glass from the base and rinsing the two pieces under a stream of deionized water, using the camel hair brush provided with the Makler to non-abrasively wash the semen from both surfaces. The chamber base and cover glass are then dried as mentioned previously and placed on a 37°C warming tray in preparation for the next specimen. Two chambers are available for use in the Norfolk andrology lab, with at least one of the two always clean and warming.

Once the Makler is properly prepared, the computer-assisted reading of concentration and motility may be performed. The chamber is placed on the microscope stage by using a glass microscope slide to stabilize the chamber between the stage clips of the microscope. A specialized holder to accommodate the circular shape of the Makler also works satisfactorily. The CSN program is accessed, and the main menu appears on the terminal screen; "3" is initially selected. If a parameter check has not been made, "1" should first be chosen and the parameter settings confirmed, and then "3" is entered. With the 10× objective in place for viewing on the microscope, the sperm cells are brought into focus. The cells should be in a uniform focal plane in a properly loaded chamber. The focusing should be performed while the operator is viewing the video projection of the Makler activity, rather than directly observing through the lenses of the microscope. The area of the chamber brought into focus should not include the grid, since readings are made in the space surrounding the grid rather than on the grid. Once optimal acuity is achieved on the video screen, the threshold is adjusted as explained. This threshold setting remains constant throughout the reading of the specimen, and since all of the cells are within the same focal plane, readjustment for the varied fields evaluated should be unnecessary.

The processing of the specimen proceeds by selecting ''5'' on the CSN program menu. The appropriate requested information is entered, and the first field is aligned for evaluation. During the alignment, an outline of the field of view detected by the computer appears on the digitized screen. This allows the user to see the cells which will actually be considered by the computer in making any calculations and prevents the accidental inclusion of grid lines in the fields chosen. Since it has been determined in the Norfolk laboratory that optimal accuracy in reading is obtained by close approximation to the grid without inclusion of grid lines, care must be taken when adjusting the chamber to the reading fields. Fields are selected beginning at the 12 o'clock position beyond the grid, with subsequent alignments at 3 o'clock, 6 o'clock, and 9 o'clock around the grid. A minimum of four fields must be evaluated, with these four fields including a minimum of 200 cells, as noted on the computer terminal while the analysis proceeds. If more fields must be analyzed to attain the minimum cell count, a systematic progression is made to various fields around the grid until an adequate number of sperm has been counted. When the total analysis is complete, the program is ended and the desired option as listed at the bottom of the screen is chosen. The first step is to view the results and record concentration, motility, mean linearity, and mean velocity on the data worksheet for the patient. The next step is to file the results for later transfer and retrieval from the REPORTS program, and the final, optional step is to print a hard copy of the histogram and statistical data on the specimen.

REPORTS is a program created by the Norfolk andrology lab which is interfaced with the Cellsoft program to permit generation of results in a report form suitable for mailing to clinicians. The program is designed for the placement of test orders, including general information on the patient and specimen as well as specific assays to be performed; the entry of manually performed determinations and transfer of computer-assisted data; and the printing of final reports for mailing. The concentration and motility data filed after analysis in the CSN program are the only information which may be transferred internally from CSN to REPORTS through appropriate commands. The remaining data must be entered into REPORTS directly from the data worksheet prepared for the specimen. Table 5.2 shows the format and reference information for a basic analysis as generated from REPORTS.

MORPHOLOGY EVALUATION

The final assay performed as a part of the semen analysis in Norfolk is the preparation and reading of morphology slides. With the recent emphasis upon morphology evaluation as a helpful prognostic indicator for clinicians in Norfolk, the need for efficient reporting of these results is recognized. In 1986 a transition was made in the laboratory from a Papanicolaou staining series to a hematology staining series, similar in results to a Wright-Giemsa stain, called Diff-Quik (distributed by American Scientific

Table 5.2
Format and Reference Information Generated by REPORTS Program

EVMS/ODU ANDROLOGY LABORATORY
EASTERN VIRGINIA MEDICAL SCHOOL
855 WEST BRAMBLETON AVENUE
NORFOLK, VIRGINIA 23510
(804) 446-5737

PHYSICIAN:
TEST DATE: 07/11/88

PATIENT: RICHARD   SS#:
SPOUSE: LINDA   SS#:
ACC. #: 10652   Date of Last Emission: 07/06/88

SPECIMEN: Time Collected: 07:30   Time in lab:
          Location: Lab. Facility   Collection Method: Masturbation
          Specimen was Complete

| | | | REFERENCE |
TEST	RESULT	UNITS	RANGE
			***** Indicates test not performed
SEMEN DATA: Time Analyzed—08:27			
Volume	2.70	ml	2.0–5.0
Odor	ok		ok
Color	ok		ok
Viscosity	ok		ok
Liquefaction	Complete in 30 min.		Complete in 30 min.
Agglutination	5.0%		None
pH	8.2		Basic = >7.5
Comments:			
SPERM ANALYSIS: # Sperm Analyzed—221			
Concentration	41.0	million/ml	20.0–200.0
Percent motile	33.5	% progressive	over 50
Motile sperm ejac.	37.0	million/ejaculate	25.0–250.0
Mean velocity	34.7	micron/sec	over 25
Motility index	11.6	(% motile × mean vel.)	over 10
Mean linearity	5.9	(10 = st. line; 0 = circular)	
Comments: PERCENTAGE DEAD SPERM CELLS = 34.6			

MORPHOLOGY ANALYSIS

SPERMATOZOAL MORPHOLOGY:		# Sperm Analyzed: 200	
Normal sperm	4.0%	over 13	
Small heads	1.0%	Round heads	7.0%
Large heads	0.0%	Duplicate forms	7.0%
Amorphous heads	47.5%	Tapered heads	1.0%
Neck defects	19.0%	Coiled tails	12.5%

Table 5.2.—*Continued*

Cytoplasmic droplet	1.0%		

ROUND CELL CYTOLOGY:	# Round Cells Analyzed: 100		
Neutrophils	0.0	million/ml	less than 1
Other round cells	3.3	million/ml	

Comments: SLIGHTLY ABNORMAL FORMS = 18.0%

Products, manufactured by AHS del Caribe, Inc., Aguada, Puerto Rico). This change required modification of slide preparation as well as staining and reading methods.

The most critical steps in the preparation of a satisfactory semen smear for morphology evaluation are the use of a small volume of semen on the slide and the thin distribution of that volume across the slide. The following technique is efficacious:

Apply an aliquot of semen to the unfrosted or unlabelled end of a clean microscope slide (Fig. 5.2). Three to a maximum of five microliters of semen should be applied.

As shown in Figure 5.3, touch the edge of another slide to the drop of semen by placing it in front of the drop (*#1*) and drawing it back (*#2*) into the droplet (*#3*). Allow the specimen to distribute along the edge at the interface between slides. Hold the upper slide at approximately a 30° angle to the bottom slide (Fig. 5.4). Slowly draw the specimen toward the labelled end of the slide, observing a constant distribution of semen across the width of the upper slide and a residue of semen along the areas of the bottom slide over which the passage has been made. Once the labelled end is reached, lift the upper slide directly off the lower. The resultant smear should be air dried and stored to avoid accumulation of dust on the surface until stained (Fig. 5.5).

The preparation of four morphology slides per patient is the routine procedure in Norfolk. This allows for maintenance of an unstained slide file in the event that a repeat analysis of a particular specimen is needed or if an insufficient number of cells is found on a single slide. Such a file is also useful for practice purposes when someone is learning the technique for reading morphology.

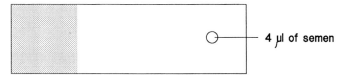

Figure 5.2.   Postion a 4-μl drop of semen on a slide.

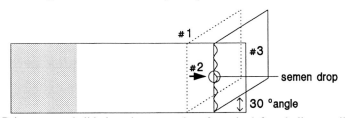

Figure 5.3.   Bring a second slide into the semen drop from the left and allow capillary action to spread the semen along the edge of the second slide (by moving the second slide from position no. 1 to position no. 3).

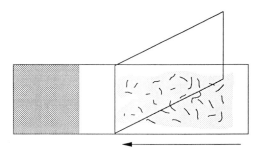

Figure 5.4.   Draw the semen across the first slide by moving the second slide to the left.

The staining of morphology slides is rapid and simple, involving three methanol-based components. The first step is a fixation, the second a predominantly cytoplasmic stain (xanthene dye), and the third a predominantly nuclear stain (thiazine dye mixture of azure A and methylene blue stains). Slides prepared as described above are placed in a holder and dipped into the fixative for 12 to 15 1-second dips. They are removed and blotted on paper towels, then placed into the xanthene dye for 12 to 15 1-second dips. They are removed, blotted, and placed in the thiazine dye for 8 to 10 1-second dips. The slides are then gently rinsed with deionized water, wiped dry on the back surface, and set on the slide warmer or bench top to dry prior to reading.

An oil immersion lens is required for accurate reading of the morphology slides after staining. A properly stained slide should appear as in Figure 5.6 (1000 × magnification). The lightened area on the head represents the acrosomal region, and the darkened area to which the tail connects represents the nuclear region. The tail does not often display distinct color characteristics but should be clearly visible. A minimum of background material is ideal, although some staining of seminal plasma components is expected. An ocular reticle micrometrically calibrated for size determination is helpful, particularly when one is first learning the technique. A minimum of 200 sperm counted and categorized by shape from fields across the entire slide gives a completed morphology analysis. Once the morphology results are calculated, recorded, and entered into the computer, the basic analysis is complete. With the inclusion of all accumulated semen parametric data in the REPORTS program, the printed report is sent to the physician.

Exceptional Evaluation

The aforementioned techniques for concentration and motility determination are applicable to the analysis of semen specimens which have concentrations of 20 to 200 × 10^6 sperm/per milliliter. In cases of oligozoospermia or polyzoospermia, modifications must be made. Oligozoospermic specimens are not evaluated using the computer, although the Makler chamber is used. The concentration of the specimen is determined by

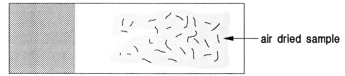

air dried sample

Figure 5.5.   Allow the semen to dry in air on a slide-warmer tray.

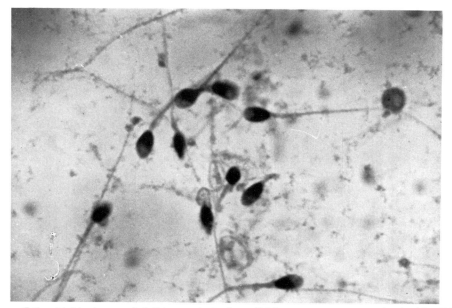

Figure 5.6. Light micrograph (oil immersion) of one field on a semen smear stained with a Diff-Quik white blood cell staining kit

counting the sperm on the entire Makler grid, reading directly through the microscope rather than on the video screen. The number of cells counted on the grid is then divided by 10 to obtain the concentration in millions per milliliter.

This alternative is used because the tendency to hunt for cells rather than to select fields is greater when the concentration is low, particularly when few cells are moving. Because the computer system is not designed to accept evaluation of a field void of cells (empty fields often being present is severely oligozoospermic specimens), it is impossible to obtain an accurate result. Since certain areas with cells must then be deliberately selected on the chamber and evaluated, the results are skewed toward a higher-than-actual concentration. Consistently more accurate results are obtained by performing several loadings and readings of the Makler without computer assistance and averaging the results for a reported concentration.

The motility evaluation for oligozoospermic specimens may be performed in a manner similar to the concentration evaluation. When one is counting the sperm cells on the grid of the Makler, one tallies the motile and non-motile sperm observed. This may then be expressed as a percentage of motile sperm for the specimen. Another technique used for motility determination in oligozoospermia is evaluation of a 25- to 40-μl aliquot wet mount of semen, using the $40\times$ or $45\times$ magnification objective. Quick progressive, sluggish progressive, and non-progressive cells are counted and percentages obtained for each category. Addition of the quick and sluggish cell fractions gives the percentage of total progressive sperm.

The difficulty encountered with polyzoospermic specimens is the inability of the computer system to handle the number of cells in each field in such highly concentrated ejaculates. Either the computer will cease the analysis and jam after several frames, or it will indicate an overload message on the screen, specifying that too many objects are present for analysis. The simplest alternative in these cases is to centrifuge an aliquot of the patient's semen, pipette off the seminal plasma, and use it as a diluent with an aliquot of the whole semen. A 1:1 dilution is most frequently used, and the diluted specimen is usually brought within the appropriate concentration range for computer evaluation. The resultant computer concentration is then doubled to give the theoretical original concentration, which is reported to the clinician. Although motility may be affected by this technique, no corrective factor is considered. Whenever such exceptional measures are necessary to perform the computerized portion of the semen analysis, a notation is given to the doctor explaining the procedure and its rationale.

Another type of specimen which may not be analyzed by computer is the azoospermic specimen. When such a specimen is received, it is initially evaluated as any other, although it is frequently noted as free of sperm cells early in the analysis due to rapid liquefaction and translucency. Once the specimen is in fact determined to be apparently free of sperm after the scanning of several aliquots on Makler and microscope slides, the specimen is centrifuged and the pellet inspected. If no sperm cells are observed in the pellet, it is reported that no sperm cells were observed in the fresh or concentrated specimen.

Regardless of sperm cell concentration, a difficulty periodically encountered is specimen viscosity. An excessively viscous specimen is not only laborious to pipette but also is impossible to conform to the crucial thin-smear morphology slides. In Norfolk the technique employed to break up the viscosity is syringe aspiration and expulsion. An 18-gauge needle is attached to a 5-cc syringe, and the specimen is flushed through the needle five to 10 times until the specimen appears less viscous. This technique usually produces bubbles in the specimen, but it is still possible to obtain aliquots free of bubbles if the specimen is allowed to settle for 5 to 10 minutes after the procedure. This aspiration greatly simplifies the seemingly impossible task of morphology slide preparation from a viscous specimen. The reading of the specimen slides is facilitated as well, because areas of viscosity on a stained slide obscure the tails of the sperm and prevent accurate reading, whereas aspiration of the specimen aids the dispersion of cells in such areas. A comparison has been made between morphology of sperm before and after this procedure to determine whether structural damage is observable; no significant difference was detected. For specimens with even moderate viscosity, this technique is of considerable assistance and its use is encouraged.

One final exceptional situation that must be considered is an excessive concentration of round cells. "Excessive" is defined as any concentration greater than 10^6 cells per milliliter. The determination of round cell concentration is made concurrently with the determination of sperm concentration. Since round cells in a specimen are perceived by the computer in the same manner as sperm cells, through phase contrast optics, the computer will analyze most round cells within a certain size range as sperm cells. This fact makes it advisable to analyze a semen specimen containing excessive round cells by the manual or direct Makler reading technique rather than the computer-assisted technique. In this way, sperm cell concentration and round cell concentration can be independently determined by the observer, whereas the computer cannot make the distinction.

Once the concentration of round cells is determined, it is helpful to assess the type of round cells. In Norfolk a peroxidase stain is used to distinguish neutrophils, basophils, and eosinophils from other round cells, including germinal cells and any other leukocytes. Although this procedure does not make distinctions among the round cells other than granulocytes, it does allow for a clearer representation of these cells than other

Table 5.3.
Peroxidase Stain for White Blood Cells in Semen

Reagents

Benzidine-cyanosine stock
a. Dissolve 125 mg of benzidine (Sigma, B-3503) in 50 ml of 96% methanol (48 ml of methanol + 2 ml of H_2O).
b. Dissolve 150 mg of cyanosine (phloxine B; Sigma, P-2759) in 50 ml of H_2O.
c. Add solution a to solution b. Store in a dark bottle at 4°C.
Working solution
a. Add 40 ml of 5% H_2O_2 (hydrogen peroxide) to 500 ml of stock.
b. The working solution can be used for 1 day.

Procedure

Add 2 drops of freshly liquefied semen to 2 drops of working solution in a microfuge tube. Vortex the mixture. Place 1 drop of mixture onto a microscope slide and apply a coverslip. After 8 minutes examine at 400× magnification.

Interpretation

a. Brown cells: peroxidase-containing neutrophils, basophils, and eosinophils
b. Other cells stain either pink or light green.
c. Calculate the percentage of round cells which stain brown. Multiply this percentage by the number of round cells per milliliter to determine the number of neutrophils per milliliter of semen.

WARNING!
Benzidine is a suspected carcinogen. When preparing stock or working solution, be very careful. Use a hood and gloves.

staining techniques. The primary disadvantage to this technique is the toxicity of the chemicals necessary for preparation of the stocks and working solutions. Table 5.3 presents the reagents, as well as procedures for preparation of the solutions, slide preparation, and interpretation, with a brief precautionary statement.

Section A2:

BASIC SEMEN ANALYSIS:
THE TYGERBERG EXPERIENCE

ROELOF MENKVELD, PH.D., AND THINUS F. KRUGER, M.D.

A semen analysis is the most important factor in the investigation of male fertility potential. It is therefore extremely important that a semen analysis should be performed skillfully and properly. If the necessary background data are obtained and the results interpreted correctly and intelligently, a wide spectrum of information can be obtained, especially if a short personal and medical history is also taken with the first semen analysis.

Collection of the Semen Sample

Patients are encouraged to produce their semen samples at the laboratory. Only when the patient has a real problem in doing so are arrangements made for him to bring the sample to the laboratory. The advantages for producing samples at the laboratory are many: samples are produced by masturbation; there is no time loss or loss of any part of the sample; coagulation and the time for liquefaction can be observed.

INITIAL VISIT

On the patient's first visit, he is interviewed by a clinical technologist or medical scientist. The clinic and laboratory procedures are explained to him, and a short questionnaire on his personal and medical history is completed. Questions include date of birth, occupation, date of marriage, and years of primary or secondary infertility. Questions on his medical history include whether he has had any medication, anesthesia, or infections or illnesses (such as a cold or flu) with fever in the past 3 months; whether he has any history of operations of the urogenital tract, especially Y-V plasty, orchidectomy, varicocelectomy, or testicular biopsy; or whether he has had any severe injuries of the testicles, or orchitis. A note is also made about his smoking and drinking habits.

Patients who are referred to our unit for full investigation and treatment are given three more semen analysis appointments at 4-week intervals. With the third analysis, the first two analyses are checked, and if any of the parameters are not within our normal range, blood is drawn for hormone evaluations (Table 5.4).

In cases of azoospermia, oligozoospermia ($<10 \times 10^6$/ml), or when the percentage of morphologically normal sperm is $\leq 10\%$, blood is also drawn for chromosome analysis. An appointment is arranged for a medical examination and consultation. In cases of azoospermia and normal FSH values, arrangements are made for a bilateral testicular biopsy or, in the case of a varicocele, for a varicocelectomy.

Table 5.4.
Normal Semen Parameter Values: Tygerberg Hospital

Parameter	Value
Sperm concentration	$\geq 10 \times 10^6$/ml
Motility (% motile)	$\geq 30\%$
Speed of forward progression (0–4)[a]	≥ 2.0
Morphology (% normal)	$\geq 20\%$

[a]On a scale of 1 to 4.

ABSTINENCE

All semen analyses are done by appointment. A patient is asked to be at the laboratory at between 7:45 and 8:30 in the morning. The patient is advised to have a period of 3 or 4 days of abstinence, as this period will, in most cases, give the optimal semen quality and corresponds to the intercourse frequency in most marriages (1, 2).

SEMEN ROOM

All samples are produced in a specially equipped room. On arrival the patient is accompanied to the room by a clinical technologist. This allows an opportunity for discussion and puts the patient at ease, since tension or emotional stress can have a marked inhibitory effect on semen parameters (3) such as volume, count, and motility. This effect is usually more severe with a patient's first analysis.

The semen room is equipped with air conditioning and heating, which is of great importance in the winter months to make the environment more comfortable for the patient and to avoid cold shock.

The patient is asked the precise period of abstinence, as well as the occurrence of any infections or illnesses in the last 3 months (if it is the first visit) or since his previous semen analysis.

METHOD OF COLLECTION

Semen samples are produced by masturbation into clean plastic containers which were sterile-packed at shipment. The patient is instructed to first urinate and then to wash his hands with soap and the glans of the penis without soap. In cases where samples for culture of aerobic and anaerobic organisms are taken, sterile gauze is used for drying off the hands and glans of the penis. For these samples, individually packed and sterilized containers are used.

The patient is informed that after producing the sample by masturbation he can leave the container on the shelf and that when he leaves the room he should switch off a little red light that is also burning in the laboratory so that an indication is given when he leaves the room.

CONTAINERS

Plastic containers of 90-ml capacity (75 mm × 45 mm in diameter), made of polypropylene with a tight-fitting plastic or metal cap, are used. Experience has indicated that plastic containers made of polystyrene may cause an increased viscosity, especially if the sample has been in the container for more than an hour.

The patient's name and all relevant information obtained from the patient is recorded on the semen container.

Examination of the Sample

When the patient leaves the semen room, he switches off the red light that is also burning in the laboratory. The time is recorded on the container, and the sample is then brought to the laboratory by the person handling the patients.

PHYSICAL CHARACTERISTICS

Semen parameters are characteristics which describe the appearance of the sample; they include color, volume, pH, coagulation, liquefaction, and viscosity (4, 5).

Coagulation

On arrival in the laboratory, the sample is examined to see whether coagulation has occurred. Coagulated semen appears as a thick, heterogeneous mass, mainly in a semisolid state, with a small portion in a liquid state, which can differ in color (5). The sample is then placed in an incubator at 37°C until liquefaction has occurred.

Liquefaction

The sample is checked at regular intervals until complete liquefaction has occurred (usually within 10 to 20 minutes). After complete liquefaction, the sample appears homogeneous in composition and color (6). Small, roundish particles may still be present in some samples; however, these can be regarded as normal and usually dissolve within an hour.

Volume

After complete liquefaction, the sample is transferred to a 15-ml graduated plastic centrifuge tube (Falcon 2099). This is used to measure the volume to the nearest 0.1 ml. If sufficient care and time are taken, an insignificant residue will remain in the container.

Color and Odor

After the volume and the color are noted, the appearance of the sample (transparent or opaque) and the presence of small particles are recorded. Only when an uncharacteristic odor is present is it noted; this is usually associated with an infection or a long period of abstinence (7).

pH

The pH is then determined with the aid of a pH meter (Metrohn, Herisan, Switzerland). It is important to do this as soon as possible because the pH decreases with time.

Viscosity

The viscosity is determined by means of a modified pipette (8). The semen is drawn into a Pasteur pipette and slowly released by drops. The viscosity is regarded as normal when single drops are released within a distance of 20 mm from the point of the pipette. If threads of 20 to 40 mm are formed, the viscosity is regarded as slightly increased, 40 to 80 mm as increased, and >80 mm as grossly increased. It is important not to confuse increased viscosity with delayed liquefaction.

In cases of increased viscosity, the semen sample is drawn into a 10-ml syringe and forced out through a number 18 or 19 needle. This can be repeated several times until the viscosity is normal, which is slightly higher than that or water. This method increases the air bubbles, but these disappear later. A normal viscosity is of the utmost importance because an increased viscosity adversely influences the determination of the other semen parameters.

SEMEN BIOCHEMISTRY

If the volume of a semen sample is $\geq$2 ml, an aliquot of 0.5 to 1.0 ml is taken from the sample directly after the determination of the physical parameters, placed in a Wassermann tube, and stored in the freezer compartment of a refrigerator until all the samples are received. The samples are then centrifuged at 3000 $\times$ g for 30 minutes to obtain a clean seminal plasma without sperm. The plasma is sent on ice to the biochemistry department for determination of zinc, acid phosphatase, and fructose.

MICROSCOPIC EXAMINATION

After the physical examination, the centrifuge tube is placed on a laboratory rotator (Hetorotator, Instruments AB, Sweden) and rotated through 360° for the duration of all subsequent procedures. After 10 minutes of rotation, a drop of semen is placed on a pre-cleaned slide kept at 37°C until use. The drop is covered with a 20 $\times$ 40-mm coverslip and left for a few minutes to stabilize before examination.

General Appearance

All examinations of wet preparations are done with phase contrast optics and 100 $\times$ (LPF) of 400 $\times$ (HPF) magnification. The examination starts with scanning through 10 fields on low power to get a general impression of the sample. This impression dictates the subsequent procedures. For instance, the performance of a mixed antiglobulin reaction (MAR) test or a supravital staining test will depend on the presence of enough motile sperm or enough total sperm to make an accurate determination of the motility and speed of forward progression.

Concentration

An estimation of the number of sperm per HPF is made to determine the dilution of the sample necessary for the determination of sperm concentration. If there are $\leq$10 sperm per HPF, a 1:10 dilution will be prepared. If there are 11 to 20 sperm per HPF, a 1:20 dilution will be prepared, and if there are >20, a 1:100 dilution will be prepared.

Agglutination and Cells

The sample is also examined for the presence of agglutinated sperm. Two types of agglutination are possible. The first can be non-specific agglutination, where sperm adhere to cells in the seminal plasma. The second is specific agglutination, caused by antisperm antibodies (9). Agglutination is described as negative ($-$), occasional ($\pm$), slight ($+$), moderate ($++$), or severe ($+++$). The presence of other cells, such as round cells, and the presence of spermine phosphate crystals are recorded as well. The presence of any microorganisms is also recorded.

Motility and Speed of Forward Progression

Evaluation of motility (quantitative) and speed of forward progression (SFP) or grade of motility (qualitative) (10) is done by scanning through 10 HPF. An estimate of the average percentage of motile sperm on these fields is reported to the nearest 10% (11). The average SFP is reported, as well as the range according to the method of Hotchkiss (12) and MacLeod (2) on a scale of 0 to 4, where 0 indicates no movement and 4 indicates a fast linear progressive movement. The average SFP is regarded as the type of movement shown by most sperm observed.

The slide is kept at room temperature in a petri dish on moist gauze and re-examined after 1.5 hours. After this, the petri dish with the slide is incubated at 37°C and examined every 2 to 4 hours. Although not physiological, the purpose of this step is two-fold. The first purpose is to monitor motility and SFP as a function of time under laboratory conditions. Normal sperm show a gradual loss of motility and SFP but still exhibit some motility after 8 hours. The second is to better observe certain aspects, such as agglutination, the forming of spermine phosphate crystals, and the presence of micro-organisms. In the presence of metabolic abnormalities or antisperm antibodies, the motility loss will be exhibited much sooner.

MIXED ANTIGLOBULIN REACTION (MAR) TEST

A MAR test is routinely included in all semen analyses if a sufficient number of motile sperm are present. We use the method described by Jager (13) (also see part 1, section E of this chapter), which screens for the presence of sperm-bound antibodies.

For this test, a suspension of sensitized R_1R_2-erythrocytes (Rh antigens 1 and 2) is needed. The erythrocytes are sensitized by washing the type O Rh-positive erythrocytes three times with a phosphate-buffered saline (PBS) solution, pH 7.5. This suspension is mixed 5:1 with a strong, incomplete anti-D serum (Behring ORRA 20/21) and incubated at 37°C for 30 minutes. After incubation the suspension is again washed three times in PBS and suspended to a hematocrit of 5% to 10% (13).

A drop of semen is placed on a clean glass slide, followed by a drop of undiluted monospecifc antiserum to human immunoglobulin G (IgG) (Behring ORCM 04/05) and a drop of sensitized R_1R_2-erythrocyte suspension. Care should be taken that the drops do not touch each other, as this can influence the outcome of the test. The drops are thoroughly mixed with a coverslip and then covered by the same slip. The test is read after 10 minutes. No interpretation is made if no red blood cell agglutination is observed. The test is negative if no motile sperm are incorporated in the red cell agglutinates; as doubtful when <10% of motile sperm are incorporated; as positive if 10% to 90% of motile sperm are incorporated, and as strongly positive if >90% of motile sperm are incorporated in the red cell agglutinates. In all cases of a positive MAR test (>10%), blood and seminal plasma are obtained for subsequent testing; an immunobead test (14) will also be done with the next semen analysis.

SUPRAVITAL STAINING

A supravital staining (SVS) test is also performed on every sample if the concentration is ≥1.0 × 10^6/ml. We use the method of Dougherty (15) modified by Eliasson (16). A drop of semen is placed on a spotplate and mixed with one drop of a 1% aqueous eosin Y solution; after 15 seconds two drops of a 10% aqueous nigrosin solution are added and thoroughly mixed. A drop of this mixture is transferred to a clean glass slide; a thin smear is made and air dried. The smears are examined with a $100\times$ oil magnification. Live sperm appear white and dead sperm pink. If possible, 200 sperm are counted and the result expressed as the percentage of live sperm. This percentage should be higher than the estimated percentage of motile sperm, as there can be live but non-motile sperm present (16).

DETERMINATION OF SPERM CONCENTRATION

The method used for the determination of sperm concentration is as described by van Zyl (17, 18) and Menkveld (19). Instead of a white blood cell pipette, a standard glass tuberculin syringe (Super Eva Glass, Micromatic, Padova, Italy) is used.

According to the estimated number of sperm per LPF, a 1:10, 1:20, or 1:100 dilution is prepared. An aliquot of 0.2 ml of semen is transferred to a small Wassermann tube (75 $\times$ 13 mm). In a separate tube, 1.5 ml of dilution fluid is placed. The semen is drawn to the 0.05- or 0.1-ml mark for a 1:20 or 1:10 dilution, respectively. Then the syringe is filled to the 1.0-ml mark with the dilution fluid. The syringe is emptied into a clean tube. The suspension is left for 5 minutes at room temperature so that the sperm can become immobilized. For a 1:100 dilution, a 1:10 dilution of a 1:10 dilution is made. Although this requires more work, the accuracy of the counting procedure is increased. As Belding (20) has shown, the probability will be high that the measured concentration will consistently be lower than the true concentration in cases where high concentrations of sperm are not sufficiently diluted.

After standing for the desired time, the suspension is again thoroughly mixed and transferred to an improved Neubauer hemocytometer with double rulings (Assistent, West Germany) by means of a Pasteur pipette. Special high-quality coverslips are used. One white blood cell block, consisting of 16 small blocks, is counted on opposite locations on each side of the chamber to compensate for possible filling defects (21). Counts are performed in the standard fashion. The sperm concentration is calculated using the formula of Freund (4). Two dilutions are made for every sample; the average concentration is calculated and taken as the concentration for the sample (22). If the difference between the two samples is $>10\%$ for a concentration of $<60 \times 10^6$/ml and $>20\%$ for a concentration of $>60 \times 10^6$/ml, the dilutions are repeated (8).

The tuberculin syringe method has one disadvantage: a correction must be made for the extra volume that is drawn up into the tip of the syringe. The result must be multiplied by 0.8, 0.7, and 0.64 for 1:10, 1:20, and 1:100 dilutions, respectively. Despite this disadvantage, very accurate determinations are obtained, compared with the white blood cell pipette method and the Makler method (19).

MORPHOLOGY EVALUATION

We divide the morphology evaluation into two categories: the evaluation of sperm and the evaluation of semen cytology. Therefore, two slides are prepared: one thick smear for cytology and one thin smear for sperm evaluation.

Morphological Evaluation of Sperm

The morphological evaluation of sperm is done as described by Menkveld (1) and Kruger (23). Slides are thoroughly cleaned before use by washing in a detergent, rinsing in clean water, rinsing in alcohol, and drying (24). Coverslips are also washed with alcohol. For the sperm evaluation smear, a small drop of semen is used so that a very thin smear is prepared and so that all the sperm will be in one focus level. Each sperm can be visualized separately, and no more than 5 to 10 sperm will be present per visual field at oil magnification. The thickness of the smear can be controlled by altering the size of the semen drop and by adjusting the angle and speed of the slide used to make the smear (8, 12). The slides are left to air dry and are fixed in alcohol before staining. A modification of the Papanicolaou method is used.

Because there is still much controversy concerning the definition of a normal sperm, we use our own strict criteria based on the form of sperm found in good periovulatory cervical mucus drawn from the upper endocervical canal after coitus. Based on this, a normal sperm is defined as one with an oval form, a smooth contour, and an acrosome comprising 40% to 70% of the distal part of the head, without any abnormalities of the neck, midpiece, or tail, and with no cytoplasmic droplets of more than half of the sperm head, as described by Eliasson (8). We also use the dimensions described by Eliasson.

Our morphological classification is based on the methods of MacLeod (25, 26) and Eliasson (8). To be classified as normal, the whole sperm must appear to be normal. The other classes used are: too large, too small, tapering, and duplications. Sperm that cannot be placed in one of these groups are classified as amorphous. We added one class: a normal head with other abnormalities, such as an abnormal tail or neck, or with a cytoplasmic droplet. These abnormalities are recorded per 100 sperm. Precursors are also included in this group.

If possible, 200 sperm are evaluated. In case of any doubt about the dimensions of a sperm, the size is measured with a micrometer. All sperm should be evaluated not in one area but in several areas: the corners and the middle of the slide. This will increase the accuracy of the evaluation.

Evaluation of Semen Cytology

For the evaluation of the semen cytology, by which is meant the investigation of the sample for the presence of different cells and microorganisms, a thicker smear is prepared. A small drop of egg albumin is added to ensure a better adherence of the cells to the slide. The slide is fixed immediately in a 1:1 mixture of ether alcohol and stained together with the slides for the sperm evaluation.

The slides are screened at a low magnification ($15 \times$); if any cells or organisms are observed, a $40 \times$ objective is used to make a better diagnosis. Cells especially looked for are white blood cells (polymorphs), epithelial cells, histiocytes, and ghost cells. The presence of these cells is recorded separately with the following symbols: $-$, no cells; $\pm$, occasional; $+$, 1 to 5/HPF; $++$, 5 to 10/HPF, and $+++$, >10/HPF.

Interpretation of Results

It must be stressed that the results of a semen analysis cannot be correctly interpreted if the background data are not known. Even more conclusions can be drawn if information on personal habits and medical history is also available. It is important to remember that certain general sources of variation (seasonal, occupational, stress, and illness) may play a role; some of these sources are discussed below. Because of these variations, care should be taken not to make a diagnosis based on only one semen analysis.

Table 5.5.
Average Semen Parameter Values of a Group of 4455 Men Seen Over a Period of 15 Years at Tygerberg Hospital

Semen Parameter	Average Values
Sperm concentration ($\times 10^6$/ml)	43.98
Volume (ml)	3.03
Motility (% motile)	48.70
Speed of forward progression[a]	2.54
Supravital staining (% live)	60.10
Morphology (% normal)	44.10

[a]On a scale of 1 to 4.

The evaluation of a semen specimen must be based on an overall picture that relates seminal volume, sperm concentration, quantitative and qualitative motility, morphological evaluation, the results of additional tests, such as the MAR test, and biochemical results. Even when results are far below the normal values of a laboratory, conception can still occur, although the time required to reach this goal may be longer.

A distinction should be made according to the reason for which the semen analysis was requested. Results of an analysis which may give a bad prognosis for in vivo fertilization may still be adequate for in vitro fertilization. Calculating an index of the total concentration of morphologically normal motile sperm may be useful for IVF but of little relevance for in vivo fertilization, since volume plays an important part in these calculations. It is known that oligozoospermia is frequently associated with large volume, which must be regarded as an abnormal parameter and therefore cannot be used to calculate such an index. Much has been written about interrelationships of semen parameters (7, 25) and their compensating interactions.

Although there may be a tendency for high sperm concentrations to be associated with higher percentages of motility and normal morphology (25), we have seen many exceptions, especially in morphology (1). In cases where the volume is within the normal range, some compensating interaction may occur but will be limited. In calculating normal and minimal values for conception based on the occurrence of conception in an infertile population, we observed that a single constantly abnormal parameter could be associated with no or only sporadic conception in apparently normal women (27).

SOURCE OF VARIATION

Many sources of variation are known, but only some of those that can cause major variations in semen parameters, such as abstinence or illness, and those that are less obvious are discussed. (For a comparison with our average semen values, see Table 5.5).

Decreasing Semen Parameters

Since the publication of the article by Nelson and Bunge (28) in 1974, there has been much discussion about whether the overall sperm counts of fertile and infertile populations are decreasing. This is supported by many researchers (29–31) and opposed by others (32, 33).

Mortimer (7) warned that one must be cautious in making such a statement, as numerous factors other than an evolutionary biological shift may be involved, not the least being technical error, statistical analysis of data, and the difference in reference populations.

We have found no decrease in sperm concentration, motility, and sperm fertilizing potential over a 15-year period (34). We did, however, find a decrease in the percentage of morphologically normal sperm: from 61.3% and 68.5% for our white and black populations in 1968 to 28.7% and 29.0%, respectively, in 1982. The Pearson correlation coefficients of -0.3403 and -0.4156 for the white and black populations were statistically significant. The decrease was attributed to the incorporation of stricter evaluation criteria and to a real decrease due to possible environmental and socioeconomic changes. The decline was much stronger in the black population, in which greater socioeconomic changes occurred.

Abstinence

Today it is an accepted fact that abstinence has a pronounced effect on semen parameters (7, 35–37). This is because the production of sperm and of secretions of the accessory glands that form the seminal plasma is a continuous process. The effect of abstinence can vary from a small change, or none, to a statistically significant difference in morphology, vitality, motility, concentration, and volume (7, 35–37).

We have found similar effects (1). There was a nearly linear increase of 0.34 ml/day in the volume, from 2.53 ± 1.8 ml with 1 day of abstinence to 3.98 ± 1.9 with 5 days.

The influence on sperm concentration was also marked. Although a small decrease was seen with 1 to 2 days of abstinence, concentration thereafter increased with every day the abstinence increased, up to 6 to 9 days. The average sperm concentration with 1 day of abstinence was $30.16 \pm 33.1 \times 10^6$/ml; for 6 to 9 days of abstinence, the concentration was $55.75 \pm 64.0 \times 10^6$/ml.

There was a decrease in the percentage of motile sperm. The best motility, $50.6 \pm 13.3\%$, was found in men with 1 day of abstinence; it decreased to $40.7 \pm 14.9\%$ for men with ≥ 21 days of abstinence. There was no change in the SFP.

The percentage of morphologically normal sperm followed an unexpected pattern. There was a drop in the percentage of normal forms if the abstinence increased from 1 to 2 days. After that, the percentage of normal forms increased when abstinence increased to 3 to 4 days, where the highest value, $44.8 \pm 18.2\%$, was found. With every additional day of abstinence, the percentage of normal forms also decreased. We concluded that optimal semen parameters are obtained with abstinence of 3 to 5 days, in agreement with the 2 to 5 days suggested by Mortimer (7).

Seasonal Influences

It is generally accepted that the human is not a seasonal breeder and that spermatogenesis is a continuous and active process throughout the year; however, some authors have investigated a possible seasonal influence (11, 38–40), mainly from increased summer temperatures which affect sperm concentration and/or morphology. The article of Tjoa (39) is the only one in which distinct differences are found; his study was done in an area known for its high daytime temperatures, averaging up to 28.9°C. Bornman (41) found a decrease but only in the percentage of normal forms. His study was done in the Pretoria area of South Africa, where summer daytime temperatures can reach up to 34°C. We found only a small tendency for a higher median sperm concentration in the late winter and early spring, with the highest median concentration, 40.16×10^6/ml, in

September. The temperatures in the Cape Town area are very mild, with an average maximum summer temperature of 26.3°C in January.

Occupational Influences

Men in certain occupations have impaired fertility potential. Lancranjan (42) found decreased fertility in men exposed to lead. The greater the exposure, the more severe was the impairment, which was noted in all semen parameters. Other investigations have been done on men working in dibutyl phthalate (DBP) plants (43) and on lorry (truck) drivers (44). Higher incidences of impaired parameters were found in these groups.

In an analysis of our patients, we also found that lorry drivers, metal workers, electricians, and military men had a lower incidence of fertility based on our criteria (Table 5.4): 59.1%, 56.4%, 58.3%, and 58.6% respectively, compared to an overall incidence of 64.5%.

Couples in the lower socioeconomic groups had a higher incidence of primary infertility (80.0% to 86.4%) than the overall incidence, 77.0%.

Couples in the higher socioeconomic groups, especially clergy, engineers, and attorneys, had a higher incidence of secondary infertility (38.5%, 31.1%, and 48.6%, respectively) than the overall incidence, 23.0%. The incidence of infertile males in these groups, however, was not higher than the average overall incidence. Increased environmental stress with increasing job demands may play a substantial role in this phenomenon.

Influence of Illness

Mention is often made in the literature on male infertility that a common cold, a bout of influenza, or some other febrile illness affects sperm concentration, and questions regarding illness should be included in the questionnaire to be completed with the first or every semen analysis (6, 7).

MacLeod (45, 46) demonstrated the effect of a viral infection with fever and the effect of chicken pox on semen quality. He found an effect on sperm concentration, motility, SFP, and morphology.

We have often seen the same effect in our patients. Because the effect can be quite drastic and is an important factor in evaluating the semen analysis results, two cases are presented to illustrate it (Tables 5.6 and 5.7). From these cases, it appears that the motility, SFP, and percentage of morphologically normal sperm are the parameters first showing the negative effects of illness. It takes longer for the negative effect to be reflected in a reduction of sperm concentration because there is already a supply of sperm in the genital tract. This would also suggest that sperm morphology and movement can be altered in the genital tract. The fact that the negative effect of illness on sperm morphology is the slowest to be detected and is the longest lasting may indicate that spermatogenesis and spermiogenesis are very sensitive.

Conclusion

Valuable information can be obtained from a semen analysis if the analysis is done correctly and skillfully. It is of utmost importance to obtain as much background data as possible. The adverse environmental effects investigated in our studies (1) seem to have their most pronounced effects on the percentage of normal morphology; these include the

Table 5.6.
Influence of Viral Infection with Increased Temperature on Semen Parameters: Case 1

Date of Semen Analysis	Abstinence (days)	Semen Parameters				
		Volume (ml)	Count ($\times 10^6$/ml)	Motility (% motile)	Forward Progression[a]	Morphology (% normal)
13-6-85	1	2.5	52.64	60	3.0	20
23–6 to 27–6–85	Viral infection. Temperature 39.4°C					
1-7-85	2	2.5	109.44	50	3.0	18
8-7-85	2	3.0	101.12	40	2.5	9
15-7-85	2	3.0	35.84	30	2.0	4
23-7-85	3	2.6	60.74	30	2.0	5
5-8-85	2	2.5	67.80	40	3.0	6
13-8-85	3	2.5	107.88	40	3.0	8
7-9-85	2	2.2	73.60	60	3.0	23

[a]On a scale of 1 to 4.

Table 5.7.
Influence of Viral Infection with Increased Temperature on Semen Parameters: Case 2[a]

Date of Semen Analysis	Abstinence (days)	Semen Parameters				
		Volume (ml)	Count ($\times 10^6$/ml)	Motility (% motile)	Forward Progression[b]	Morphology (% normal)
17-5-82	4	2.9	158.72	50	3.0	51
14-6-82	2	1.2	37.66	<10	1.5	46
19-7-82	4	2.9	96.96	50	3.0	27
9-8-82	4	3.1	74.08	60	3.0	47

[a]The illness occurred just before the first semen analysis.
[b]On a scale of 1 to 4.

effects of smoking and varicocele. We concluded that morphology is a very sensitive parameter that will reflect any adverse influence on the body, especially the testes, in a short time. Any illness or infection will cause a temporary decrease in the percentage of morphologically normal forms, after which the percentage will return to its original value. However, if the testes are repeatedly attacked by adverse influences or conditions, these will cause histological changes in the lamina propria and basal membrane. This will influence spermatogenesis, as reflected first in a gradual lowering of the percentage of normal forms, an increase in the percentage of elongated sperm, and in increase in the number of immature forms, then by a decrease in sperm concentration (1).

References

1. Menkveld R: An investigation of environmental influences on spermatogenesis and semen parameters (Ph.D. Dissertation). Faculty of Medicine, University of Stellenbosch, South Africa, 1987
2. MacLeod J: The semen examination. Clin Obstet Gynaecol 8:115, 1965
3. Hellinga G: Clinical Andrology. London: William Heinemann, 1976
4. Freund M: Semen analysis. In Behrman SJ, Kistner RW (eds): Progress in Infertility. Boston: Little, Brown & Co., 1968, p. 593
5. Zaneveld LDJ, Polakoski KL: Collection and the physical examination of the ejaculate. In Hafez ESE (ed): Techniques of Human Andrology. Amsterdam: Elsevier, 1977, p. 147
6. Schirren C: Practical Andrology. Berlin: Verlay Brüder Hartman, 1972, p. 10

7. Mortimer D: The male factor in infertility. I. Semen analysis. Cur Probl Obst et Gynecol Fertil 8:4, 1985
8. Eliasson R: Standards for the investigation of human semen. Andrologie 3:49, 1971
9. Rose N, Hjort T, Rümke P, Harper MJK, Vyazox O: Techniques for detection of iso- and auto-antibodies to human spermatozoa. Clin Exp Immunol 23:175, 1976
10. World Health Organization: Laboratory Manual for the Examination of Human Semen and Semen-Cervical Mucus Interaction, 2nd ed. Cambridge: Cambridge University Press, 1987, p. 6
11. MacLeod J, Heim LM: Characteristics and variation in semen specimens in 100 normal young men. J Urol 54:474, 1945
12. Hotchkiss RS: Fertility in men. London: William Heinemann, 1945
13. Jager S, Kremer J, Van Slochteren-Draaisma T: A simple method of screening for antisperm antibodies in the human male: detection of spermatozoal surface IgG with the direct mixed antiglobulin reaction carried out on untreated fresh human semen. Int J Fertil 23:12, 1978
14. Clarke GN, Stojanoff A, Cauchi MN: Immunoglobulin class of sperm-bound antibodies in semen. In Branatov K (ed): Immunology of Reproduction: Proceedings of the Fifth International Symposium on Immunology of Reproduction. Sofia: Bulgarian Academy of Sciences, 1982, p. 482
15. Dougherty KA, Emilson LVB, Cockett ATK, Urry RL: A comparison of subjective measurements of human sperm motility and viability with two live-dead staining techniques. Fertil Steril 26:700, 1975
16. Eliasson R: Supravital staining of human spermatozoa. Fertil Steril 28:1257, 1977
17. van Zyl JA: A review of the male factor in 231 infertile couples. S Afr J Obstet Gynaecol 10:17, 1972
18. van Zyl JA: The infertile couple. II. Examination and evaluation of semen. S Afr Med J 57:485, 1980
19. Menkveld R, van Zyl JA, Kotze TJvW: A statistical comparison of three methods for the counting of human spermatozoa. Andrologia 16:544, 1984
20. Belding DL: Fertility in the male. II. Technique of the spermatozoa count. Am J Obstet Gynecol 27:25, 1934
21. Chamberlain AC, Turner FM: Errors and variations in the white-cell counts. Biometrics 8:55, 1952
22. Berkson J, Magath TB, Hurn M: Error of estimate of the blood cell count as made in the hemocytometer. Am J Physiol 128:309, 1940
23. Kruger TF, Menkveld R, Stander FSH, Lombaard CJ, Van der Merwe JP, van Zyl JA, Smith K: Sperm morphologic features as a prognostic factor in in vitro fertilization. Fertil Steril 46:1118, 1986
24. World Health Organization: Laboratory Manual for the Examination of Human Semen and Semen-Cervical Mucus Interaction, 1st ed. Singapore: Press Concern, 1980
25. MacLeod J, Gold RZ: The male factor in fertility and infertility. IV. Sperm morphology in fertile and infertile marriages. Fertil Steril 2:394, 1952
26. MacLeod J: A possible factor in etiology of human male infertility. Fertil Steril 13:29, 1962
27. van Zyl JA, Menkveld R, Kotze TJvW, Van Niekerk WA: The importance of spermiograms that meet the requirements of international standards and the most important factors that influence semen parameters. In: Proceedings of the 17th Congress of the International Urological Society, V. 2. Paris: Diffusion Doin, 1976, p. 263
28. Nelson CMK, Bunge RG: Semen analysis: evidence for changing parameters of male fertility potential. Fertil Steril 25:503, 1974
29. Smith KD, Steinberger E: What is oligospermia? In Troen P, Nankin HR (eds): The Testis in Normal and Infertile Men. New York: Raven Press, 1977, p. 489
30. James WH: Secular trend in reported sperm counts. Andrologia 12:381, 1980
31. Leto S, Frensilli FJ: Changing parameters of donor semen. Fertil Steril 36:766, 1981
32. MacLeod J, Wang Y: Male fertility in terms of semen quality: a review of the past, a study of the present. Fertil Steril 31:103, 1979
33. David G, Jouannet P, Martin-Boyce A, Spira A, Schwartz D: Sperm counts in fertile and infertile men. Fertil Steril 31:453, 1979
34. Menkveld R, van Zyl JA, Kotze TJvW, Joubert G: Possible change in male fertility over a 15-year period. Arch Androl 17:143, 1986
35. MacLeod J, Gold RZ: The male factor in infertility and fertility. V. Effect of continence on sperm quality. Fertil Steril 3:297, 1952
36. Mortimer D, Templeton AA, Lenton EA, Coleman RA: Influence of abstinence and ejaculation of suspected infertile men. Arch Androl 8:251, 1982
37. Schwartz D, Mayaux MJ, Guihard-Moscato ML, Spria A, Jouannet P, Czyglik F, David G: Study of sperm morphologic characteristics in a group of 833 fertile men. Andrologia 16:423, 1983

38. Mortimer D, Tempelton AA, Lenton EA, Coleman RA: Annual patterns of human sperm production and semen quality. Arch Androl 10:1, 1983

39. Tjoa WS, Smolensky MH, Hsi BP, Steinberger E, Smith KD: Circannual rhythm in human sperm count revealed by serially independent sampling. Fertil Steril 38:454, 1982

40. Hotchkiss RS: Factors in stability and variability of semen specimens: observations on 640 successive samples from 23 men. J Urol 45:875, 1941

41. Bornman MS, Schullenburg GW, Boomkar D, Van der Merwe CA, Reif S: Ambient temperature and semen quality (Abstract). Reproductive Biology Workshop, Faculty of Medicine, University of Pretoria, South Africa, 1987

42. Lancranjan I, Popescu HI, Gavanescu O, Klepsch I, Serbanescu M: Reproductive ability of workmen occupationally exposed to lead. Arch Environ Health 30:396, 1975

43. Whorton JD, Meyer CR: Sperm count results from 861 American chemical/agricultural workers from 14 separate studies. Fertil Steril 42:82, 1984

44. Sas M, Szöllösi J: Impaired spermiogenesis as a common finding among professional drivers. Arch Androl 3:57, 1979

45. MacLeod J: The clinical implications of deviations in human spermatogenesis as evidenced in seminal cytology and the experimental production of these derivations. In: Proceedings of the Fifth World Congress on Fertility and Sterility, Stockholm, 1965. Excerpta Medica International Congress Series 133, 1966, p. 563

46. MacLeod J: Effect of chicken pox and of penumonia on semen quality. Fertil Steril 2:523, 1951

Section A3:

BASIC SEMEN ANALYSIS: CLINICAL IMPORTANCE OF MORPHOLOGY

THINUS F. KRUGER, M.D., ANIBAL A. ACOSTA, M.D., ROELOF MENKVELD, PH.D., AND SERGIO OEHNINGER, M.D.

Today in vitro fertilization (IVF) not only plays an important role in the management of infertile couples but also has led to a better understanding of the basic physiological principles of, for example, ovulation induction and male infertility (1). Several categories of male infertility can be encountered: severe oligozoospermia, oligoteratozoospermia, pure teratozoospermia, asthenoteratozoospermia, asthenozoospermia, and oligoasthenoteratozoospermia (2). It is very important to recognize that one of the problems in the evaluation of male infertility is that, when patients are not categorized as mentioned above, the investigative results are often confusing and difficult to interpret. One category of great interest to us is pure teratozoospermia: normal spermatozoa concentration and motility but a low percentage of normal sperm morphology.

Sperm Morphology

EVALUATION

Evaluation of the percentage of normal sperm morphological features is subjective and difficult to compare among the laboratories of the world, and different means of assessing these features have been described (3, 4). Furthermore, the role of sperm morphology as a predictor of penetration capacity in the hamster zona-free oocyte sperm penetration assay (SPA) (5) and of fertilization potential in human IVF programs (6) has been questioned by some researchers. Although it is difficult to compare morphological features, the critical issue is what these features tell us in an IVF program.

Spermatozoa are considered normal when the head has a smooth, oval configuration, with a well-defined acrosome involving about 40 % to 70% of the sperm head; absence of defects in the neck, midpiece, and tail; and no cytoplasmic droplets of more than half the size of the sperm head. Kruger (4) counts borderline forms as abnormal, in contrast to Eliasson (3).

In a study of sperm morphology, at least 200 cells per slide were evaluated. All male patients selected for study were required to have a concentration of $>20 \times 10^6$ sperm per milliliter and a normally motile sperm fraction of $>30\%$ (7, 8) in the basic semen analysis to minimize the impact of these two variables on the fertilization rate (8).

PREDICTIVE ROLE OF BASIC SEMEN ANALYSIS

In a prospective study of 129 male patients in 190 cycles, Kruger (4) divided the patients into four groups based on their percentage of normal morphology. According to criteria set by van Zyl (7), all patients had a sperm concentration of $>20 \times 10^6$/ml, with a normal motility of $>30\%$. Group 1 had a normal morphology of 0 to 14%; group 2, 15% to 30%; group 3, 31% to 45%; and group 4, 46% to 60%. In group 1, 104 oocytes were obtained; of these, 37% fertilized. In group 2 there were 324 oocytes, with a fertilization rate of 81%. In group 3, 309 oocytes produced a fertilization rate of 82%, and in group 4, 69 oocytes produced a fertilization rate of 91%.

A clear threshold of 14% normal sperm morphology was observed. No pregnancy was achieved in the group with $<14\%$ normal morphology. A pregnancy rate per embryo transfer of 25.8% was seen in the group with $>14\%$ normal morphology if three or more oocytes were retrieved; the rate was 11.4% if one or two oocytes were retrieved.

In a similar study at the Jones Institute, Kruger (8) used the same threshold, with a fertilization rate of 49.4% in the group with $<14\%$ normal morphology and a rate of 88.3% in the group with $>14\%$ normal morphology ($P<0.0001$). To select an accurate threshold, stricter criteria of normal morphology than those of the World Health Organization were used. Borderline forms were classified as abnormal, contributing to the low percentage of normal morphology. With the possibilities offered by evaluating egg-sperm interaction in vitro, a much better understanding of the meaning of normal morphology can be obtained.

Patterns in Patients with <14% Normal Morphology

Although there is severe impairment in the fertilization rate of patients with $<14\%$ normal morphology, some can still fertilize the human egg. Researchers at the Jones

Institute (9) studied 45 patients with <14% normal morphology to seek a morphological pattern which would differentiate the subgroup who fertilize from the subgroup who do not. All male patients had a sperm concentration of >20 × 10^6/ml and a motile sperm fraction of ≥30% in the basic semen analysis to minimize the impact of these two variables on the fertilization rate. They were divided into two groups. Group 1 consisted of those who had fertilized no oocytes; group 2 consisted of those who had fertilized at least one oocyte. There was a significant difference between their percentages of normal morphology: 1.8% (standard error, 2.4) in group 1 and 7.7% (standard error, 3.3) in group 2 ($P<0.0001$) (9). The percentage of slightly amorphous head abnormalities was 14.8% (9.7) in group 1 and 28.4% (7.8) in group 2 ($P<0.0001$). The predictive value ($R^2=0.44$) of normal morphology was better than that of slightly amorphous forms ($R^2=0.36$). No other sperm abnormalities showed a significant difference between the two groups. When the percentage of normal morphology and the percentage of slightly amorphous abnormalities were added and analyzed by multiple regression, there was a highly significant regression relationship ($P<0.0001$), with an even better predictive value ($R^2=0.56$). The combined percentage of slightly amorphous and normal forms (morphology index) was 19.7% (standard error 11.7) in group 1 and 42% (standard error, 7.8) in group 2.

The Statistical Analysis System (SAS) general linear model was used with the number of embryos as the dependent variable to determine a threshold at which the chances of fertilization were significantly impaired. A threshold of <4% was indicated for normal morphology; <30% was indicated for the morphology index (combined percentage of normal morphology and slightly amorphous forms) (9). The fertilization rate per oocyte in group 1 (morphology index <30%, normal morphology <4%) was 7.1%; in group 2 (>30%, >4%), 60.7%. The mean number of embryos in the 13 patients in group 1 was 0.4; for the 32 patients in group 2 it was 2.6. These means were significantly different ($P<0.0001$). The ongoing pregnancy rate in group 1 was 1 in 13, or 7.6%; in group 2 it was 6 in 32, or 18.75%, with 3 abortions and 1 ectopic pregnancy (9).

Our results indicate that severe impairment of fertilization takes place at a level of <4% normal morphology, based on the strict criteria explained above. Results also indicate that by adding the slightly amorphous and normal forms, a morphology index can be established with a cut-off figure of 30%. Patients with a value of <30% have a significantly smaller chance to fertilize than patients with a level >30% ($P<0.0001$). None of the other semen parameters evaluated were of any help in predicting a patient's chance to fertilize.

The advantage of strict morphology evaluation is that it is reproducible between patients and between technicians (10). It also allows the clinician to classify the patient into one of two specific groups (<14% and >14% normal morphology), providing a reliable criterion for counseling the patient and planning the approach in future IVF cycles (4, 8).

Based on the significant differences between normal morphology and the slightly amorphous forms in groups 1 and 2, we propose that two patterns can be observed in the <14% group. The P pattern (poor prognosis) has a mean normal morphology of <4%, and the G pattern (good prognosis) has 5% to 14% normal morphology. The G pattern gives the patient a significantly better chance to fertilize ($P<0.0001$) than the P pattern.

The evaluation of sperm morphology is a controversial issue. Results in fertilization rates differ among IVF units (4, 8, 11, 12). Do we look at the same spectrum of

Table 5.8.
Fertilization Rate of Patients with Teratozoospermia

	P Pattern (<4% Normal Forms)	G Pattern (4% to 14% Normal Forms)
Metaphase I oocytes	7 of 29 (24%)[a]	68 of 155 (43.8%)[b]
Metaphase II oocytes	3 of 15 (20%)[a]	65 of 112 (58.04%)[b]

[a]Not significant.
[b]$P<0.01$.

abnormalities, explaining the difference in results, or is our classification of abnormal and normal sperm morphology in need of revision? We believe that the latter is true and needs urgent attention (4, 8, 9).

Manipulation of Gametes In Vitro to Improve the Fertilization Rate

Once fertilization and cleavage have occurred in the group of patients with <14% normal morphology, their chance of a pregnancy is good. This is perhaps more applicable to the G pattern (10). Increasing the concentration of spermatozoa in vitro from 100,000/ml to 500,000/ml improves the fertilization rate significantly (13). However, the pregnancy outcome in the P-pattern group was 4.1%, compared to 17.8% in the G-pattern group (9).

Another factor of utmost importance in handling patients with teratozoospermia—and perhaps all male factor patients—is the maturity of the oocytes. Patients were divided into two groups: those with <4% normal forms (P pattern) and those with 5% to 14% normal forms (G pattern). Oocytes were classified into metaphase I and II, according to the criteria of Veeck (14), 6 hours after retrieval and were fertilized at that time with 100,000 sperm per milliliter. The fertilization rate in the P-pattern group was 7 of 29 metaphase I oocytes (24.1%) and 3 of 15 metaphase II oocytes (20%) (Table 5.8). In the G-pattern group, the fertilization rate was 68 of 155 metaphase I oocytes (43.8%) and 65 of 112 metaphase II oocytes (58.04%) ($P<0.01$). The conclusion was drawn that, in the G-pattern group, selection of oocytes according to the criteria of Veeck (14) can influence the prognosis of fertilization and pregnancy outcome. In the P-pattern group, the fertilization rate did not differ significantly; although the numbers were small, it is well known that the prognosis of these patients is very poor (9). The delayed insemination principle reported by Trounson (15) is questionable when we treat male infertility, and specifically those with teratozoospermia.

It is also important to note that the oocyte classification which we used in the past, derived from the work of Testart (16), did not distinguish between metaphase I and II, although a so-called mature oocyte was retrived. In a study by Stander (unpublished data), this fact was pointed out. Kruger (17) used a grading system with an 8-point scale to indicate oocyte maturity, with >6 of 8 indicating a mature oocyte. This system was correlated with metaphase I and II oocytes in patients with all semen parameters normal and with a sperm morphology of >14% normal forms. In the metaphase I group, 66 oocytes had a score of ≥6; in the metaphase II group 71 had this score. No correlation was found between the scoring system and the metaphase stage of the oocyte. The oocytes were evaluated 6 hours after retrieval; soon afterward, insemination was performed. The fertilization rate in both groups was good, 87.9% in the metaphase I group and 98.6% in the metaphase II group.

Although the fertilization rate was good in the fertile group, the same observation was not made in the group with <14% normal morphology. In that group, the quality of the oocytes, particularly the distinction between metaphase I and II oocytes, became extremely important.

Thus, a clear trend was observed. Not only the recognition of the specific male problem was important but also the ability to distinguish between metaphase I and II oocytes. By doing this and by increasing the concentration of the spermatozoa to 500,000/ml for in vitro insemination, the fertilization rate will be signficantly improved.

Summary

It has been pointed out in this chapter that if sperm morphology is classified according to the strict criteria we have laid down, this parameter can be used as a predictor of fertilization. Swim-up morphology can also be used to distinguish between different categories of patients with poor prognosis in vitro.

We advocate that failure of fertilization in vitro can often be attributed to a a morphological problem of the spermatozoa. Patients with a sperm morphology <14% normal sperm fertilize fewer eggs in vitro when we use 100,000 sperm per milliliter and can be divided into two groups (P pattern and G pattern) according the fertilization rate and prognosis. By increasing the concentration of spermatozoa to 500,000/ml and taking into consideration the *maturity* of the oocyte, the prognosis of these patients can be significantly improved.

References

1. Acosta AA, Chillik CF, Brugo S, Ackerman S, Swanson RJ, Pleban P, Yuan J, Haque D: In vitro fertilization and the male factor. Urol 28:1, 1986
2. De Kretser DM, Yates C, Kovacs GT: The use of IVF in the management of male infertility. Clin Obstet Gynaecol 12(4): 767–773, 1985
3. Eliasson R: Standards for investigation of human semen. Andrologia 3:49, 1971
4. Kruger TF, Menkveld R, Stander FSH, Lombard CJ, Van der Merwe JP, van Zyl JA, Smith K: Sperm morphology as a prognostic factor in in vitro fertilization (IVF). Fertil Steril 46:1118, 1986
5. Aitken RJ, Best FSM, Richardson DW, Djahanbakhch O, Mortimer D, Templeton AA, Lees MM: An analysis of sperm function in cases of unexplained infertility: conventional criteria, movement characteristics, and fertilizing capacity. Fertil Steril 38:212, 1982
6. Hirch I, Gibbons WE, Lipshultz LI, Rossavik KK, Young RL, Dodson MG, Findley WE: In vitro fertilizaiton in couples with male factor infertility. Fertil Steril 45:659, 1986
7. van Zyl JA, Menkveld R, Kotze TJvW, Van Niekerk WA: The importance of spermiograms that meet the requirements of international standards and the most important factors that influence semen parameters. In: Proceedings of the 17th International Society of Urology. Paris: Diffusion Doin, 2:263, 1976
8. Kruger TF, Acosta AA, Simmons KF, Swanson JR, Matta JF, Veeck LL, Morshedi M, Brugo S: A new method of evaluating sperm morphology with predictive value for IVF. Urol 30:248, 1987
9. Kruger, TF, Acosta AA, Simmons KF, Swanson RJ, Matta JF, Oehninger S: Predictive value of abnormal sperm morphology in in vitro fertilization. Fertil Steril 49:112, 1988
10. Kruger TF, Ackerman SB, Simmons KF, Swanson RJ, Brugo S, Acosta AA: A quick reliable staining technique for sperm morphology. Arch Androl 18:275, 1987

11. Mahadevan MM, Trounson AO: The influence of seminal characteristics on the success rate of human in virto fertilization. Fertil Steril 42:400, 1984
12. Alper MM, Lee GS, Seibel MM, Smith D, Oskowitz SP, Ransil BF, Taymor ML: The relationship of semen parameters to fertilization in patients participating in a program of in vitro fertilization. J In Vitro Fertil Embryo Trans 2:217, 1985
13. Oehninger S, Acosta AA, Morshedi M, Veeck L, Swanson RJ, Simmons K. Rosenwaks Z: Corrective measures and pregnancy outcome in in vitro fertilization in patients with severe sperm morphology abnormalities. Fertil Steril 50:283, 1988
14. Veeck LL, Maloney M: Insemination and fertilization. In Jones HW Jr, Jones GS, Hodgen GD, Rosenwaks Z (eds): In Vitro Fertilization—Norfolk. Baltimore: Williams & Wilkins, 1986, p 168
15. Trounson AO, Mohr LR, Wood C, Leeton JF: Effect of delayed insemination on in vitro fertilization culture and transfer of human embryos. J Reprod Fertil 64:285, 1982
16. Testart J, Frydman R, De Mouzon J, Lassale B, Belaisch-Allart JC: A study of factors affecting the success of human fertilization in vitro. I. Influence of ovarian stimulation upon the number and condition of oocytes collected. Biol Reprod 28:415, 1983
17. Kruger TF, Stander FSH, Smith K, Van der Merwe JP, Lombard CJ: The effect of serum supplementation on the cleavage of human embryos. J In Vitro Fertil Embryo Trans 4:10, 1987

Section B:

SPERMATOZOA MOTILE FRACTION SEPARATION

THINUS F. KRUGER, M.D., ROELOF MENKVELD, PH.D., RICHARD T. SCOTT, M.D., RAJASINGAM S. JEYENDRAN, D.V.M., PH.D., LOURENS J.D. ZANEVELD, D.V.M., PH.D., AND MARIE-LENA WINDT, M.S.

In our laboratory, washed semen is used for artificial insemination by husband (AIH), in vitro fertilization (IVF), and gamete intrafallopian transfer (GIFT). Trounson's method of preparation (1) is used.

Liquefied semen samples obtained by masturbation after 3 days of abstinence are mixed with 2 ml of Ham's F-10 medium plus 10% human serum (midcycle from wife). The mixture is centrifuged at 1500 rpm for 10 minutes. This is repeated once with 10 ml of Ham's F-10 plus 10% serum. The resultant pellet is overlaid with 0.5 to 1 ml of Ham's F-10 plus 10% serum and incubated at 37°C for 30 to 60 minutes. Motile sperm swim up into the layer of medium, which is then pipetted off for use in AIH, IVF, or GIFT.

In all cases, an estimated count, motility, and forward progression are noted in the samples before the wash procedure. A slide for morphology evaluation is also prepared. Slight modifications are made, depending on the procedure to be carried out.

Methods of Sperm Wash

FOR AIH

For intrauterine insemination, the whole semen sample is mixed with 2 ml of Ham's F-10 plus 10% serum and centrifuged at 1500 rpm for 10 minutes; the supernatant is discarded. The pellet is washed once more with 2 ml of Ham's F-10 plus 10% serum. The final pellet is overlaid with 0.8 ml of Ham's F-10 plus 10% serum and incubated for 1 hour at 37°C to allow sperm swim-up. Then 0.5 to 0.7 ml of the top layer is aspirated; the count, motility, and forward progression are noted and used for insemination. A morphology slide of the swim-up sample is prepared for later evaluation.

FOR IVF AND GIFT

In the wash procedure for IVF and GIFT, 1 ml of semen is washed twice with 2 ml of Ham's F-10 plus 10% serum and centrifuged at 1500 rpm for 10 minutes. The final sperm pellet is overlaid with 1 ml of Ham's F-10 plus 10% serum. The sperm are allowed to swim up for 30 minutes at 37°C in an incubator with 5% CO_2 in air. The top layer containing the swim-up sperm is aspirated and investigated for concentration, motility, and forward progression; a slide is made for morphology. A count for the determination of the final swim-up sperm concentration is performed, and the appropriate volume is added to the ova to obtain the recommended number of sperm per ovum.

For GIFT, the resultant swim-up samples are diluted to a sperm concentration of 4 $\times$ 10^6/ml and 20 $\times$ 10^6/ml to get a final count of 100,000 and 500,000 sperm in normal males (>14% morphologically normal sperm) and in teratozoospermic males (<14% morphologically normal sperm), respectively.

We have found that when we use sperm preparations as described, we obtain improved semen samples. The resulting swim-up samples contain a high proportion of motile sperm (80% to 100%), with improved forward progression and free of any foreign cells or debris. Sperm survival is usually very good, up to 72 hours. We have also found an increased percentage of morphologically normal sperm in the swim-up samples.

FOR ANTISPERM ANTIBODIES

Our studies have shown that washed, swim-up sperm from men with antisperm antibodies do not differ from unwashed samples in terms of sperm-bound antibodies. Swim-up procedures are exactly the same as for AIH preparation, and antibodies are detected with the immunobead test (IBT) and sperm cervical mucus contact (SCMC) test before and after sperm separation. However, the semen parameters—morphology, forward progression, and motility—are all improved by the wash and swim-up procedures (2).

We also did a study on washed semen samples obtained by the method of Boettcher (3) and Harrison (4). Semen samples were ejaculated in 15 ml of Ham's F-10 plus 10% serum, mixed thoroughly, and incubated until liquefication was completed. The mixture was centrifuged at 1500 rpm for 10 minutes. Pooled pellets were washed once more, and the final pellet was covered with 1 ml of medium to allow swim-up. After 10 to 60 minutes at 37°C, the top layer was aspirated and analyzed. Results again showed no significant differences in sperm-bound antibodies between washed and unwashed samples, as detected by the IBT and SCMC tests. Resultant sperm parameters were again improved, as in the normal wash procedure (5).

Our results suggest that patients can achieve pregnancy despite antisperm antibodies (2, 5). Improvement in sperm parameters (2, 5), minimizing the distance between sperm and ova, and bypassing the cervical mucus may be reasons for the relatively high pregnancy rate.

Comparison of Sperm Morphology before and after Swim-Up for IVF

The correlation of sperm morphology using strict criteria and IVF fertilization rates is based on evaluations of morphology in the initial specimen. Since specimens undergo a double swim-up before insemination, the sperm used for insemination may not be accurately reflected by the sperm morphology of the initial specimen. Previous evaluations using the criteria of the World Health Organization have documented an improvement in sperm morphology following the double swim-up preparation (6). That study used less rigid criteria and did not correlate the magnitude of the improvements with the degree of abnormality in the initial specimen. Therefore, sperm morphology was analyzed before and after swim-up and was correlated with the percentage of improvement and morphology patterns.

The initial specimens of 73 consecutive IVF patients were evaluated for sperm morphology. The double swim-up was performed by standard techniques. The specimens were coded, randomized, and read in a double-blind manner. Statistical evaluations were performed using paired data analysis and contingency table analysis, as indicated.

Of the 73 patients, 62 showed an improvement in their normal forms ($P<0.001$). The mean percentage of normal forms in the pre- and post-swim-up specimens was 19.8% and 23.4%, respectively. This represents an 18% difference, which is statistically significant ($P<0.05$).

Of the 73 patients, 27 had abnormal morphology ($\leq14\%$ normal forms) upon evaluation of their initial specimens. Of these, 18 (67%) showed an improvement in normal forms, eight (30%) were unchanged, and only one (4%) showed a decline in the percentage of normal forms. The mean improvement in normal forms was from 8.2% to 20.0%, an increase of 243.9% ($P<0.005$).

These data support our observation that the double swim-up preparation enhances sperm morphology. The most substantial benefit seems to be in patients with abnormal morphology in their initial specimens.

Predictive Role of Swim-Up Morphology

In a study at the Reproductive Biology Unit of Tygerberg Hospital (Grobler, unpublished data), the role of swim-up morphology as a predictor of fertilization was studied in 122 IVF cycles of patients with $<14\%$ normal morphology by basic semen analysis. A sperm morphology slide was prepared after swim-up. The fertilization rate was 5.1%, or 3 of 58 oocytes, in the group with $<14\%$ normal swim-up morphology, and 35.2%, or 179 of 508 oocytes, in the group with $>14\%$ normal swim-up morphology ($P<0.01$). It was concluded that if, after swim-up, the normal sperm morphology is $<10\%$, the chance of fertilization is small; this fact can be used as a predictor of IVF outcome.

Glass Wool Filtration

Many techniques have been developed to recover viable sperm from an ejaculate for artificial insemination, IVF, and GIFT. However, many of these techniques yield a poor recovery of sperm or do not produce consistent results, particularly when the ejaculate is oligozoospermic, asthenozoospermic, or viscous. A technique that yields a high recovery of viable sperm from these ejaculates is therefore desirable. Glass wool filtration, as described by Jeyendran (7–8), is such a method.

Using the filtration technique, it was shown that all or almost all viable sperm in samples following centrifugation (washed sperm) or 50% to 70% of the viable sperm present in the unwashed ejaculate were recovered (7–9). The repeatability of the filtration technique was good, as assessed by determining the recovery of viable sperm from different aliquots of the same ejaculate. The reliability of the technique was tested by mixing known numbers of frozen-thawed sperm with untreated sperm prior to filtration. The relationship between the expected and observed sperm recovery was high ($r = 0.86$, $n = 12$) (10). The recovery of viable sperm by this filtration technique is much better than that obtained by swim-up procedures, especially in cases of viscous and/or oligozoospermic ejaculates (8), or asthenozoospermic ejaculates (11). A higher recovery of motile and hypo-osmotic swelling (HOS)-positive sperm is obtained from asthenozoospermic ejaculates by glass wool filtration than by a two-layer Percoll density gradient centrifugation technique (9).

The main purpose of treating an ejaculate is to select viable and potentially fertile sperm so that the sperm population has a higher fertilizing potential than the original ejaculate. Glass wool filtration has been criticized for causing latent injury to the membrane and acrosome of sperm heads (12), which may be detrimental to the fertilizing capacity of the sperm. These observations were based on an electron microscopic study of five ejaculates, during which some evidence of membrane damage was found. However, the sperm obtained by filtration survived cryopreservation as well as, or better than, those obtained from the unfiltered ejaculates. Also, the glass wool-filtered sperm survived storage at 22°C for 12 hours, better than sperm in the original ejaculate. Therefore, the functional studies do not support the electron microscopic observations. Another study did not find ultrastructural changes after glass wool filtration (10). Other data also argue against the occurrence of significant damage to the sperm membranes.

The filtration technique results in a significantly increased percentage of sperm with intact membranes as determined by the dye exclusion (viability) test and the HOS test (7). Sperm obtained by glass wool filtration have already been shown to be fertile. Seventy-six percent of the sperm samples ($n = 64$) obtained by glass wool filtration fertilized intact human oocytes (8). Of these, 11 resulted in pregnancies after embryo transfer. Paulson and Comhaire (13) and Jeyendran and Perez-Pelaez (14) reported pregnancies resulting from artificial insemination with glass wool-filtered sperm. Therefore, no good evidence exists that glass wool filtration leads to significant functional changes in the sperm.

Sperm recovered after glass wool filtration penetrate denuded hamster oocytes more successfully than untreated sperm, even after the samples are adjusted so that they contain the same number of motile sperm as unfiltered samples (15). Sperm in the first fraction of the filtrate were of higher quality than those of subsequent fractions or the original ejaculate, based on motility, velocity, hypo-osmotic swelling, acrosin activity, and the ability to penetrate denuded hamster oocytes (16).

In view of these data, filtering sperm through glass wool produces a much higher yield of viable sperm than the swim-up technique, possibly than other methods, particularly when the ejaculate is asthenozoospermic and/or oligozoospermic. Sperm recovered by glass wool filtration are fertile. Therefore, the technique is useful for the preparation of sperm for IVF, GIFT, or for intrauterine insemination. Some glass wool fibers may appear in the filtrate even after the column has been rinsed extensively. It is important to assure the absence of fibers by light microscopic observations before using glass wool-filtered sperm for artificial insemination.

References

1. Trounson AO, Mohr LR, Wood C, Leeton JF: Effect of delayed insemination on in vitro fertilization culture and transfer of human embryos. J Reprod Fertil 64:285, 1982
2. Windt M-L, Menkveld R, Kruger TF, Van der Merwe JP, van Zyl JA: The effect of sperm washing and swim-up on antibodies bound to sperm membrane: use of immunobead/sperm cervical mucus contact tests. Arch Androl 22:55, 1989
3. Boettcher B, Kay DJ, Fitchett SB: Successful treatment of male infertility caused by antispermatozoal antibodies. Med J Aust 2:471, 1982
4. Harrison KL, Hennessey JF: Treatment of male sperm autoimmunity by in-vitro fertilization with washed spermatozoa. Med J Aust 141:498, 1984
5. Windt M-L, Menkveld R, Kruger TF, Lombard JC: The effect of rapid dilution of semen on sperm-bound autoantibodies. Arch Androl (in press)
6. McDowell JS, Veeck LL, Jones HW Jr: Analysis of human spermatozoa before and after processing for in vitro fertilization. J In Vitro Fertil Embryo Trans 2:23, 1985
7. Jeyendran RS, Perez-Pelaez M, Crabo BG: Concentration of viable spermatozoa for artificial insemination. Fertil Steril 45:132, 1986
8. Van der Ven HH, Jeyendran RS, Tunnerhoff A, Hoebbel K, Al-Hasani S, Perez-Pelaez M: Glass wool column filtration of human semen: relation to swim-up procedure and IVF outcome. Human Reprod 3:85, 1988
9. Rhemrev J, Jeyendran RS, Zaneveld LJD: Selection of viable spermatozoa by glass wool filtration or Percoll density gradient centrifugation. J Androl 9:23, 1988
10. Jeyendran RS, Van der Ven HH, Perez-Pelaez M, Al-Hasani S, Diedrich K: Separation of viable spermatozoa by standardized glass wool column. Presented at the 12th World Congress on Fertility and Sterility, Singapore, 1986
11. Van der Ven HH, Tunnerhoff A, Al-Hasani S, Perez-Pelaez M, Diedrich K, Jeyendran RS: Effectiveness of concentrating viable spermatozoa by two sperm separation techniques from normal and asthenozoospermic semen. J Androl 7:5, 1986
12. Sherman JK, Paulson JD, Lin KC: Effect of glass wool filtration on ultrastructure of human spermatozoa. Fertil Steril 36:643, 1981
13. Paulson JD, Comhaire F: Filtration of human semen in glass wool column. In Negro-Vilar A (ed): Male Reproduction and Fertility. NY: Raven Press, 1983, p 319
14. Jeyendran RS, Perez-Pelaez M: Pregnancy following insemination with glass wool filtered spermatozoa. Rev Lat Am Esteril Fertil 1:150, 1987
15. Holmgren WJ, Jeyendran RS, Neff MR, Perez-Pelaez M: Ability of glass wool filtration to isolate fertile sperm fractions. J Androl 8:39, 1987
16. Jeyendran RS, Bielfeld P, Vantman D, Rachagan SP, Perez-Pelaez M, Zaneveld LJD: Selection of viable spermatozoa by glass wool column filtration. In: Proceedings of the IVth Annual Meeting of the European Society of Human Reproduction and Embryology, Barcelona, Spain, 1988, p 92

Section C:

MICROBIOLOGY AND LEUKOSPERMIA (MALE ACCESSORY GLANDS INFECTION)

FRANK H. COMHAIRE, M.D., AND AUK HINTING, M.D., PH.D.

Male Accessory Glands Infection

ROLE IN INFERTILITY AND IN VITRO FERTILIZATION

Some authors have reported that male accessory glands infection (MAGI) occurs twice as frequently in the male partners of infertile couples as in men with recently proven fertility. Others have suggested that the treatment of MAGI improves semen quality and fertility in subfertile men. However, double blind prospective trials with doxycycline treatment in our laboratory did not reveal any significant effect on pregnancy rate of subfertile couples with MAGI (1).

Although 13% of male partners of infertile couples fulfill the criteria for MAGI, in our study (1) MAGI with abnormal semen quality was the only demonstrable abnormality in only 1.6% of all infertile couples studied. Indeed, two-thirds of the female partners of these men presented abnormalities which impaired their fertility. Hence, MAGI with abnormal semen quality is rarely the only abnormality in infertile couples.

On the other hand, the presence of white blood cells, bacteria, or mycoplasmata and ureaplasmata has been reported to exert a disastrous effect on semen for in vitro fertilization (IVF) (2).

TREATMENT

For many years, doxycycline and co-trimoxazole have been advocated as the treatment of choice for chronic MAGI. Indeed, the concentration of doxycyline in the human prostate gland obtained during surgery was found to be elevated (3), and therefore this drug was thought to be efficient for the treatment of bacterial or mycoplasma prostatitis. Long-term treatment with co-trimoxazole was reported to improve the fertility of men suffering from prostato-vesiculitis and abnormal semen quality (4). However, no beneficial effect could be detected from either doxycycline or erythromycin in double blind prospective studies (1, 5). These discrepancies can be explained by the fact that changes in the pH of prostatic secretory fluid, due to chronic inflammation and functional impairment of the glandular epithelium, result in decreased concentration of doxycycline in the chronically infected prostate (6).

Improvement of sperm quality, particularly of sperm motility, also occurs during placebo treatment, suggesting spontaneous regression of the disease. The improved sperm characteristics, however, are not reflected in an improved fertilizing potential, as pregnancy rates remain unsatisfactory.

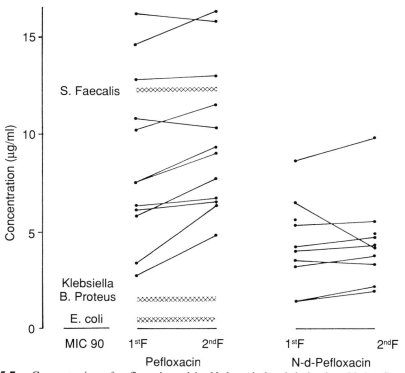

Figure 5.7.   Concentration of pefloxacin and its N demethylated derivative (N-d-pefloxacin) in fractions 1 (*1st F*) and 2 (*2nd F*) of split ejaculates of patients with male accessory gland infection. Minimal inhibitory concentrations (*MIC 90, crossed lines*) of pefloxacin for more common aerobic urinary tract pathogens also are shown. (From Comhaire FH: Concentration of pefloxacine in split ejaculates of patients with chronic male accessory gland infection. J Urol 138:828–830, 1987.)

Recently, substances of the quinolone group with antibacterial properties have been developed for the treatment of urinary tract infection. Whereas tissue penetration of so-called first and second generation quinolones was poor, substances of the third generation appeared to perform better in this respect. In view of the latter, several studies have been performed to measure the concentration of those quinolone derivatives in split ejaculates of patients with chronic MAGI. Our own study includes 12 men presenting with infertility or complaints suggestive of MAGI who fulfilled the criteria for MAGI. Split ejaculates were obtained before initiation of treatment and after 3 to 4 weeks of continuous intake of 400 mg of pefloxacin twice daily. The concentrations of pefloxacin and its *N*-demethylated derivative (norfloxacin) were assessed by single blind coded samples using high-pressure liquid chromatography. The concentrations were similar in both fractions of the split ejaculate, and there was a strong correlation between the concentration of either substance in fractions 1 (*1st F*) and 2 (*2nd F*) (Fig. 5.7).

The antibacterial activity of norfloxacin equals that of pefloxacin. Therefore, the therapeutic index (the sum of the concentration of pefloxacin + norfloxacin, divided by the minimal inhibitory concentration 90) in fraction 1 of the split ejaculate, which had a predominantly prostatic origin, and in fraction 2, which still originated from the seminal vesicles, was approximately 30 for *Escherichia coli* and *Klebsiella* species, more than 100 for *Proteus* species, and equal to 1 for *Streptococcus faecalis*.

On the basis of these findings, we concluded that pefloxacin and norfloxacin are excreted by the prostate and seminal vesicles of patients with chronic inflammation of these glands. Since the antibacterial activity of the secretory fluids is many times the minimal inhibitory concentration 90 for the more common aerobic bacteria involved in the pathogenesis of MAGI, these substances may be suitable for the treatment of prostatovesiculitis. Preliminary data on the clinical effectiveness of this treatment sustain this presumption.

EFFECT OF TREATMENT

Up to now, studies performed with antibiotics such as doxycycline, erythromycin, and co-trimoxazole have not revealed any effect on fertility superior to that of placebo. In spite of the improvement in sperm motility and sperm morphology, the pregnancy rate observed within the follow-up period of these studies was low and comparable to the expected non-treatment pregnancy rate (7, 8). It is speculated that treatment of infection remains ineffective because of irreversible impairment of both spermatogenesis and male accessory gland secretory function, once these have been damaged. As yet, no controlled prospective studies have been performed with the new quinolone derivatives, which seem to be more efficient in clearing infections. It should be stressed that it is difficult to find suitable couples for such studies, since MAGI with abnormal semen quality is rarely the only demonstrable abnormality in infertile couples.

Prevention of chronic MAGI appears to be the more logical approach. Indeed, in the majority of cases, chronic MAGI with abnormal semen quality is the consequence of poorly treated acute cysto-urethritis. During urethritis, bacteria invade the prostate and remain there in spite of treatment with urinary antiseptics or conventional antibiotics. Bacterial infestation may remain oligo- or asymptomatic for many years and become manifest only through male infertility. Adequate treatment of trivial cysto-urethritis with sufficiently high doses of the new quinolones, given for at least 10 days, can be expected to prevent development of chronic infection resulting in infertility.

ANTIBIOTIC TREATMENT FOR IN VITRO FERTILIZATION

Considering the detrimental effect of white blood cells and bacteria on the fertilizing potential of semen in vitro (9), all male partners of couples undergoing IVF should be investigated for MAGI. Semen analysis should include specific staining for white blood cells and bacterial cultures, including culture for mycoplasma and ureaplasma. Men harboring these infections should be treated with third generation quinolones in adequate doses for at least 10 days. Two weeks after interruption of the treatment, a new semen analysis, including culture, should be performed. Patients in whom bacterial infection is not cleared should undergo long-term treatment, but IVF can be attempted while the patient is still taking medication. Under these circumstances, spermatozoa should be isolated from the seminal plasma as soon as possible after ejaculation, using swim-up techniques.

ADDITION OF ANTIBIOTICS DURING SPERM MANIPULATION AND OOCYTE CULTURE

Some authors have reported that semen preparation techniques reduce bacterial contamination in human semen. The absence of bacteria after preparation is not due to a simple dilution effect of the medium (9). Among the techniques for semen preparation, only Percoll gradient is able to eliminate bacterial contamination without any addition of antibiotics to the medium (10). With antibiotic supplementation, however, the most commonly used method, washing and swim-up, is sufficiently effective in eliminating bacteria present in the untreated semen (11). Therefore, addition of antibiotics to the medium for sperm preparation and oocyte culture is recommended. Penicillin and streptomycin are generally used. These antibiotics have a wide spectrum of activity and remain stable in culture medium at 37°C for up to 3 days.

References

1. Comhaire FH, Rowe PJ, Farley TMM: The effect of doxycycline in infertile couples with male accessory gland infection: a double blind prospective study. Int J Androl 9:91, 1986
2. Cohen J, Edwards R, Fehilly C, Fishel S, Hewitt J, Purdy J, Rowland G, Steptoe P, Webster J: In vitro fertilization: a treatment for male infertility. Fertil Steril 43:422, 1985
3. Oosterlinck W, Wallijn E, Wijndaele JJ: The concentration of doxycycline in human prostate gland and its role in the treatment of prostatitis. Scand J Infect Dis 9:85, 1976
4. Fortune A: Co-trimoxazole in the treatment of prostatovesiculitis associated with a diagnosis of male infertility. Br J Sex Med 7:16, 1980
5. Baker HWG, Straffon WGE, McGowan MP, Burger HC, de Kretser DM, Hudson B: A controlled trial of the use of erythromycin for men with asthenospermia. Int J Androl 7:383, 1984
6. Comhaire F, Pieters O, Debrock M, Vermeulen L, Rowe P, Farley T: Importance of male accessory gland infection in fertility disorders. In Weidner W, Brunner H, Krause W, Rothauge CF (eds): Therapy of Prostatitis. Munich: W Zuckschwerdt, 1986, p 223
7. Collins JA, Wrixon W, Janes JB, Wilson EH: Treatment-independent pregnancy among infertile couples. N Engl J Med 309:1201, 1983
8. Comhaire FH: Simple model and empirical method for the estimation of spontaneous pregnancies in couples consulting for infertility. Int J Androl 10:671, 1987
9. Forman R, Guillett-Rosso F, Fari A, Volante M, Frydman R, Testart J: Importance of semen preparation in avoidance of reduced in vitro fertilization results attributable to bacteria. *Fertil Steril* 47:527, 1987
10. Sun LS, Gastaldi C, Peterson EM, de la Maza LM, Stone SC: Comparison of techniques for the selection of bacteria-free sperm preparations. *Fertil Steril* 48:659, 1987
11. Wong PC, Balmaceda JP, Blanco JD, Gibbs RS, Asch RH: Sperm washing and swim-up technique using antibiotics removes microbes from human semen. *Fertil Steril* 45:97, 1986

Section D1:

BIOCHEMISTRY: ACROSIN

LOURENS J. D. ZANEVELD, D.V.M., PH.D., RAJASINGAM S. JEYENDRAN, D.V.M., PH.D., JOANNE M. KAMINSKI, PH.D., AND PATRICIA PLEBAN, PH.D.

It is generally accepted that the activity of acrosin, a unique serine proteinase associated with the acrosome of spermatozoa, is essential for fertilization. In animal species, acrosin appears to be involved in the acrosome reaction as well as the capability of spermatozoa to bind to and penetrate the zona pellucida (1). The enzyme is primarily present in an inactive form, called proacrosin, which becomes activated during the fertilization process (2–6). Part of the proacrosin becomes activated during the acrosome reaction, with the resultant acrosin being involved in the dispersion of the outer sperm membranes. Subsequently, the proacrosin that remains bound to the inner acrosomal membrane may become activated during the penetration of the spermatozoon through the zona pellucida, the acrosin aiding in the formation of the penetration slit and the passage of the spermatozoon.

Evidence is accumulating that acrosin is also important for human fertilization. Inhibitors of acrosin and/or proacrosin prevent the penetration of human spermatozoa into zona-free hamster oocytes (4, 7, 8). Although the zona pellucida is absent from such oocytes, the acrosome reaction is required before penetration can occur. Direct evidence for a role of acrosin in the human acrosome reaction was recently provided by showing that 4-acetamidophenyl 4′-guanidinobenzoate (AGB), a potent acrosin inhibitor, prevents the calcium ionophore A-23187- or the dibutyryl cyclic adenosine monophosphate (cAMP)-induced acrosome reaction of human spermatozoa (9). When added to human spermatozoa, AGB rapidly passes through the membrane and inhibits sperm acrosin as well as the conversion of proacrosin to acrosin (10, 11). AGB also prevents the penetration of human spermatozoa through the human zona pellucida in the "hemi-zona assay" (Fulgham D, Burkman L, Alexander N, and Hodgen G: unpublished observations). These experiments indicate that decreased acrosin activity results in decreased fertilizing ability. Therefore, the amount of acrosin associated with spermatozoa should be another indicator of their functional activity.

Measurement of acrosin is not only important to qualify the activity of the enzyme itself but may also provide a more sensitive indicator of the acrosomal status (integrity/ damage) than morphological observations (12–15). An intact acrosome is essential for fertilization. For instance, acrosomeless spermatozoa that are almost devoid of acrosin are unable to fertilize even if they are motile and possess an intact plasma membrane (16, 17).

A number of techniques are available to measure the acrosin activity or content of human spermatozoa (see Chapter 4, Part 1, Tests of Sperm Function: Acrosin). The acrosin content is most accurately evaluated by immunological techniques, and the acrosin activity by extraction and measuring its interaction with substrate. From a clinical standpoint, it is most likely preferable to measure the acrosin activity rather than the acrosin content of the spermatozoa because it is the available activity that determines the ability of the spermatozoa to function. For instance, it is conceivable that proacrosin conversion to acrosin cannot take place, which would not alter the total acrosin content but would greatly decrease the amount of active acrosin available to the spermatozoa.

Most of the assays used to measure the acrosin activity of human spermatozoa are rather complicated, require large numbers of spermatozoa and/or are time consuming (18, 19), or are not sufficiently quantitative, like the substrate (gelatin) film test (10, 18, 20, 21) and gelatin-sodium dodecylsulfate (SDS)-polyacrylamide electrophoresis (22). A simple assay was recently developed (23, 24) that can be readily applied clinically (see Chapter 4, Part 1, Tests of Sperm Function: Acrosin). The assay consists of three steps. First, the spermatozoa are washed free of seminal plasma by centrifugation over Ficoll to remove the soluble proteinase inhibitors in semen that can interfere with acrosin activity (18, 25). The sperm pellet is subsequently suspended in buffer that has: (*a*) a detergent which facilitates disruption of the acrosomes and releases the acrosomal enzymes; (*b*) a basic pH which allows activation of proacrosin into enzymatically active acrosin; and (*c*) a synthetic arginine amide substrate which, when hydrolyzed, releases a chromophoric product. Finally, the total amount of color developed after a 3-hour incubation period is measured spectrophotometrically. The assay is repeatable, linear with increasing sperm concentration, and sensitive to a lower limit of 2×10^6 spermatozoa unless microtechniques are employed; the results correspond to those obtained with a standard acrosin extraction and assay technique (19). All the activity can be inhibited by benzamidine, a proteinase inhibitor. This technique measures the total acrosin activity of the spermatozoa, i.e., the free (non-zymogen) acrosin plus the acrosin that is generated by conversion of proacrosin to acrosin. Separate measurement of proacrosin and the non-zymogen acrosin is probably not important from a clinical standpoint. Leukocytes show no or minimal activity in the assay, i.e., leukocyte contamination of the ejaculate will not alter the assay results significantly.

A problem with measuring the amidase or esterase activity of spermatozoa or sperm extracts is that other serine proteinases besides acrosin can hydrolyze these substrates. However, no good evidence is available that spermatozoa possess other sperm serine proteinases besides acrosin. Although several publications have appeared that claim the presence of other serine proteinases (26, 27), it is likely that these represent different forms of acrosin. Until the presence of different proteinases is firmly established, it must be assumed that acrosin is the only or primary benzamidine-sensitive serine proteinase associated with the sperm acrosome. Additionally, even if other serine proteinases are present which hydrolyze the same substrates as acrosin, it is likely that they have the same function. Therefore, measurement of the total benzamidine-sensitive amidase or esterase activity of spermatozoa would still be valid as a fertility indicator.

Argument is present in the literature regarding the storage of the ejaculate if acrosin measurements cannot be performed immediately after ejaculation. Freezing at $-20°C$ (28; Goodpasture JC: unpublished observations) or cryopreservation (15, 28, 29) of human spermatozoa causes a large reduction in their acrosin activity. In contrast to these observations, some studies have indicated that freezing the ejaculate before analysis does not alter the acrosin activity of human spermatozoa and can actually increase the acrosin activity (30–32). However, these results were probably obtained because the investigators did not adequately allow proacrosin conversion to acrosin to occur before assay, so that primarily the non-zymogen acrosin was measured. The non-zymogen acrosin represents only a small fraction of the total acrosin. Freeze-thaw procedures damage the acrosome so that more acrosin and/or proacrosin is released. Even though a significant proportion of the acrosin and/or proacrosin is lost or destroyed by freeze-thawing, the remaining activity may still be the same as or higher than that of spermatozoa which are unfrozen if proacrosin activation is not part of the assay. Therefore, for accurate measurement of the total acrosin activity, ejaculates cannot be frozen or cryopreserved, and proacrosin activation should be induced. Acrosin is more unstable to cryopreservation than any of the other acrosomal enzymes measured (15). Measurement of the acrosin activity before and after cryopreservation may be useful as an additional indicator of the success of cryopreservation.

Although ejaculates should not be stored by freezing, they can be kept refrigerated or at 22–24°C for 24 hours without loss of acrosin activity (unpublished results). In order to prevent bacterial contamination, antibiotics should be added. Storage at $\geq37°C$ causes changes in acrosin activity within 6 hours, so that such high temperatures should be avoided.

It is becoming increasingly clear that the standard semen parameters (sperm number, motility, and morphology) are often insufficient for diagnostic purposes. Therefore, it is important that new assays be developed for the functional activity of spermatozoa that, together with the standard semen parameters, will provide a better indication of the fertilizing capacity of ejaculated spermatozoa. One such test, the hypo-osmotic swelling (HOS) test, is described in this chapter. The acrosin assay may be another such test, not only because it measures the activity of an enzyme that is important in the fertilization process but also because it indicates the integrity of the sperm acrosome (see above).

Since fertility involves two individuals, it is very difficult to prove that a sperm assay is useful as an indicator of fertility/infertility. First of all, it has to be shown that the assay measures a different parameter than an already existing test. This is the case for acrosin, since Goodpasture (33) showed that the total acrosin activity of ejaculates cannot be predicted from sperm concentration, sperm motility, and sperm morphology measurements. Secondly, its association with fertility/infertility has to be shown. In regard to acrosin, spermatozoa from apparently normal, asymptomatic men possess approximately three times as much enzyme activity as those from symptomatic men showing semen abnormalities (34, 35). In addition, Koukoulis (36) recently concluded that sperm acrosin measurements can identify subpopulations of infertile or subfertile patients that are not recognized by the standard semen parameters.

Additional data support the use of acrosin as a fertility indicator. It is generally accepted that the first portion of a split ejaculate, mostly consisting of prostatic fluid and spermatozoa, is more fertile on artificial insemination than the last portion, which mostly contains seminal vesicle fluid and less viable spermatozoa. The acrosin activity of the spermatozoa in the first portion is also approximately twice as high as that of the last portion (34). Similarly, cryopreserved spermatozoa are generally less fertile on artificial insemination than spermatozoa from the same ejaculate that have not been frozen. As presented in a previous paragraph, such cryopreserved spermatozoa also possess two- to three-fold lower acrosin activity (15, 28). In addition, more successfully cryopreserved sperm populations (as indicated by their ability to penetrate zona-free hamster oocytes) generally also possess a higher acrosin activity than poorer cryopreserved sperm samples (29). Finally, spermatozoa prepared by a "swim-up" technique generally represent a much better quality sperm population than that of the original ejaculate (37). Such selected sperm populations also average approximately a two-fold higher acrosin activity than the spermatozoa in the ejaculate (24).

In order to determine if the acrosin activity of ejaculated spermatozoa is related to their ability to fertilize oocytes, the acrosin activity can be correlated with the outcome of human in vitro fertilization (IVF). A relationship between the sperm acrosin content and successful IVF was first suggested by Burkman (38). More recently, we explored this relationship by using sperm populations that were not selected (e.g., by a swim-up procedure) before IVF, so that the composition of the spermatozoa added to the oocytes reflected that of the original ejaculate (24). Ejaculates were classified as "fertile" if the spermatozoa fertilized one or more oocytes and as "infertile" if none of the oocytes became fertilized. It is realized that false negatives are associated with this test because lack of fertilization may be associated with oocyte factors rather than sperm factors. Acrosin activity was assessed by the clinical assay (see Chapter 4, Part 1, Tests of Sperm Function: Acrosin). The acrosin activity of the ejaculates in the "fertile" group varied from 14 to 60 μIU/10^6 spermatozoa, with a mean $\pm$ SEM of 34.4 $\pm$ 2.9 μIU/10^6 spermatozoa. The activity of the ejaculates in the "infertile" group varied from 7 to 35 μIU/10^6 spermatozoa with a mean $\pm$ SEM of 20.3 $\pm$ 3.2 μIU/10^6 spermatozoa. These differences are statistically significant. With two exceptions, all the spermatozoa that possessed an acrosin activity of ≥ 25 μIU/10^6 spermatozoa fertilized oocytes. No fertilization occurred when the spermatozoa contained less than 14 μIU of acrosin per 10^6 spermatozoa. Based on these observations, we have tentatively designated an acrosin activity of ≥ 25 μIU/10^6 spermatozoa in the clinical acrosin assay as normal and of ≤ 14 μIU/10^6 spermatozoa as abnormal. It should be noted that these values only apply to the clinical acrosin assay because different methods may give different values. In addition, these ranges only apply to ejaculates and not to selected sperm populations because the acrosin activity of such populations differs (see above).

In summary, much evidence is available for an essential role of acrosin in the fertilization process. The usefulness of acrosin as an indicator of sperm quality is becoming increasingly clear. Therefore, it is important to include sperm acrosin measurements as a standard assay in the semen analysis. Together with the standard parameters and other new indicators, e.g., the HOS test, this should improve the diagnosis of fertility/infertility.

References

1. Rogers BJ, Bentwood B: Capacitation, acrosome reaction and fertilization. In Zaneveld LJD, Chatterton RT (eds): Biochemistry of Mammalian Reproduction. New York: John Wiley & Sons, 1982, p 203
2. Green DPL: The activation of proteolysis in the acrosome reaction of guinea pig sperm. J Cell Sci 32:153, 1978
3. Goodpasture JC, Reddy JM, Zaneveld LJD: Acrosin, proacrosin and acrosin inhibitor of guinea pig spermatozoa capacitated and acrosome reacted in vitro. Biol Reprod 25:44, 1981
4. Kennedy WP, Van der Ven HH, Strauss JW, Bhattacharyya AK, Waller DP, Zaneveld LJD, Polakoski KL: Gossypol inhibition of acrosin and proacrosin, and oocyte penetration by human spermatozoa. Biol Reprod 29:999, 1983
5. Huneau D, Harrison RAP, Flechon JE: Ultrastructural localization of proacrosin and acrosin in ram spermatozoa. Gamete Res 9:425, 1984
6. Nuzzo N, Zaneveld LJD: Correlation between proacrosin activation, acrosin release and the acrosome reaction of guinea pig spermatozoa. Biol Reprod 30: 135A, 1984
7. Berger T, Marrs RP, Kletzk OA, Moyer DL: The effect of inhibition of acrosome reaction and in vitro sperm aging on the hamster penetration test. Biol Reprod 26:148A, 1982
8. Van der Ven HH, Kaminski J, Bauer L, Zaneveld LJD: Inhibition of human sperm penetration into zona-free hamster oocytes by proteinase inhibitors. Fertil Steril 43:609, 1985
9. DeJonge C, Mack SR, Zaneveld LJD: The effect of various modulators on the human sperm acrosome reaction. J Androl 9:46P, 1988
10. Kaminski JM, Smith D, Reid DS, Kennedy W, Jeyendran RS, Zaneveld LJD: Effect of aryl 4-guanidinobenzoates on the acrosin activity of human spermatozoa. Biol Reprod 36:1170, 1987
11. Kaminski JM, Mack SR, Zaneveld LJD: Interaction of aryl 4-guanidinobenzoates (AGB) with human proacrosin. Biol Reprod 36:147A, 1987
12. Froman DP, Amann RP, Riek, PM, Olar TT: Acrosin activity of canine spermatozoa as an index of cellular damage. J Reprod Fertil 70:301, 1984
13. Froman DP, Schenk JJ, Amann RP: Sperm bound amidase activity as a marker for acrosomal integrity in bull spermatozoa. J Androl 8:162, 1987
14. Cechova D, Zelezna B, Petlikova J, Panlok P: Board proacrosin: Correlation between total proacrosin content and sperm fertilizing capacity. Andrologia 16:171, 1984
15. Mack SR, Zaneveld LJD: Acrosomal enzymes and ultrastructure of unfrozen and cryotreated human spermatozoa. Gamete Res 18:375, 1987
16. Florke-Gerloff S, Topfer-Peterson E, Muller-Esterl W, Mansouri A, Schatz R, Schirren C, Schill W, Engel W: Biochemical and genetic investigations of round-headed spermatozoa in infertile men including two brothers and their father. Andrologia 16:187, 1984
17. Jeyendran RS, Van der Ven HH, Kennedy W, Heath E, Perez-Pelaez M, Sobrero AJ, Zaneveld LJD: Acrosomeless sperm: a cause of primary male infertility. Andrologia 17:31, 1985

18. Fritz H, Schleuning WD, Schiessler H, Schill W-B, Windt V, Winkler G: Boar, bull and human sperm acrosin—isolation, properties and biological aspects. In Reich E, Rifkin DB, Shaw E (eds): Proteases and Biological Control. Cold Spring Harbor: Cold Spring Harbor Laboratory, 1975, p 715

19. Goodpasture JC, Polakoski KL, Zaneveld LJD: Acrosin, proacrosin, and acrosin inhibitor of human spermatozoa: extraction, quantitation, and stability. J Androl 1:16, 1980

20. Gaddum P, Blandeau RJ: Proteolytic reaction of mammalian sperm on gelatin membranes. Science 170:749, 1970

21. Ficsor G, Ginsberg LC, Oldford GM, Snoke RE, Becker RW: Gelatin substrate film technique for detection of acrosin in single mammalian sperm. Fertil Steril 39:548, 1983

22. Siegel MS, Polakoski KL: Evaluation of the human sperm proacrosin-acrosin system using gelatin dodecylsulfate-polyacylamide gel electrophoresis. Biol Reprod 32:713, 1985

23. Kennedy WP, Reid DS, Kaminski JM, Jeyendran RS, Zaneveld LJD: Development and evaluation of a clinical assay for the determination of the acrosin activity of human spermatozoa. Presented at the 41st Annual Meeting, American Fertility Society, 1985

24. Van der Ven HH, Kennedy WP, Kaminski JM, Jeyendran RS, Zaneveld LJD: Human sperm acrosin as a fertility marker. J Androl 8:20P, 1987

25. Zaneveld LJD, Schumacher GFB, Fritz H, Fink E, Jaumann E: Interaction of human sperm acrosomal proteinase with human seminal plasma proteinase inhibitors. J Reprod Fertil 32:525, 1973

26. Johnson RA, Jakobs KH, Schultz G: Extraction of the adenylate cyclase activating factor of bovine sperm and its identification as a trypsin-like protease. J Biol Chem 260:114, 1985

27. Siegel MS, Bechtold DS, Willand J, Polakoski KL: Partial purification and characterization of human sperminogen. Biol Reprod 36:1063, 1987

28. Goodpasture JC, Zavos PM, Cohen MR, Zaneveld LJD: The acrosin system of human spermatozoa: effects of various conditions of semen storage. J Reprod Fertil 63:397, 1981

29. Jeyendran RS, Van der Ven HH, Kennedy W, Perez-Pelaez M, Zaneveld LJD: Comparison of glycerol and a zwitter ion buffer system as cryoprotective media for human spermatozoa. J Androl 5:1, 1984

30. Schill W-B, Wolff H: Ultrastructure of human sperm acrosome and determination of acrosin activity under conditions of semen preservation. Int J Fertil 19:217, 1974

31. Schill W-B: Quantitative determination of acrosin activity in human spermatozoa. Fertil Steril 25:703, 1974

32. Schill W-B: Acrosin activity of cryo-preserved human spermatozoa. Fertil Steril 26:711, 1975

33. Goodpasture JC, Zavos PN, Zaneveld LJD: Relationship of human sperm acrosin and proacrosin to semen parameters. II. Correlations. J Androl 8:267, 1987

34. Goodpasture JC, Zavos PM, Cohen MR, Zaneveld LJD: Relationship of human sperm acrosin and proacrosin to semen parameters. I. Comparisons between symptomatic men of infertile couples and asymptomatic men, and between different split ejaculates. J Androl 3:151, 1982

35. Mohsenian M, Syner FN, Moghissi KS: A study of sperm acrosin in patients with unexplained infertility. Fertil Steril 37:223, 1982

36. Koukoulis G, Vantman D, Dennison L, Sherins RJ: Consistently low acrosin activity in sperm of a subpopulation of men with unexplained infertility. J Androl 9:46P, 1988

37. Russell LD, Rogers BJ: Improvement in the quality and fertilizing potential of a human sperm population using the rise technique. J Androl 8:25, 1987

38. Burkman LJ, Syner FN, Moghissi KS, Acosta A: Sperm acrosin content and semen parameters for successful in vitro fertilization: "normal" and oligospermic groups. Fertil Steril 41:102S, 1984

Section D2a:

BIOCHEMISTRY: ATP

FRANK H. COMHAIRE, M.D., LUTGARDE VERMEULEN, Industrial Engineer in Chemistry, AUK HINTING, M.D., PH.D., AND FRANK SCHOONJANS, B.S.

Accuracy of Traditional Sperm Characteristics and ATP in Assessing Fertilizing Potential of Human Sperm In Vivo and In Vitro

Many tests have been advocated to evaluate the function of sperm and to estimate the capacity of sperm to fertilize. The functional characteristics which determine the fertilizing potential of sperm in vivo (after intercourse or artificial insemination) are different from those in vitro.

For in vivo fertilization, sperm motility is of crucial importance, since the sperm must swim up into and/or through the female genital tract, mostly by means of their own motility. The proportion and concentration of sperm with type *a* motiliity is the best discriminant to separate the semen of fertile men from that of subfertile men (1). Type *a* motility is defined by rapid, progressive movement following a straight or nearly straight track. All tests which directly or indirectly measure this parameter will reflect one aspect of sperm function. Counting sperm with type *a* motility using the conventional method recommended by the World Health Organization (WHO) (2) gives results which are reasonably reproducible. However, methods for the objective assessment of swimming speed and especially the velocity of linear progression give more precise and reliable information.

Using a simple, single-step procedure for the objective assessment of sperm motility (Autosperm, AMSATEN Corp., De Pinte, Belgium), we found that the concentration of type *a* sperm with linear progression >22 μm/sec is 90% accurate in classifying semen as fertile or subfertile (3). Measurements using automatic methods are subject to many errors and should be interpreted with caution (4).

Tests which *indirectly* measure the proportion or concentration of type *a* motile sperm will also give information on the functional quality of semen, though it has not been proven that any of these tests more accurately assess fertilizing potential. Different sperm migration tests are available, including the postcoital test and the in vitro migration test into human or standard bovine cervical mucus (Penetrak, Serono Diagnostics, Norwell, Mass.) in capillary tubes (5, 6) or on a slide (7). Those tests which evaluate the interaction of sperm and the cervical mucus of the female partner are probably the most useful.

The amount of adenosine triphosphate (ATP) per milliliter of semen, but not the concentration of ATP per spermatozoon, is significantly correlated with the concentration of type *a* motile sperm. Hence ATP per milliliter of semen can be used as a marker of

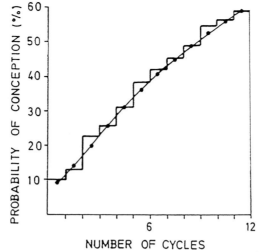

Figure 5.8. Observed life-table curve (*solid line*) in case of insemination with semen selected on the basis of the number of motile sperm after freezing-thawing. The observed life-table analysis curve (step-wise) overlaps with the curve for a constant probability of conception of 7.2% per cycle (*closed circles*).

sperm fertilizing capacity. Its performance in discriminating between fertile and subfertile semen is similar to that of the concentration of type *a* sperm, as estimated by the WHO method (2), but it has less discriminating power than objectively assessed type *a* motile sperm concentration (8).

In contrast with the situation in vivo, the most important sperm characteristic for defining the fertilizing potential in vitro is sperm morphology. Indeed, it is the number of sperm per ejaculate with regularly outlined oval heads which is the best discriminant between semen that will or will not fertilize in vitro (9). The concentration and percentage of sperm with type *a* motility needed for successful fertilization in vitro is much less than that needed for fertilization in vivo.

Advantage of Selecting Donor Semen on the Basis of Its ATP Content

Selection of frozen-thawed donor semen for artificial insemination (AID) is traditionally made on the basis of the concentration of motile sperm per milliliter. At least 5 $\times 10^6$ sperm with progressive motility are given per intracervical insemination. Using this selection criterion, AID results in a relatively low probability of conception (approximately 7% per cycle), corresponding to slightly less than 60% pregnancies after 12 months of trial (Fig. 5.8).

In an attempt to improve the success rate of AID, we have evaluated whether the ATP content of frozen-thawed donor semen can more adequately estimate the relative fertilizing potential. Semen was frozen after dilution with a cryoprotectant medium containing egg yolk or HEPES buffer and glycerol. The 0.25-ml straws were first left at $-80°C$ for 8 to 10 minutes in the vapor of liquid nitrogen before being immersed in the liquid nitrogen. Measurement of ATP was performed immediately after rapid thawing of the semen, which had been cryopreserved for at least 7 days.

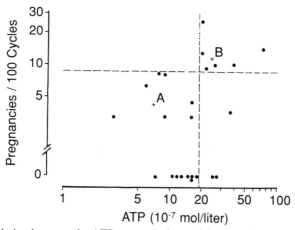

Figure 5.9. Correlation between the ATP concentration and the rate of pregnancy per 100 cycles. *A*, Mean value of ATP and pregnancy rate of donors with ATP <1.7 μmol/liter who attained conception. *B*, Mean value of ATP and pregnancy rate of donors with ATP >1.7 μmol/liter who attained conception.

The relative fertilizing potential of the thawed semen was calculated by dividing the number of pregnancies by the number of insemination cycles (P/C) and was expressed as a percentage. The ATP content was measured in 84 semen donations of 24 donors (at least 3 different donations for each donor), and the mean ATP concentration was calculated per donor. The semen was used for the insemination of 198 women during 1225 cycles.

Insemination of the frozen-thawed semen of the 24 donors resulted in 14 pregnancies, with a P/C rate of 3% to 16% (mean 7.6%). The mean value was similar to the observed P/C rate of 7.2% in our original population. The ATP concentration of the thawed semen of the donors achieving pregnancies was 0.4 to 7.5 μmol/liter. The important variability of ATP content stands in contrast to the fact that sperm concentration and the proportion of sperm with progressive motility were similar in all samples. Insemination with semen of the residual 10 donors did not result in pregnancies. The ATP content in their semen was significantly lower (0.7 to 2.6 μmol/liter).

In fact, 50% of the donors with ATP content in thawed semen <1.7 μmol/liter failed to produce pregnancies, and for those who did, the mean P/C was only 5%. Of the donors with ATP content >1.7 μmol/liter, 30% failed to produce pregnancies; for those who did, the mean P/C rate was 12%. There was a significant linear correlation between the ATP concentration and the P/C rate (Fig. 5.9).

Considering these results, we decided to select frozen-thawed donor semen on the basis of its ATP content rather than its concentration of motile sperm. Insemination with frozen-thawed semen selected in this way resulted in an increased success rate of AID (Fig. 5.10), with 70% pregnancies in 12 cycles. Remarkably, the curve of cumulative probability of conception was found to consist of two components. During the first six cycles, the P/C was approximately 13%, whereas it dropped dramatically to only 2.5% in cycles 7 to 12. It was suspected that the latter drop was due to female factors rather than to the limitation of semen quality. Therefore, women not attaining conception after 6 months of trial were submitted to laparoscopy and treatment, if indicated, including ovulation induction with gonadotropins. As a result, the cumulative success rate of AID

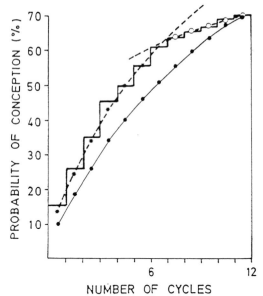

Figure 5.10.   Observed life-table curve (*solid line*) in couples inseminated with frozen-thawed donor semen selected on the basis of an ATP content >1.7 μmol/liter. The life-table curve depicting a constant probability of conception of 9.6% per cycle (*closed circles*) differs from the observed curve (*dashed line*), which appears to consist of two components.

increased to 85% in 12 cycles, corresponding with a probability of conception of 13.7% per cycle (Fig. 5.11).

Conclusion

Assessment of ATP concentration in semen is simple and gives reproducible results. The ATP concentration of fresh semen has a reasonable power to discriminate between semen of fertile and subfertile men as far as fertilization in vivo is concerned. In this respect, it is equivalent to the proportion of sperm with type *a* motility estimated by conventional methods. The ATP measurement, however, is less discriminative than the objectively assessed concentration of type *a* motile sperm. The fertilizing potential of semen in vitro depends primarily on the number of sperm with normal head morphology per ejaculate.

Measurement of the ATP content of frozen-thawed donor semen is useful in selecting semen with high fertilizing potential. Insemination of frozen-thawed donor semen with an ATP content >1.7 μmol/liter results in an increased probability of conception per cycle and enhanced overall success rate of AID.

References

1. Comhaire FH, Vermeulen L, Schoonjans F: Reassessment of the accuracy of traditional sperm characteristics and adenosine triphosphate (ATP) in estimating the fertilizing potential of human semen in vivo. Int J Androl 10:653, 1987
2. World Health Organization: Laboratory Manual for the Examination of Human Semen and Semen-Cervical Mucus Interaction. Cambridge: Cambridge University Press, 1987, p 52

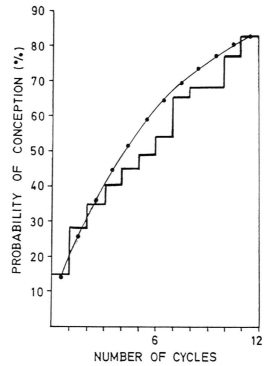

Figure 5.11.   Observed life-table curve (*solid line*) in couples inseminated with frozen-thawed semen with elevated ATP, in whom induction of ovulation was performed if no conception was attained in six cycles.

3. Hinting A, Schoonjans F, Comhaire F: Validation of a single-step procedure for the objective assessment of sperm motility characteristics. Int J Androl 11:277, 1988
4. Knuth UA, Yeung C-H, Nieschlag E: Computerized semen analysis: objective measurement of semen characteristics is biased by subjective parameter setting. Fertil Steril 48:118, 1987
5. Kremer J, Jager S: The sperm-cervical mucus contact test: a preliminary report. Fertil Steril 27:335, 1976
6. Alexander N: Evaluation of male infertility with an in vitro cervical mucus penetration test. Fertil Steril 36:201, 1981
7. Moghissi KS: Post-coital test: physiological basis, technique and interpretation. Fertil Steril 27:117, 1976
8. Hinting A, Comhaire F, Schoonjans F: Capacity of objectively assessed sperm motility characteristics in differentiating between semen of fertile and subfertile men. Fertil Steril 50:635, 1988
9. Comhaire FH, Vermeulen L, Hinting A, Schoonjans F: Accuracy of sperm characteristics in predicting in vitro fertilizing capacity of semen. J In Vitro Fertil Embryo Trans 5:326, 1988

Section D2b:

BIOCHEMISTRY:
ATP, THE NORFOLK EXPERIENCE

MAHMOOD MORSHEDI, PH.D.

For years, infertility was considered to be a female problem. Our attention, research, and efforts were therefore focused on female infertility. In recent years, however, the nearly equal contribution of the male to infertility has been recognized, and progress has been made in elucidating the causes of male infertility. With the advent of assisted reproduction such as in vitro fertilization (IVF), assessment of semen quality has become an important factor in establishing the suitability of couples for these procedures. However, disagreement exists as to which semen characteristics most strongly influence fertilization and the pregnancy outcome of these techniques (1).

Because various semen characteristics are interrelated, each one must be evaluated in association with the others, as well as by itself. The result could be a different categorizing of the influence of each factor and could allow us to determine which factors are most important for prediction of fertilization potential or pregnancy outcome. It might also help to identify certain semen parameters in samples which did poorly in IVF, for example, compared to samples with more successful results (1).

Since many semen characteristics are interrelated and patient populations are not comparable, variations in the ordering of the importance of specific characteristics by different investigators is not surprising, especially if the chosen characteristics lack strength. For example, sperm count and motility are accepted by many to be among the most important parameters related to the success of fertilization and resulting pregnancy. Nevertheless, some investigators have reported pregnancy rates of about 30% in partners of men with semen parameters, including count and motility, below normal levels (2). At the same time, about 25% of infertile males show no abnormality in basic semen parameters (3). This brings into question the value of this type of gross evaluation of semen quality. Assessment of sperm count based on the total number of sperm rather than the type of movement and energy used (or required) to maintain that movement may give spurious data.

In response to the urgent need for more definite results, newer approaches for evaluation of semen samples have been developed. Attention has recently been focused on the use of adenosine triphosphate (ATP) as a possible marker of semen quality and sperm fertilizing potential. Although other sources of energy, such as creatine phosphate, have been implicated in the sperm metabolic system (reserve energy), the role of ATP as the major source of immediate energy required for many important functions cannot be disputed. Unfortunately, findings implicating the quantity of sperm ATP as a sensitive factor in male infertility have not been consistent. Several lines of evidence indicate major sources of error in evaluating the role of ATP in infertility.

Semen samples from fertile donors, as well as numerous tests, such as the sperm penetration assay (SPA), have been used to evaluate the role of ATP in infertility. The major problem with fertile donors is that data rarely exist on the true fertility of the specific sample being used as a reference. While IVF procedure obviates this problem, it places one more demand on the IVF team to salvage a portion of each sperm sample for simultaneous laboratory testing, a demand not always fulfilled because of time limitations and the number of sperm available. When ATP values cannot be obtained from the same sample used in an IVF procedure, most researchers rely on correlating ATP with other tests of sperm function, most commonly SPA. Starting with a fertile donor and adding a passing SPA score does not mean that the ATP assay has been run on a truly fertile semen sample, since SPA results are not always consistent and do not always correlate well with human ova fertilization and pregnancy.

In vivo, human cervical mucus serves as a barrier to seminal fluid and semen elements other than sperm. In most IVF procedures, swim-up samples are used for the insemination of oocytes. ATP studies using whole semen or washed semen samples may contain seminal elements such as round cells, which contain high levels of ATP. Compared to swim-up samples, washed samples may exhibit extreme variation in the percentage of motility and possibly in the number of good sperm.

It is known (4–6) that the ATP content of sperm declines with time. We have observed that the decline is more significant in some samples than in others and that there is a possibility of significant decline even 1 hour after ejaculation with certain patients (unpublished observation). These findings suggest that sample processing for preparation of swim-up and for determination of ATP must be carried out within 30 to 45 minutes after ejaculation. To correlate ATP values with IVF results, ATP in swim-up samples must be determined at the time of oocyte insemination.

Other sources of error, such as improper use of instrumentation, inadequate amount of enzyme in the assay procedure, and improper units used to report ATP concentration (molar units rather than the amount of ATP per specific number of sperm), have also been identified in many ATP studies. The first portion of the light output in an ATP assay is very unstable and sensitive to many assay conditions. To obtain more predictable results, elimination of this portion of light is necessary. In some investigations the volume of luciferin-luciferase mixture has not been high enough to keep ATP as a limiting reagent at all ATP concentrations. Since sperm count varies tremendously from sample to sample, reporting ATP concentration based on the amount of ATP per certain number of sperm reduces the effects of sperm count variation on ATP values.

In light of these facts, it is essential to correct both assay and instrumentation inadequacies and to evaluate both semen and swim-up preparations for the study of infertile males. The ultimate method of validating andrological assays and their usefulness in the evaluation of male infertility is to correlate assay values of the semen samples of infertile males with human oocyte fertilization, cleavage, embryo development, and resulting pregnancy (or lack of it) initiated by the same samples. Under these conditions, reproducibility studies can also be carried out to determine if ATP is of value in screening patients for IVF.

Methodology

A variety of methods such as spectrophotometry, luminometry (chemoluminescence), fluorometry, radioimmunometry (radioimmunoassay, RIA), and enzyme immunometry (EA) are available for detecting, monitoring, or analyzing biological compounds. Chemoluminescence is one of the safest, simplest, and most sensitive methods for many applications.

Chemoluminescence is the chemical production of light, often confused with fluorescence. The difference between these two is the source of energy which produces molecules in an excited state. In fluorescence, an incident light source is needed to excite the molecules to the singlet state, after which they return to the ground state, emitting light of a higher wavelength. This process is temperature-independent and has a very short life span. In contrast, in chemoluminescence the creation of an excited state is through an enzyme-catalyzed (chemical) reaction, and the decay from the excited state to the ground state is accompanied by emission of light which is temperature-dependent, long-lasting, and measurable by a special photometer (Fig. 5.12).

REAGENTS AND EQUIPMENT

Reagents

1. 0.5-M TRIS acetate-0.02-M EDTA buffer, pH 7.75;
2. Luciferin-luciferase (LKB Instruments, Gaithersburg, Md.);
3. ATP standards (LKB Instruments);
4. High-performance liquid chromatography (HPLC)-grade water used in all reagent preparations.

Equipment

1. ATP luminometer, integrating photometer model 3000 (Biospherical Co., San Diego, Calif.);
2. pH meter (Corning model 5);
3. Boiling water bath.

ASSAY

Extraction

1. To 730 to 740 μl of boiling TRIS-EDTA buffer in cryotubes, add 20 or 10 μl, respectively, of whole semen or swim-up sample in duplicate.
2. Place immediately in boiling water for 15 minutes.
3. Assay immediately or store at $-20°C$ for no longer than 48 hours.

Procedure

1. Thaw the extracts.
2. Add 1.1 ml of TRIS-EDTA buffer.
3. Add 150 μl of luciferin-luciferase; mix well for 15 seconds.
4. Register the first 1-minute light output (B).
5. Immediately add 100 μl of 50×10^{-7} dilution of ATP standard; mix well for 15 seconds.
6. Register the second 1-minute light output (C).
7. Calculate ATP from: ($B \times$ concentration of standard)/($C - B$) (in mol/liter), or use a standard curve.
8. Adjust for sample volume, divide by semen or swim-up count in millions, and report in picomole/10^6 sperm.

Results

In our evaluation of the ATP assay, we studied patients randomly chosen from Norfolk series 27 and 30. To reduce the number of variables for correlation studies,

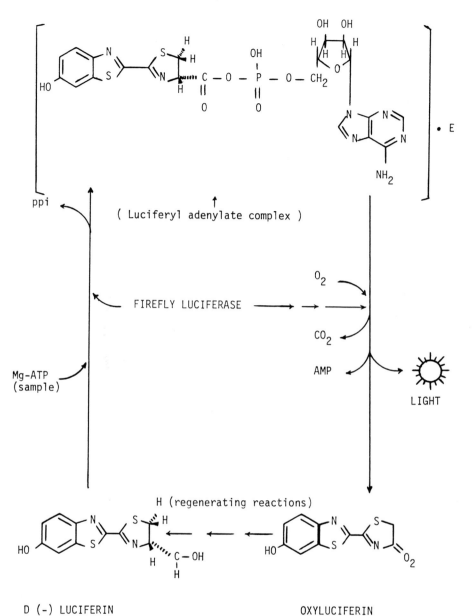

Figure 5.12.   Reactions in chemoluminescence determination of ATP.

normal sperm count ($\geq 20 \times 10^6$/ml) and motility ($\geq 40\%$) and a round cell count of $\leq 1 \times 10^6$/ml were included in this study. No sample with non-morphological abnormalities was included. All female partners of these patients (except one with two healthy prophase I oocytes) had at least one healthy metaphase II oocyte recovered. The statistical general linear model of the Statistical Analysis System (SAS) was used with the fertilization rate per oocyte and the pregnancy rate as the dependent variables to determine a threshold of ATP concentration and to indicate where the chances of fertilization or pregnancy were significantly ($P<0.05$) impaired. A threshold of 41 pmol/10^6 sperm for the swim-up samples was indicated. A reliable threshold for the fresh semen samples could not be established. With these findings we categorized swim-up samples into low-ATP (≤ 40 pmol/10^6 sperm) and high-ATP (>40 pmol/10^6 sperm) groups. Discriminant function analysis was used to identify seminal variables (parameters) contributing most significantly to IVF outcome. It was also used to devise formulas for predicting the pregnancy outcome of IVF. The major purpose of discriminant function analysis was to find out the best combination of independent variables to maximize differences (discriminate) between groups (pregnant versus non-pregnant).

STUDIES ON NORFOLK IVF SERIES 27

Seventy-eight patients in this series were included in a blind study. With the exception of samples with abnormal count and motility, the selection of patients was random. Statistical analysis indicated no specific threshold for seminal (whole semen) ATP below which the chances of fertilization or pregnancy could be impaired, although no pregnancy resulted from samples with seminal ATP <65 pmol/10^6 sperm. Based on the ATP results obtained from the swim-up samples, two groups could be identified: patients with low swim-up ATP and those with high swim-up ATP (Table 5.9). When compared with the IVF outcome, all patients with low swim-up ATP had a significantly lower fertilization rate per oocyte and a lower pregnancy rate. Both groups had similar swim-up count and percent of motility. The average number of preovulatory oocytes retrieved was higher in patients receiving semen samples with low ATP concentrations. These results may indicate that differences in fertilization rate per oocyte and the pregnancy rate observed between the two groups are not due to differences in count, percent of motility, or the number of preovulatory oocytes recovered. There were no differences in the average number of embryos transferred per patient and the cleavage rate between the two groups. Although not statistically significant ($P<0.06$), the number of cells per embryo was lower in the group with low swim-up ATP (Table 5.9). Seminal ATP determinations showed no significant correlation with the IVF outcome.

In a further study of the relationship between sperm morphology and seminal or swim-up ATP, 70% of patients with poor (P) pattern of sperm morphology had low (≤ 40 pmol/10^6 sperm) swim-up ATP but slightly higher whole semen (seminal) ATP, compared to the other two morphology groups. In contrast to the semen samples with P-pattern morphology, only 33% of semen samples with a good (G) pattern of morphology showed low swim-up ATP. Seminal ATP in this group was similar to that seen in those with normal morpology. Only 6% of semen samples with normal morphology had low swim-up ATP.

STUDIES ON NORFOLK IVF SERIES 30

To obtain more data and to ascertain whether the significant results found in series 27 could be repeated, we randomly chose patients from Norfolk IVF series 30. Semen and swim-up creatine kinase (CK) were determined to evaluate these in predicting the IVF outcome. ATP results obtained from semen evaluations showed no significant correlation with series 30 IVF outcome ($P<0.057$). Swim-up results, however, showed a similar trend and level of significance as was observed in series 27 (Table 5.10). Although the fertilization rate per oocyte was higher in patients with low ATP, pregnancy results remained low, as in Series 27. No pregnancy was achieved in the group with low ATP. As in Series 27, the significant difference in pregnancy rate between two groups

Table 5.9.
Correlation Between Swim-Up ATP[a] and Human IVF Results (Series 27)[b]

	ATP≤40 (n = 13)	ATP>40 (n = 65)	Significance
Mean swim-up ATP/10^6 sperm	35.3	101.1	$P<0.01$
Mean swim-up count/% motility	19/86	27/87	NS[c]
Fertilization rate per oocyte	54.6	93.8	$P<0.04$
Pregnancy rate per cycle	0.0	30.8	$P<0.001$
Pregnancy rate per transfer	0.0	31.3	$P<0.001$
Ongoing pregnancy rate	0.0	24.6	$P<0.008$
Abortion rate	—	20.0	—
Average preovulatory oocytes per patient	4.5	3.3	$P<0.05$
Average embryos transferred per patient	2.2	3.3	NS
Cleavage rate	96.3	94.8	NS
Number of cells per embryo	3.8	4.2	NS

[a]ATP concentration in pmol/10^6 sperm.
[b]No patient with primary male factor infertility other than morphology included.
[c]NS = no significance.

may not be related to differences in swim-up count, motility, or average number of embryos transferred per patient. The number of cells per embryo transferred was lower (3.8 and 3.6) for low-ATP groups of Series 27 and 30, respectively, compared with groups with high ATP (4.2 and 4.4). The difference, however, was not significant ($P<0.06$).

RESULTS FROM IVF SERIES 27 AND 30, COMBINED

When patients of IVF Series 27 and 30 were combined and grouped, based on their swim-up ATP concentrations, some interesting results were observed (Table 5.11). In addition to pregnancy rates which were significantly different ($P<0.001$) between the

Table 5.10.
Correlation Between Swim-Up ATP[a] and Human IVF Results (Series 30)[b]

	ATP≤40 (n = 5)	ATP>40 (n = 50)	Significance
Mean swim-up ATP/10^6 sperm	31.2	108.3	$P<0.001$
Mean swim-up count/% motility	16.3/88	19.4/92	NS[c]
Fertilization rate per oocyte	100.0	74.0	$P<0.05$
Pregnancy rate per cycle	0.0	30.0	$P<0.005$
Pregnancy rate per transfer	0.0	30.6	$P<0.006$
Ongoing pregnancy	0.0	30.0	$P<0.006$
Abortion rate	—	0.0	$P<0.001$
Average preovulatory oocytes per patient	4.4	1.0	$P<0.03$
Average embryos transferred per patient	3.0	3.0	NS
Cleavage rate	92.9	93.8	NS
Number of cells per embryo	3.6	4.4	NS

[a]ATP concentration in pmol/10^6 sperm.
[b]No patient with primary male factor infertility other than morphology included.
[c]NS = no significance.

Table 5.11.

Comparison of Seminal and Swim-Up Variables in Patients with Low and High Swim-Up ATP (Series 27 and 30 Combined)[a,b]

Variable[c]	Low ATP			High ATP			
	Mean	(SEM)	(n)	Mean	(SEM)	(n)	Significance
COUNT 1	93.5	(13.6)	(18)	134.3	(10.5)	(106)	$P<0.05$
% MOT 1	51.8	(5.6)	(18)	67.1	(1.7)	(106)	NS
%NORMAL	4.8	(0.8)	(21)	10.2	(0.6)	(118)	$P<0.05$
VELO 1	39.6	(1.9)	(16)	41.1	(0.7)	(114)	NS
LINE 1	5.8	(0.3)	(16)	5.8	(0.1)	(114)	NS
ATP 1	111.6	(20.7)	(20)	124.5	(6.5)	(105)	NS
COUNT 2	16.5	(3.7)	(13)	27.5	(2.0)	(97)	$P<0.05$
MOT 2	89.2	(3.0)	(13)	98.0	(7.3)	(97)	NS
VELO 2	59.2	(2.2)	(11)	63.9	(1.1)	(82)	NS
LINE 2	5.2	(0.3)	(11)	7.3	(1.0)	(82)	$P<0.05$
ATP 2	30.2	(1.7)	(21)	89.6	(3.5)	(119)	$P<0.001$
% PREG	0.0	(0.0)	(21)	30.3	(4.2)	(119)	$P<0.001$

[a]Low ATP, swim-up ATP ≤ 40 pmol/10^6 sperm; High ATP, swim-up ATP >40 pmol/10^6 sperm.
[b]No patient with primary male factor infertility (other than morphology) included.
[c]Number 1 after each variable denotes "seminal"; 2 denotes "swim-up". MOT, % motility; VELO, velocity in μm/sec; LINE, linearity; COUNT, sperm count in 10^6/ml semen or swim-up. %PREG, pregnancy rate; NS, no significance.

two groups, other variables also exhibited significant differences. Semen and swim-up counts (not percent of motility) of these two groups were significantly different ($P<0.05$), and the percentage of normal sperm was different ($P<0.05$).

Another interesting finding was the significant difference ($P<0.05$) between swim-up linearity of the low-ATP group compared with the high-ATP group. Sperm in swim-up samples with low swim-up ATP were less linear (5.2) than those with high swim-up ATP (7.3). Although not significantly different, sperm mean linear velocity was also slightly lower in the group with low swim-up ATP. This may indicate that the lower linearity observed in swim-up samples with low ATP was not due to hyperactivation of sperm, which normally leads to lower linearity. Grouping patients based on pregnancy results exhibited a similar trend (Table 5.12).

Discussion

With the advent of IVF and other clinical techniques, it is important to use the best sperm available from a semen sample. To achieve this goal, many centers use swim-up preparations. Many reports indicate an increase in the percentages of motile forms and normal morphology. However, other sperm functions and characteristics must be considered concurrently. For example, a sperm swimming from point A to point B may use an amount of energy significantly different from that of another sperm, although both may contribute equally to the measured percent of motility and the mean velocity. Since many important sperm functions are active processes, determination of levels of available (ATP) and reserve (CK total and CK isoenzymes) energy is of great importance. This determination, however, is valuable only if all major technical and procedural errors are eliminated.

Table 5.12.
Comparison of Seminal and Swim-Up Variables in Pregnant and Non-Pregnant Patients of Series 27 and 30 Combined[a]

Variable[b]	Pregnant			Non-Pregnant			Significance
	Mean	(SEM)	(*n*)	Mean	(SEM)	(*n*)	
COUNT 1	125.9	(13.3)	(29)	125.1	(10.9)	(101)	NS
% MOT	64.1	(3.6)	(29)	64.6	(1.9)	(101)	NS
NORMAL	10.5	(0.6)	(39)	6.9	(0.6)	(112)	$P<0.05$
VELO 1	38.2	(1.5)	(28)	41.7	(0.7)	(96)	NS
LINE 1	5.7	(0.2)	(28)	5.8	(0.1)	(96)	NS
ATP 1	138.6	(12.5)	(30)	121.6	(7.7)	(100)	$P<0.056$
COUNT 2	26.3	(3.4)	(26)	26.2	(2.2)	(84)	NS
MOT 2	91.6	(1.6)	(26)	98.6	(8.5)	(84)	NS
VELO 2	63.9	(1.9)	(22)	61.7	(1.2)	(71)	NS
LINE 2	5.7	(0.2)	(22)	7.4	(1.1)	(71)	$P<0.05$
ATP 2	97.2	(7.4)	(36)	75.0	(3.8)	(104)	$P<0.03$

[a]No patient with primary male factor infertility (other than morphology) included.
[b]Number 1 after each variable denotes "seminal"; 2 denotes "swim-up." MOT, % motility; NORMAL, mean percentage of normal sperm; VELO, velocity in μm/second; LINE, linearity; ATP, in pmol/10^6 sperm; NS, no significance.

The method of measuring ATP described above is more accurate and reproducible. We have modified the Comhaire procedure (7) and eliminated all factors which have been shown to affect the results. We have found that swim-up ATP is more valuable than seminal ATP in correlation with the pregnancy outcome of an IVF program. The value of swim-up ATP is even greater in patients with G and P patterns of sperm morphology. Semen samples of the G or P pattern with normal swim-up ATP can be used to inseminate oocytes at 50,000 sperm/oocyte/ml of medium, a finding that must be further studied.

The pregnancy outcome of IVF can be predicted through the formulas devised during our study. Our criteria for the selection of samples must be kept in mind: normal count and motility, with a normal number of round cells. The contribution of oocytes to IVF outcome has not been determined, since we studied only patients with at least one recovered, healthy metaphase II oocyte. Our data may not be reproducible in other centers because there is no standard procedure for sperm capacitation and the swim-up technique. Temperature, pH, osmolarity, duration of pre-insemination capacitation, time lapse between ejaculation and processing for IVF, the exact volume inseminated, and the exact number of capacitated sperm in the insemination dish vary from team to team. Also, in many studies one knows little about the correlations between IVF results and the characteristics of the ejaculate. A study of such correlation might be helpful in determining whether our definition of the lower limits beyond which successful IVF is unlikely can be repeated.

Of 11 patients evaluated for swim-up ATP before IVF, no pregnancy resulted from three samples with low swim-up ATP. More reproducibility studies are needed to confirm findings in patients before and after IVF. Studies must also be carried out to determine the contribution of oocytes to the outcome of IVF with a particular stimulation protocol. The contribution of seminal and swim-up ATP, CK, and hypo-osmotic swelling (HOS) testing and sperm morphology to IVF outcome using samples with abnormal count, motility, and number of round cells must also be evaluated. Why an increased number of sperm cells per oocyte in an insemination dish increases the fertilization rate but does not improve the pregnancy rate is another matter for investigation, of particular importance because of recent interest in micromanipulation techniques.

References

1. Talbert LM, Hammond MG, Halme J, O'Rand M, Fryer JG, Ekstrom DE: Semen parameters and fertilization of human oocytes in vitro: a multivariate analysis. Fertil Steril 48:270, 1987
2. Jeulin C, Feneux D, Serres C, Jouannet P, Guillet-Rosso F, Belaisch-Allart J, Frydman R, Testart J: Sperm factors related to the failure of human in vitro fertiliztion. J Reprod Fertil 76:1, 1986
3. George FW, Silxon JD: Sex determination and differentiation. In Knobil E, Neill JF (eds): The Physiology of Reproduction, vol 1. New York: Raven Press, 1988, p 3
4. Caldini AL, Orlando C, Fiorelli G, Cuomo S: ATP and ADP content of human ejaculated spermatozoa. II. Time-dependent changes after ejaculation. Int J Androl 5:579, 1982
5. Singer R, Barnet M, Savig M, Allalouf D, Landan B, Servadio C: ATP content of human semen, seminal plasma, and isolated sperm at time intervals after ejaculation. Int J Biochem 15:105, 1983
6. Morshedi M, Acosta A, Ackerman S, Pleban P, Yuan J: Seminal ATP and its significance in male infertility (Abstract). Joint meeting of the American and Canadian Fertility Societies, Toronto, 1986
7. Comhaire F, Vermeulen L, Ghedira K, Mas J, Irvine S, Callipolitis G: Adenosine triphosphate in human semen: a quantitative estimate of fertilizing potential. Fertil Steril 40:500, 1983

Section E:

IMMUNOLOGY

NANCY J. ALEXANDER, PH.D., STEVEN B. ACKERMAN, PH.D., AND MARIE-LENA WINDT, M.S.

The female reproductive tract, through sexual activity, undergoes periodic inoculation with hundreds of millions of highly specialized, immunologically alien spermatozoa. Yet only rarely do women develop an immune response to these cells. Similarly, the presence in the male's reproductive tract of sperm-associated antigens, which arise at puberty and after the establishment of tolerance to self-antigens, only occasionally invokes autoimmune stimulation.

Several mechanisms have been postulated to account for the formation of antisperm antibodies. The structural integrity of the epithelial linings of both the male and female reproductive tracts provides a barrier to the penetration of sperm antigens into the lymphatic and systemic circulations. It is well recognized that, in men, injury or infection of the testes or epididymides and vasectomy often invoke a potent antisperm antibody response. Both seminal fluid and sperm factors have been demonstrated to be capable of activating T suppressor/inducer cells which may, in normal individuals, elicit immunosuppression to sperm antigens within the confines of the reproductive systems of either sex (1). The lack of such immunosuppressive factors in ejaculatory secretions or the reduced ability to respond to such factors may allow for the generation of antisperm immunity. Alternatively, enhanced responsiveness to genital tract components by antigen-processing cells, T helper cells, or B cells may overwhelm immunosuppressive mechanisms and invoke antisperm responses. Evidence from animal models suggests that some women who develop antisperm antibodies are genetically predisposed to mount higher magnitudes of immune responses. Factors in semen which have been postulated to abnormally activate immune cells within the reproductive tract include bacteria, viruses, increased numbers of seminal epithelial cells or lymphoid cells, and the presence on sperm membranes of antibodies or aberrant surface antigens.

Antisperm antibodies may adversely affect sperm function in a number of ways. Numerous laboratories around the world are conducting excellent research projects investigating these phenomena in order to elucidate the mechanisms of immunological infertility, as well as delineate normal reproductive processes (2–4). Antibodies which agglutinate, immobilize, or opsonize sperm impair penetration through the female reproductive tract and significantly reduce the number of sperm at the fertilization site. Likewise, antibodies binding to surface-bound macromolecules may interfere with the normal processes of sperm differentiation, capacitation, cumulus-penetration, acrosome reaction, zona-penetration, and/or sperm-oocyte membrane interactions. The development of newer methods of assisted human reproduction, such as in vitro fertilization (IVF) and gamete intrafallopian transfer (GIFT), has allowed for the incidental study of the role of human immunological infertility. Various anecdotal cases of men and women with antisperm antibodies undergoing IVF or GIFT have been reviewed by Clarke (4). Currently it is not possible to analyze these results definitively, since the incidence of immunological infertility is low among patients of assisted reproduction programs, and the methodologies of antibody analysis differ among laboratories. Fertilization and pregnancy rates generally seem to be adversely affected in patients with high titers of antisperm antibodies; yet pregnancies have occurred. In the Norfolk IVF program, 15 patients (6 male, 9 female) with systemic and/or local antisperm antibodies had a total pregnancy rate of 34.7% per cycle and an ongoing pregnancy rate of 21.7% per cycle. In Tygerberg the GIFT procedure produced an ongoing pregnancy rate of 27.2% per cycle for 16 patients with antisperm antibodies. For both programs, these results were comparable among patients with or without antisperm antibodies.

Methodology

Antisperm antibodies in serum, seminal plasma, or cervical mucus have been implicated as an etiological factor of infertility. Although the incidence of such antibodies is increased in subfertile individuals, the exact nature of their effects on sperm function has yet to be fully elucidated (5, 6). Serological tests developed to detect and quantitate isoantibodies and autoantibodies to sperm may be categorized into three groups based on the nature of the antigen source: (*a*) ''sperm extract'' assays such as immunodiffusion or immunoelectrophoresis; (*b*) ''fixed sperm'' assays such as immunofluorescence, mixed agglutination tests, enzyme-linked immunoassays, and radioimmunoassays; (*c*) ''live sperm'' assays such as macroagglutination, microagglutination, cytotoxicity, immobilization, or sperm/cervical mucus interaction tests (7–9). Only several of the more ''traditional'' live sperm assays (e.g., macroagglutination, microagglutination, and immobilization) and several of the newer fixed sperm assays (e.g., mixed agglutination tests and enzyme immunoassays) are routinely performed by diagnostic laboratories and appear to correlate well with the clinical entity of immunological infertility.

It has become increasingly clear that antibodies which do not agglutinate or immobilize sperm may nevertheless interfere with fertilization. Traditional assays for sperm antibody detection based on measurement of sperm agglutination or immobilization can therefore not be conclusive (10). A number of factors can also complicate the interpretation of sperm agglutination tests. These factors include variations in ionic strength or divalent cations, serum proteins in combination with steroid hormones, 3'5'-cyclic adenosine monophosphate (3'5'-cAMP) and adenosine triphosphate (ATP), all of which can cause head-to-head agglutination of sperm (11). Additional assays are therefore needed which will detect the full range of immunoglobulin reactivity with spermatozoa. Enzyme-linked immunosorbent assays (ELISAs), a radioimmunoassay (RIA), and an immunobead binding test (IBT) for sperm antibody detection have recently been developed to meet this need.

MACROAGGLUTINATION

In 1952 Kibrick (12) described a macroscopic procedure for identifying antibodies to mammalian sperm in serum. Since the work of Rumke in 1954 (13), numerous investigators have used this assay to demonstrate the presence of antisperm antibodies in the sera of infertile patients. This test, also known as gelatin agglutination test (GAT), is performed by suspending semen from a donor without antisperm antibodies with the complement-inactivated serum of the suspected subfertile patient in a gelatin mixture in a small glass tube. After incubation for 60 minutes at 37°C, the formation of large agglutinated clumps of sperm toward the bottom of the tube and clearing of the homogeneous suspension of sperm in the upper portion of the tube indicate that antisperm antibodies were present in the serum sample. Microscopic observation of the clumps of sperm indicates that tail-to-tail agglutination predominates in the GAT, especially when the sera of men are being tested. (As with any serologic assay, both positive and negative control procedures must be performed simultaneously with the testing of patient specimens.)

The GAT is simple to perform; however, agglutination may occasionally occur due to factors unrelated to antisperm antibodies. Sperm agglutination has been reported to be associated with the presence of bacteria, fungi, or debris in seminal plasma and with non-immunoglobulin serum proteins or pregnancy-related steroids in serum (3). Yet this assay continues to be a mainstay of testing for immunological infertility. In a review of 17 investigations wherein over 7000 unexplained infertile patients were tested by GAT, an average of 7% were positive for sperm agglutinins (14).

MICROAGGLUTINATION

In 1964 Franklin and Dukes (15) introduced the tube slide agglutination test (TSAT), also called the Franklin and Dukes (F&D) test. In this assay, a mixture of donor semen and complement-inactivated patient serum is incubated at 37°C for 60 minutes. An aliquot is pipetted onto a microscopic slide for observation of sperm agglutination, which is generally of the head-to-head type. Because of technical difficulties involved in this assay, we have revised it in the following ways: (*a*) Donor semen from an individual previously shown not to have antisperm antibodies in his serum or on his sperm is subjected to a swim-up separation procedure; therefore, sperm used in this assay are free of seminal plasma, semen debris, and dead, non-motile sperm. (*b*) Patients' sera are diluted with a pool of serum previously shown to be negative for antisperm antibodies in order to obviate the effects of low protein concentrations which would occur if sera were diluted in buffer. (*c*) Positive and negative control sera are tested simultaneously to assure the quality of test conditions. (*d*) Since the use of undiluted serum has been shown to produce false-positive results, patients' sera are screened initially at 1:4 dilutions and, if positive, retested in a dilution series from 1:4 to 1:1024.

The TSAT has been extensively employed to detect antisperm antibodies, especially in serum of infertile females; yet results from different investigations have varied widely. We reviewed 26 studies using the TSAT; percentages of women positive for antibodies ranged from 9% to 78% (14). Such discrepancies may be related to technical problems or to the criteria used to select infertile patients for immunological infertility testing. Using our modified TSAT, the incidence of sera positive for antisperm antibodies from patients suspected of immunological infertility (i.e., with spontaneous sperm agglutination or increased incidence of spontaneous abortions) or with idiopathic infertility averages 5% to 10%.

Friberg (16) has introduced another microagglutination assay which is simpler to perform than the TSAT. This assay, the tray agglutination test (TAT), uses microliter amounts of reagents and avoids the need for transfer of material from the tube to a microscope slide, which is required by the TSAT. In the TAT, donor sperm and patients' sera are incubated in a flat-bottom tissue-typing tray, and agglutination is observed using an inverted microscope. This technique enables a technician to test several hundred serum specimens in a single day, using sperm from a single donor (17). The TAT is apparently more sensitive than the GAT technique, not only for detecting head-to-head agglutination but also for tail-to-tail agglutination (18). This difference in sensitivity is most prominent in the case of female sera, probably because the microscopic examination can detect small agglutinates commonly found with such sera. Comparative investations have demonstrated that the sensitivity of TAT for the sera of men was comparable to that of GAT (19).

IMMOBILIZATION

The interaction of antisperm antibody molecules with their appropriate antigens may activate the complement system and disrupt the integrity of the cell membrane. The ultimate effects of such processes may be the immobilization and/or death of the sperm (8). Fixation of complement and initiation of the cascade sequence is possible only if the antibodies are of the immunoglobulin G (IgG) or immunoglobulin M (IgM) classes, not with IgA immunoglobulins (20). Although both sperm cytotoxicity and immobilization assays have been devised for the measurement of complement-dependent antisperm antibodies, only immobilization tests have found widespread acceptance. Most laboratories currently use the sperm immobilization tests (SIT) proposed by Isojima (21, 22) or a modification of this assay. The SIT is considered more specific than any of the agglutination assays, since, if it is properly performed, only complement-fixing antibodies can produce positive results (17). Since fewer sera are shown to be positive by the SIT than by the agglutination tests, the sensitivity of the SIT is considered by some investigators to be lower than the agglutination assays (23). However, this is probably due to the high rate of false positives in agglutination tests. The major disadvantage of the complement-mediated immobilization and cytotoxicity assays is their inability to detect IgA antibodies and antibodies directed against sperm-head antigens which may not result in immobilization (20). Such undetected antibodies may interfere with other sperm functions such as acrosome reactions, capacitation, and sperm-egg interactions (24). In spite of these drawbacks, the SIT remains a reliable and clinically useful assay which has repeatedly been shown to correlate well with the patient's fertility status.

The SIT procedure is initially similar to the TSAT, since donor semen is incubated with dilutions of patient serum for 30 minutes at 37°C. Then small volumes of fresh rabbit or guinea pig serum are added as a source of complement, and the mixture is allowed to incubate for an additional 30 minutes before microscopic evaluation. The percentages of freely motile sperm and non-motile sperm are determined for each patient's serum and a negative control serum. A patient is considered positive for immobilizing antibodies if the percentage of motile sperm is less than half that of the negative control. In a review of nine studies using the SIT on over 1000 infertile patients, positive sperm-immobilizing antibodies were detected in approximately 8% of sera tested (14).

MIXED AGGLUTINATION REACTION

Although the incidence of antisperm antibodies is higher among infertile individuals than in fertile ones, the relationship between systemic (humoral) and local (in reproductive tract or on sperm membranes) secretions remains unclear (5). Several assays have been developed which can demonstrate the binding of antibodies directly to the sperm surface. These assays can be adapted to identify autoantibodies produced by men and adsorbed to sperm in the ejaculate (direct test) or can be used to demonstrate and/or quantitate antisperm antibodies in body fluids such as serum, cervical mucus, and seminal plasma (indirect test). The original concept for the mixed agglutination assays was provided by Coombs (25) in investigating IgG antibodies to thrombocytes. These antibodies were demonstrated by a mixed agglutination reaction between the thrombocytes with antibodies attached and indicator cells, group O Rh-positive human erythrocytes sensitized by incubation in human serum containing a high titer of incomplete anti-Rh. The two cell types, thrombocytes and erythrocytes, were agglutinated using an antiglobulin (anti-human immunoglobulin), and the assay was called mixed antiglobulin reaction (MAR). The MAR was also adapted to detect antisperm antibodies by Edwards and Coombs (27). With several modifications, the MAR test has become one of two mixed agglutination assays routinely used to demonstrate membrane-bound antibodies on sperm. The other assay, more recently devised, employs immunoglobulin-coated latex particles as an indicator source but also uses antiglobulin to produce a mixed agglutination between antibody-bound sperm and the indicator. These assays not only demonstrate the presence of antibody but can indicate the regionalization of binding on the sperm surface and can be modified to determine the class and/or subclass of immunoglobulin involved (28–30).

The MAR test has not been shown to correlate well with sperm agglutination assays performed on seminal plasma (31). However, strong positive reactions in the MAR test were found in ejaculates from patients with sperm agglutination titers of $\geq 1:32$ in their serum (32). Shortcomings of the direct MAR test include: (*a*) More than 1×10^6 sperm per milliliter of semen with adequate motility are required for this assay, and it cannot be applied to men with azoospermia or severe oligozoospermia (33). (*b*) Due to the progressive reduction in sperm motility which occurs as semen sits at room temperature, the MAR test must be performed within 30 to 60 minutes after ejaculation (32). (*c*) This assay is not quantitative. (*d*) Interference by debris, mucus, or microbial factors may occur (34). (*e*) Since some surface antigens may not be crucial to sperm function, the presence of membrane-bound immunoglobulin may not correlate with the patient's fertility status. However, with all of these shortcomings, the MAR test is a simple method for screening for sperm antibodies which may impair male reproductive abilities (35).

IMMUNOBEAD TEST

Traditionally the identification of patients with immunological infertility has depended on tests for antisperm antibodies in circulating blood serum. It is now recognized that some individuals possess antibodies in local secretions of the reproductive system (seminal plasma or cervical mucus) or bound to the plasma membranes of sperm, without the presence of detectable systemic antibodies (36, 37). Therefore assays such as the immunobead test (IBT) have been developed to allow for the demonstration of membrane-bound antibodies, reflective of local immunity to sperm antigens (38–40). Adeghe (37) stated that it is no longer sufficient to demonstrate sperm antibodies without determining their isotype, surface specificity, and concentration. The IBT, used directly, can detect and characterize sperm membrane-bound antibodies; indirectly, it can identify and provide semiquantitative data on antisperm antibodies in reproductive tract secretions. The direct IBT is relatively simple to perform, involving only a bench centrifuge, light microscope, commercially available reagents, and minimal technician time and experience. The direct IBT takes less than 30 minutes to perform, and the indirect IBT requires only an additional 30- or 60-minute pre-incubation.

Cross-inhibition studies have demonstrated high specificity between positive IBT results and the presence of membrane-bound immunoglobulins (39, 41, 42). Good correlations have been reported between the results of the IBT and other immunoassays suggestive of antibodies attached to the sperm membrane: post-coital test (38, 42, 43), sperm-cervical mucus compatibility assay (31, 42, 44), sperm immobilization test (38, 39, 45), and mixed agglutination reaction (25, 29, 30). Poor correlations between the IBT results and sperm agglutination assays have been reported (46) but may reflect the observation that sperm agglutination may occasionally be due to non-immunological components (3). Bronson (47, 48) reported that the indirect IBT agreed with results of the ELISA method for only 47% of serum specimens tested, when glutaraldehyde-fixed sperm were used. When live sperm were incubated with test sera before fixation for ELISA, the agreement was 83% for IgG and 70% for IgA.

Direct IBT

The immunobead reagents consist of 5- to 10-μm polyacrylamide beads to which rabbit anti-human immunoglobulins of the IgG, IgA, or IgM class have been covalently bound. These beads can be purchased commercially in lyophilized form (BioRad Laboratories), are reconstituted before use, and are resuspended in 5 mg/ml of a solution compatible with sperm viability. Sperm from the patient are washed well to eliminate free immunoglobulins which may be in the seminal plasma and which, if present, would inhibit the assay. One drop of the immunobead suspension is then mixed on a microscope slide with one drop of the sperm suspension. A coverslip is applied, and the mixture is incubated in a moist petri dish for 5 to 10 minutes at room temperature. Antibodies bound to sperm membranes will react with the anti-human immunoglobulins attached to the beads, and sperm-immunobead complexes can be observed microscopically. The percentage of motile sperm with attached beads, the localization of bead attachment (head, tail, tail-tip), and the number of beads bound per sperm are recorded.

Modifications of this procedure have been developed. Choices for the reconstitution/wash/resuspension solutions have included phosphate-buffered saline, Baker's saline, Tyrode's medium, Ham's medium, and Biggers, Whitten and Whittingham's medium. These solutions are supplemented with bovine or human albumin. Sperm concentrations are generally adjusted in the final washed suspension to 10 to 25 $\times$ 10^6 motile sperm per milliliter to optimize microscopic evaluation of sperm-immunobead interactions. Adjustments are occasionally necessary if the specimen is oligozoospermic or asthenozoospermic. Separation of sperm from seminal plasma components usually involves standard centrifugation methods, although some investigators have employed glass wool filtration or swim-up procedures (24, 45, 49). Finally, there are differences in interpretation between laboratories. Clarke (36, 38, 39) reported a specimen as positive for clinically significant antisperm antibodies if >20% of motile sperm bound immunobeads, since specimens from fertile men exhibited binding up to 10% of their sperm. Bronson (24, 45) considered a specimen positive for antisperm antibodies if any motile sperm exhibited binding of beads to the head or tail regions or if >15% of motile sperm bound to the tail-tip, an area which may manifest non-specific bead binding. Adeghe (37) reported a specimen as positive if >10% of motile sperm exhibited immunobead binding.

Indirect IBT

The indirect IBT can be performed on seminal plasma of semen with too few motile sperm for a direct IBT and also on serum, cervical mucus, and follicular fluid (36, 39). Samples for the indirect IBT may be stored frozen until analyzed. Before use, the sample is heated to 56°C for 30 minutes to inactivate the complement. Aliquots of the sample are incubated with donor sperm previously proven negative for membrane-bound antibodies by the direct IBT. These sperm are washed to eliminate unreacted immunoglobulin and mixed with immunobeads, as in the direct IBT. Antisperm antibodies in the test sample will bind to the donor sperm, which then can interact with the anti-human immunoglobulin on the immunobeads.

The performance, evaluation, and interpretation of the indirect IBT vary slightly between laboratories. Although some investigators incubate the specimen with unprocessed donor semen, the use of washed sperm or an isolated motile sperm fraction is recommended (37, 45). The volumes and dilution concentrations of the test specimens vary widely depending on the laboratory's experience and the type of fluid being tested. Seminal plasma is often filtered before use, and cervical mucus is liquefied with bromelin (2 mg/ml of Tyrode's medium). The incubation of the patient specimen with donor sperm is usually performed at 37°C for 30 or 60 minutes, occasionally in 5% carbon dioxide, depending on the requirements of the diluent or wash medium. The choices of diluent or wash medium are similar to those for the direct IBT. Although the assay is most often performed as a qualitative test, Clarke (40) incubated donor sperm in serial dilutions of the patient's specimen to generate a relative titration of antibody concentration.

Commercially Available Modifications

We recently evaluated a commercially available kit for the determination of antisperm antibodies which employs IgG-coated polystyrene microspheres and anti-IgG antiserum to create a mixed agglutination reaction between the microspheres and sperm with membrane-bound antibody (50). This kit, SpermMar by Ortho Diagnostic Systems (Beerse, Belgium), was found to possess several advantages over the IBT: (*a*) It was more sensitive than the IBT and as specific as sperm-immobilization assays; (*b*) the test can be performed with fresh, unprocessed semen with fewer motile sperm than required by the IBT; (*c*) background microsphere agglutination acted as an internal control for reagents, a feature not inherent in the IBT.

ELISA

The enzyme-linked immunosorbent assay (ELISA) has been extensively adapted for the detection and quantitation of antibodies and antigens in virtually every field of medicine (51). Most often performed indirectly, ELISA uses anti-human immunoglobulin with covalently linked enzymes to detect the presence of antibodies in body fluids. ELISA combines the specificity of the antigen-antibody reaction with the continuous degradation of a chromogenic substrate by an enzyme to amplify the sensitivity of the reaction. The sensitivity of ELISA is comparable to that of radioimmunoassay, without the potential hazards, waste disposal problems, and need for expensive detection equipment (51).

In the ELISA procedure, antigen is immobilized by passive adsorption to a solid phase; test sera are incubated with this antigen to allow for antibody binding. Unbound immunoglobulin is removed by washing, and the antigen is exposed to enzyme-coupled anti-human immunoglobulin, which is fixed to the solid phase only if antibodies were present in the test sera. Following another wash, a substrate is added; the degree of color change following degradation of the substrate is directly proportional to the antibody concentration in the test sample.

Numerous materials and methods have been used for the ELISA procedure: solid phase materials (silicone rubber, glass, polyvinyl chloride, polystyrene) and carriers (test tubes, beads, disks, microtitration plates); enzymes (alkaline phosphatase, horseradish peroxidase, glucose oxidase, galactosidase), substrates (*p*-nitrophenyl phosphate, *o*-phenylene-diamine); and a wide range of wash solutions and incubation conditions.

The ELISA procedure has been adapted to detect and quantitate antisperm antibodies (52). Many different methods are used, differing mainly in the type of antigen. Most researchers use whole sperm as antigen, while some use a sperm membrane extract.

Other variables in these assays are concentration of whole sperm (as antigen), type of solid phase and carrier, type of fixation of sperm, blocking agents, serum and seminal plasma dilutions, incubation times and temperatures, type of enzyme conjugate, type of substrate, and interpretation of results.

WHOLE SPERM ELISA

Concentrations varied from 2×10^6 per well to 1×10^6 per well (10, 11, 53–55). Lynch (54) concluded that 2×10^6 sperm per well proved to have the greatest sensitivity and that the higher the concentration of sperm initially added to the wells, the greater the percentage of sperm lost. Witkin (10) also stated that the concentration of sperm is a critical factor. If the concentration is too high, a thick sperm pellet will be formed following centrifugation which will not adhere well to the solid phase and will be removed by the washing process. He found a concentration of 6×10^6 per well adequate but recommended that optimal sperm concentration be experimentally determined for particular microtiter plates (10).

Most authors agree that a sperm pool from different donors should be used, as the use of individual semen samples allows the possibility of specimen-to-specimen variability (53, 55–60). Semen samples are washed several times to remove seminal plasma and can be frozen for later use. Wolff (61) showed that there were no differences in results between previously frozen and freshly coated sperm.

SPERM EXTRACT ELISA

Alexander (58) used a 0.3-M lithium 3,5-diidosalicylate (LIS) sperm membrane antigen preparation to coat wells for performing ELISA. When other sperm membrane extracts and whole sperm cells as antigen were compared, the LIS extract was superior. Often sperm are fixed with gluteraldehyde, increasing background values as well as interassay variability. Using an antigen extract, many of the problems of the whole cell ELISA are eliminated.

The extract is made of a sperm pool of different donors; LIS selectively extracts membrane glycoproteins which have been shown to bind to sperm antibodies. Membrane extracts may contain internal antigens not associated with the fertilization process and therefore are not of real clinical value (46, 62, 63). Most authors find the sperm membrane antigen extract superior to whole cell ELISA methods, with good reproducibility, small interassay variability, and ease of performance (60, 64, 65). One hundred microliters of antigen extract (7.5 to 15 μg/ml) in bicarbonate buffer (0.05 to 0.1 M, pH 9.6), are loaded into microtiter wells, blocked, and washed; the rest is performed as for the whole cell ELISA (58, 60, 64, 65). The alkaline bicarbonate buffer activates the plastic of the microtiter plate, giving it a negative charge. Glycoprotein antigen has a positive charge and is bound to the plate by electrostatic force. The antigen extract ELISA seems to be a very useful, reproducible, and easy method for the detection of sperm antibodies in serum and seminal plasma.

SOLID PHASE CARRIER

Most researchers use microtiter plates as solid phase for the ELISA assays. These plates are primarily made of polystyrene or polyvinyl chloride (PVC). Wolff (61) compared microtiter plates of both polystyrene and PVC and concluded that PVC plates adsorbed a high percentage of sperm, whereas polystyrene plates were not able to bind sperm sufficiently unless gluteraldehyde was applied. PVC microtiter plates seem to be the most popular (53–55, 60, 64) although some authors do use polystyrene plates in combination with gluteraldehyde fixation (57). NUNC Immunoplate I (53, 55), Dynatech Immulon II (10, 11, 57, 60), and Titertek microplates (54) are some of the commercially available products.

FIXATION OF SPERM

Fixation of whole cells such as sperm is essential when performing an ELISA. Fixatives bind the sperm to the plastic of the solid phase (10) and eliminate degradation of surface antigens by proteolytic enzymes in seminal plasma, for instance (55). Fixatives also immobilize cells and stabilize surface antigens by means of crosslinking amino acids (53, 56, 60). Many different fixatives have been used, indicating that this step in the whole cell ELISA is the most problematic one. Fixatives can cause many problems— high background values (56, 58), poor repeatability (58), binding to circulating immune complexes (58), denaturation and loss of surface antigens (47, 61, 62), and breakdown of the sperm plasma membrane, leading to exposure of intracellular antigens not important in reproduction (47, 62). Gluteraldehyde is the most popular and often used fixative, but it can cause all the above-mentioned problems. Some authors use gluteraldehyde without reporting any difficulties with the fixative (10, 57). A few alternative fixatives and fixation method have been tried:

1. Cytofix pressure spray (56);
2. Positively charged PVC microtiter plates (54, 61);
3. Paraformaldehyde 2% (53, 55);
4. Immobilization with phytohemagglutinin (PHA) (60);
5. Incubation of live sperm with test sera before fixation (47).

BLOCKING AGENTS

Blocking is essential to prevent non-specific protein binding, which may result in high background values (56). Blocking is performed before the addition of the test sera. Ing (56) used a 1% human serum albumin (HSA) solution, while Yan (65) used a 1% bovine serum albumin (BSA) solution. Howe (55) and Lynch (53) used a 0.25% gelatin solution to block reactive sites on the plastic solid phase. Blocking solution was made with phosphate-buffered saline (PBS) or PBS-Tween (56, 65).

SERUM AND SEMINAL PLASMA DILUTION

Serum dilutions ranged from 1:8 to 1:100 (10, 11, 53–58, 61), while seminal plasma dilutions were much lower, ranging from 1:3 to 1:64 (54, 55, 57, 61). Howe (55) determined optimal dilution of patient sera and seminal fluid using dilutions ranging from undiluted (1:1) to 1:100. A prozone-like phenomenon or hook effect was noted at lower dilutions of both serum and seminal fluid. Optimal assay sensitivity occurred at serum dilutions of 1:20 and seminal fluid dilutions of 1:3. Most authors used PBS containing Tween 20 and HSA and BSA as diluents for sera and seminal plasma (10, 54, 56, 57, 61). Howe (55) and Lynch (53) used gelatin in their PBS-Tween diluent, while Alexander (58) applied 4% polyethylene glycol (PEG) in Tween buffer. PEG reduced the time necessary for antibody binding with antigen, and Tween 20 reduced non-specific binding of serum protein to antigen and plastic (10, 58). Frozen serum and seminal plasma samples are normally used. Wolff (61) did a study to evaluate the effect of freezing on ELISA results and concluded that there were no differences between the results for previously frozen and freshly coated sperm. To overcome the effect of immune complexes in test samples, centrifugation to sediment them was performed (1800 $\times$ g for 10 min) (53, 55). Witkin (10) also proposed pepsin treatment to circumvent the effect of immune complexes by digesting Fc regions but not affecting F(ab$'$) regions. Goloumb (57) dialyzed seminal plasma samples against PBS, followed by centrifugation. Most authors used heat-inactivated sera and seminal plasma (55, 61), although Alexander (58) stated that inactivated serum samples should not be used. Wolff (61) found no difference between heat-inactivated and non-inactivated samples, indicating that the attachment of antisperm antibodies to sperm in the ELISA is not dependent on the complement system.

INCUBATION TIMES AND TEMPERATURES

Incubation times and temperatures of sera and enzyme conjugates varied from 30 minutes to 3 hours and from 22°C to 37°C (10, 11, 53–58, 60, 61, 64, 65). Most researchers used a combination of 1 hour at 37°C or 2 hours at 25°C. For blocking, the former was most often used (11, 56). Yan (65) used a combination of 3 hours at 22°C, while Howe (55) incubated for 1 hour at room temperature. Substrate incubation depended on the type of enzyme conjugate and substrate used. Time of incubation ranged from 10 minutes to 1 hour at temperatures ranging from 22°C to 37°C (55, 60, 61, 64, 65). Peroxidase substrate reaction takes a shorter time than alkaline phosphatase substrate reaction (60, 64, 65). Sperm and antigen coating were usually performed for longer times and at lower temperatures (4° to 22°C for 16 hours) (53, 55, 58).

ENZYME CONJUGATES AND SUBSTRATES

The enzyme conjugates most often used in sperm antibody ELISAs are peroxidase and alkaline phosphatase conjugates. Pig, goat, and rabbit conjugated anti-immunoglobulin are used as conjugates with both enzymes. The substrate for peroxidase conjugates is 2,2'-azino-di-3-ethylbenzothiazoline sulphonate (ABTS) + H_2O_2 (11, 64, 65) or o-phenylene diamine + H_2O_2 (53, 55, 60). The intensity of color caused by the digestion of $ABTSH_2O_2$ is read with an ELISA reader (spectrophotometer) at 414 nm (65) or 405 nm (11). The reaction can be terminated by SDS addition (64, 65). When o-phenylene diamine + H_2O_2 is used as the substrate, readings are done at 492 nm (60) or 490 nm (53, 55). The substrate for alkaline phosphatase is p-nitrophenylphosphate (10, 46, 57, 61) and its stable yellow intensity is read at 405 nm.

Ing (56) used urease-conjugated specific anti-immunoglobulin in his ELISA method. The substrate was urea solution containing bromocresol purple and ethylenediamine tetraacetic acid (EDTA). The absorbance of the reaction product was read at 570 nm, and the reaction was stopped with thimerosal solution. Ing stated that urease has the advantage over other enzymes in that it is not present in seminal fluid. The use of this enzyme eliminates the possibility of non-specific reactions due to endogenous enzymes contaminating the antigen layer. Urease catalyzes the hydrolysis of the substrate urea; carbon dioxide and ammonia are formed. Ammonia formation results in a pH shift which is detected by color change of the bromocresol purple indicator. Urea, unlike the other substrates, is safe, non-toxic, and non-carcinogenic (56). Alexander (58) used a β-D-galactosidase-protein A conjugate with p-nitrophenyl-β-D-galactopyranoside as substrate. Optical density (OD) of the reaction product was read at 405 nm.

INTERPRETATION OF RESULTS

Results varied from author to author. Most authors used a blank well to zero the ELISA reader, as well as other control wells to obtain non-specific binding to the substrate, plastic, etc. Alexander (58) used as a blank a well filled only with substrate, while Marquant-Le Guienne (64) and Herr (11) used a well coated with antigen and substrate as zero. Howe (55) used adsorbed negative sera and seminal plasma in wells instead of test sera to zero the ELISA reader. Herr (11) and Goloumb (57) used wells without antigen to assess nonspecific antigen-free wells. The most common way of expressing ELISA results is in terms of known positive and negative controls (10, 57, 58, 61, 64). Marquant-Le Guienne (63) expressed results in ELISA units, one unit being two times the OD of the negative control. Wolff (61) considered values positive if the OD was more than twice the OD of the negative control. Witkin (10) stopped the reaction when the positive control had an OD of 1 and compared test sera with the positive control. Goloumb (57) used the same method and considered values positive when the OD was ≥2 standard deviations of the mean from the negative control. Ing (56) obtained a threshold value of 250 negative serum samples and considered samples positive when they had values >30% above the threshold and negative when they were lower than the threshold. Howe (55) used a standard reference curve to define positive results.

COMPARISON OF ELISA WITH OTHER CONVENTIONAL METHODS

Agglutination and Immobilization

Several researchers did ELISA tests on semen and seminal plasma parallel with the classic agglutination and immobilization tests. Paul (60) found, when testing antisera against human sperm, that the sensitivity of the ELISA for sperm antibodies was more than 1000-fold greater than the classic tray sperm immobilization test. Wolff (61) and Ing (56) reported that the ELISA they performed on sera was more sensitive than the GAT, SIT, and TAT, stating that the ELISAs also detect antibodies other than those causing agglutination and immobilization. Alexander (58) reported a very good correlation ($P = 0.0001$) between results obtained with a LIS-antigen extract ELISA and sperm agglutinating and immobilizing titers. The same conclusion was found in the study that Howe (55) did when comparing ELISA and agglutinating and immobilizing assays on seminal plasma. Lynch (53) found a 95% agreement between the ELISA and the SAT and TAT, with a 92% positive predictive value with respect to the SAT and SIT assay results.

Radioimmunoassay (RIA)

Both Paul (60) and Alexander (58) found that ELISA compared well to and was as sensitive as RIA. Alexander found the ELISA superior to RIA: it is easier to perform, requires less expensive equipment, and eliminates the use of radioactive material.

Indirect Immunobead Test (IBT)

Bronson (47) did a study comparing the results of the indirect IBT with those of ELISA. The two assays were comparable only when test sera were incubated with donor sperm before fixation with gluteraldehyde in the ELISA assay. When gluteraldehyde-fixed sperm were incubated with test sera, the ELISA was less sensitive than the IBT, especially where IgA was detected. He concluded that the use of living sperm in the detection of sperm-reactive antibodies is very important.

Usefulness and Superiority of ELISA

The usefulness and superiority of ELISA for the detection of antisperm antibodies compared to functional sperm antibody tests lies mainly in the fact that ELISA obviates the need for fresh, good-quality semen, is non-subjective, is quantitative, and is immunoglobulin-specific (10, 53, 55, 56, 58, 61). Other factors making the ELISA very useful are its sensitivity (10, 11, 53, 55, 56, 58, 61), relative simplicity, and rapidity (10, 58, 60). ELISA is also thought to be inexpensive and economical, especially compared to RIA and IBT (11, 56, 58). The test allows high-volume qualitative screening (56, 58, 61) and can easily be automated (58). It is also non-hazardous (10) and reproducible (53, 55, 61). Pooled semen is used as antigen. This prevents a factor from one ejaculate from being a major influence on the assay (58, 61).

Semen used in ELISA need not be of excellent quality (61), and microtiter plates coated with antigen can be stored for later use (56, 61). Some authors feel that ELISA is well suited to replace functional sperm antibody assays, as it shows excellent correlation with these assays but has a certain superiority over them (53, 55). It is also a very useful tool in research (53).

The fact that antisperm antibodies detected with ELISA include those that cause neither agglutination nor immobilization, but can still influence fertility, makes the assay an important one.

The ELISA assay for antisperm antibodies is, however, not without disadvantages. In most ELISA assays, gluteraldehyde-fixed sperm are used as antigen. This fixative can change or remove the antigenicity of the sperm, causing false-negative or -positive results. Gluteraldehyde also causes high background values (49, 61, 62). The use of sperm membrane extract solves this problem, but extracts expose intracellular antigens that play no role in reproduction (46, 62). Mathur (63) stated that ELISA assays are only reliable when purified antigen is used, as the presence of Fc receptors on sperm or binding of adsorbed microbial antigens may lead to non-specific binding of immunoglobulins to sperm cells.

A quantitative antisperm antibody ELISA is potentially useful clinically or in research and may provide convenience and accuracy not possible with functional assays.

References

1. Witkin SS: Mechanisms of active suppression of the immune response to spermatozoa. An J Reprod Immunol Microbiol 17:61, 1988
2. Alexander NJ, Ackerman S: Sperm antigens and antibodies. In Runnebaum B, et al (eds): Female Contraception. Berlin: Springer-Verlag, 1988, p 356
3. Mandelbaum SL, Diamond MP, DeCherney AH: The impact of antisperm antibodies on human infertility. J Urol 138:1, 1987
4. Clarke GN: Sperm antibodies and human fertilization. Am J Reprod Immunol Microbiol 17:65, 1988
5. Alexander NJ, Anderson DJ: Immunology of semen. Fertil Steril 47:192, 1987
6. Alexander NJ, Ackerman SB: Sperm antigens and antibodies. In Proceedings of 2nd Heidelberg International Symposium on New Aspects in Female Contraception, 1987
7. Shulman S: Reproduction and Antibody Response. Cleveland: CRC Press, 1975
8. Rose NR, Hjort T, Rumke P, Harper MJK, Vyazov OE: Techniques for detection of iso- and autoantibodies to human spermatozoa. Clin Exp Immunol 23:175, 1976
9. Haas GG, Cines DB, Schreiber AD: Immunologic infertility: identification of patients with antisperm antibody. N Engl J Med 303:722, 1980
10. Witkin SS: Enzyme-linked immunosorbent assay (ELISA) for detection of antibodies to spermatozoa. Res Reprod 15:1, 1983
11. Herr JC, Flickinger CJ, Howards SS, Yarboro S, Spell DR, Galoras D, Gallien TN: An enzyme-linked immunosorbent assay for measuring antisperm autoantibodies following vasectomy in Lewis rats. Am J Reprod Immunol Microbiol 11:75, 1986
12. Kibrick S, Belding DL, Merrill B. Methods for the detection of antibodies angainst mammalian spermatozoa: gelatin agglutination test. Fertil Steril 3:430, 1952
13. Rumke P: The presence of sperm antibodies in the serum cf two patients with oligoazoospermia. Vox Sang (Basil) 4:135, 1954
14. Wortham JWE, Ackerman SB, Acosta AA, Swanson RJ, Taylor MK: Infertility 4:115, 1981
15. Franklin RR, Dukes CD: Antispermatozoal antibody and unexplained infertility. Am J Obstet Gynecol 89:6, 1964
16. Friberg J: A simple and sensitive micromethod for demonstration of sperm agglutinating activity in serum from infertile men and women. Acta Obstet Gynecol Scand (Suppl 36): 21, 1974
17. Jager S: Immunoglobulin class of antispermatozoal antibodies and inhibition of sperm penetration into cervical mucus (Dissertation). Rijksuniversiteit, Groningen, The Netherlands, 1981
18. Ingerslev HJ, Ingerslev M: Clinical findings in infertile women with circulating antibodies against spermatozoa. Fertil Steril 33:514, 1980
19. Hellema HWJ, Rumke P: Comparison of the tray agglutination technique with the gelatin agglutination technique for the detection of sperm agglutinating activity in human sera. Fertil Steril 27:284, 1976
20. Bronson RA, Cooper GW, Rosenfeld DL: Correlation between regional specificity of antisperm antibodies to the spermatozoan surface and complement mediated sperm immobilization. Am J Reprod Immunol 2:222, 1982
21. Isojima S, Li TS, Ashitak Y: Immunologic analysis of sperm immobilizing factor found in sera of women with unexplained sterility. Am J Obstet Gynecol 101:677, 1968

22. Isojima S, Tsuchiya K, Koyama K, Tanaka C, Naka O, Adachi H: Further studies on sperm immobilizing antibody found in sera of unexplained cases of sterility in women. Am J Obstet Gynecol 112:199, 1972

23. Boettcher B, Hjort T, Rumke P, Shulman S, Vyazov OE: Auto and isoantibodies to antigens of the human reproductive system: results of an international comparative study of antibodies to spermatozoa and other antigens detected in sera from infertile patients deposited in the WHO Reference Bank for Reproductive Immunology. Acta Pathol Microbiol Scand 258 (Suppl C):1, 1977

24. Bronson RA, Cooper GW, Rosenfeld DL: Sperm specific isoantibodies and autoantibodies inhibit the binding of human sperm to the human zona pellucida. Fertil Steril 38:724, 1982

25. Coombs RRA, Marks J, Bedford D: Specific mixed agglutination: mixed erythrocyte platelet antiglobulin reaction for the detection of platelet antibodies. Br J Haematol 2:84, 1956

26. Edwards RG, Ferguson LG, Coombs RRA: Blood group antigens on human spermatozoa. J Reprod Fertil 7:153, 1964

27. Coombs RRA, Rumke P, Edwards RG: Immunoglobulin classes reactive with spermatozoa in the serum and seminal plasma of vasectomized and infertile men. In Bratanov K, Edwards RG, Vulchanov Vh, Dikov V, Somlev B (eds): Immunology of Reproduction. Sofia: Bulgarian Academy of Sciences, 1973, p 354

28. Bronson R, Cooper G, Rosenfeld D: Membrane bound sperm-specific antibodies: their role in infertility. In Jagiello G, Vogel H (eds): Bioregulators of Reproduction. New York: Academic Press, 1981, p 521

29. Comhaire F, Vermeulen L: Le test "MAR" aux particules de latex et le test spermotoxique selon Suominen: simplification et nouveauté dans l'arsenal du diagnostic immunologique. Contracep Fertil Sexualité 11 (Suppl): 381, 1983

30. Grobler S, Franken DR, Pretorius E: IgG coated latex particles and the identification of sperm antibodies. S Afr Med J 66:97, 1984

31. Jager S. Kremer J, Kuiken J, Van Slochteren-Draaisma T: Immunoglobulin class of antispermatozoal antibodies from infertile men and inhibition of in vitro sperm penetration into cervical mucus. Int J Androl 3:1, 1980

32. Kremer J, Bouman O, Tjeenk W, Willink HD: Die betekenis van de Sims-Huhner test voor de fertiliteits/prognose. Ned T Geneesk 119:653, 1975

33. Jager S, Kremer J, Van Slochteren-Draaisma T: A simple method of screening for antisperm antibodies in the human male. Int J Fertil 23:12, 1978

34. Mathur S, Williamson HD, Landgrebe SC, Smith SL, Fudenberg HH: Application of passive hemagglutination for evaluation of antisperm antibodies and a modified Coomb's test for detecting male auto-immunity to sperm antigens. J Immunol Method 30:381, 1979

35. Asbacher R: Sperm antibodies and infertility. Fertil Steril 36:446, 1981

36. Bio Rad Laboratories: Immunobead binding test (IBT) protocol for antisperm cell antibody detection. Bulletin 1170, 1987

37. Adeghe J-HA, Cohen J, Sawers SR: Relationship between local and systemic autoantibodies to sperm, and evaluation of immunobead test for sperm surface antibodies. Acta Eur Fertil 17:99, 1986

38. Clarke GN, Stojanoff A, Cauchi MN: Immunoglobulin class of sperm-bound antibodies in semen. In: Proceedings, Fifth International Symposium on Immunology of Reproduction, 1982

39. Clarke GN, Elliot PJ, Smaila C: Detection of sperm antibodies in semen using the immunobead test: a survey of 813 consecutive patients. Am J Reprod Immunol Microbiol 7:118, 1985

40. Clarke GN, Lopata A, Johnston WIH: Effect of sperm antibodies in females on human in vitro fertilization. Fertil Steril 46:438, 1986

41. Clarke GN: Induction of the shaking phenomenon by IgA class antispermatozoal antibodies from serum. Am J Reprod Immunol Microbiol 9:12, 1985

42. Clarke GN, Stojanoff A, Cauchi MN, McBain JC, Speirs AL, Johnston WIH: Detection of antispermatozoal antibodies of IgA class in cervical mucus. Am J Reprod Immunol 5:61, 1984

43. Pepperell RJ, McBain JC: Unexplained infertility: a review. Br J Obstet Gynaecol 92:569, 1985

44. Pretorius E, Franken DR, Shulman S, Gloeb J: Sperm cervical mucus contact test and immunobead test for sperm antibodies. Arch Androl 16:199, 1986

45. Bronson R, Cooper G, Rosenfeld D: Ability of antibody-bound human sperm to penetrate zona-free hamster ova in vitro. Fertil Steril 36:778, 1981

46. Franco JG, Schimberni M, Stone SC: An immunobead assay for antibodies to spermatozoa in serum: comparison with traditional agglutination and immobilization tests. J Reprod Med 32:188, 1987

47. Bronson R, Cooper G, Rosenfeld D, Witkin SS: Detection of spontaneously occurring sperm-directed antibodies in infertile couples by immunobead binding and enzyme-linked immunosorbead assay. Ann NY Acad Sci 438:504, 1984

48. Bronson R, Cooper G, Rosenfeld D: The role of sperm antibodies in infertility. Res Reprod 16:1, 1984

49. Alexander NJ, Ackerman S: Therapeutic insemination. Obstet Gynecol Clin North 14:905, 1987

50. Ackerman SB, McGuire G, Fulgham DF, Alexander NJ: Assessment of a commercially available assay for the detection of antisperm antibodies. Fertil Steril 49:1, 1988

51. Voller A, Bartlett A, Bidwell DE: Enzyme immunoassays with special reference to ELISA techniques. J Clin Pathol 31:507, 1978

52. Ackerman SB, Wortham JWE, Swanson RJ: An indirect enzyme-linked immunosorbent assay (ELISA) for the detection and quantitation of antisperm antibodies. Am J Reprod Immunol 1:199, 1981

53. Lynch DM, Leali BA, Howe SE: A comparison of sperm agglutination and immobilization assays with a quantitative ELISA for anti-sperm antibody in serum. Fertil Steril 46:285, 1986

54. Wolff H, Scill WB: Antisperm antibodies in infertile and homosexual men: relationship to serologic and clinical findings. Fertil Steril 44:673, 1985

55. Howe SE, Lynch DM: Quantitation of sperm bindable IgA and IgG in seminal fluid. Am J Reprod Immunol Microbiol 11:17, 1986

56. Ing RMY, Wang S-X, Brennecke AM, Jones WR: An improved indirect enzyme-linked immunosorbent assay (ELISA) for the detection of antisperm antibodies. Am J Reprod Immunol 8:15, 1983

57. Goloumb J, Vardinon N, Homannai ZT, Braf Z, Yust I: Demonstration of antispermatozoal antibodies in varicocele-related infertility with an enzyme-linked immunosorbent assay (ELISA). Fertil Steril 45:397, 1986

58. Alexander NJ, Bearwood D: An immunosorption assay for antibodies to spermatozoa: comparison with agglutination and immobilization tests. Fertil Steril 41:270, 1984

59. Pexieder T, Biollat E, Janecek P: Antisperm antibodies and in-vitro fertilization failure. J In Vitro Fertil Embryo Trans 2:229, 1985

60. Paul S, Baukloh V, Mettler L: Enzyme-linked immunosorbent assays for sperm antibody detection and antigenic analysis. J Immunol Methods 56:193, 1983

61. Wolff H, Scill WB: A modified enzyme-linked immunosorbent assay (ELISA) for the detection of antisperm antibodies. Andrologia 17:426, 1985

62. Bronson R, Cooper G, Rosenfeld D: Sperm antibodies: their role in infertility. Fertil Steril 42:171, 1984

63. Mathur S: Immune and immunogenetic mechanisms in infertility. Contrib Gynecol Obstet 14:138, 1985

64. Marquant-Le Guienne B, De Almeida M: Role of guinea-pig sperm autoantigens in capacitation and the acrosome reaction. J Reprod Fertil 77:337, 1986

65. Yan YC, Wang LF, Koide SS: Characterization of sperm agglutinating monoclonal antibody and purification of the human sperm antigen. Int J Fertil 31:77, 1986

Section F:

HYPO-OSMOTIC SWELLING TEST

LOURENS J. D. ZANEVELD, D.V.M., PH.D., RAJASINGAM
S. JEYENDRAN, D.V.M., PH.D., PATRICIA KRAJESKI,
B.S.N., KEVIN COETZEE, M.S., THINUS F. KRUGER, M.D.,
AND CARL J. LOMBARD, PH.D.

One of the most perplexing problems in the evaluation and treatment of the infertile male is the inability of the standard semen analysis to reliably predict the fertilizing potential of the ejaculated spermatozoa (1–6). Other assays need to be developed to evaluate different functional entities of the sperm beyond the standard parameters. Since a functional membrane is a requisite for the fertilizing ability of sperm (7), assessment of this membrane may be a useful indicator of fertility. The hypo-osmotic swelling (HOS) test assesses the functional integrity of the sperm membrane by evaluating its reaction under hypo-osmotic conditions (see Chapter 4, Part 1, Tests of Sperm Function: Hypo-osmotic Swelling Test). By combining the information obtained from the standard semen analysis with that from the HOS test and other sperm function indicators such as the acrosin assay, one can predict more accurately the fertilizing potential of a sperm population.

The HOS test is relatively new, but a number of in vitro and in vivo studies have already suggested its clinical usefulness. In fact, more studies have been performed to prove the applicability of the HOS test than of any other new semen indicator. The intra-assay variability is reasonably small; the consistency increases with an increased percentage of swollen spermatozoa (8). Variability is most likely due to the error that occurs whenever visual sperm evaluations are made. The reliability of the assay was established by heat-inactivating sperm and evaluating mixtures of treated and untreated sperm (8). A linear decrease ($r = 0.94$) occurs in the percentage of sperm swelling with increased concentrations of treated sperm. Thus the number of sperm that swell is not influenced by the number of sperm that are unable to swell.

The outcome of the HOS test cannot be predicted from the standard semen parameters (8). Although statistically significant correlations are present between the HOS test and sperm motility, sperm morphology, and the live-dead stain, the correlation coefficients ($r = 0.30$ to 0.52) are too low to be predictive. These results indicate that the HOS test measures a different entity than do the standard semen parameters.

It is very difficult to prove that a test is predictive of the fertilizing capacity of sperm. This is probably the reason that it has taken so long to understand the limitations of the standard semen parameters. In vitro studies are the easiest to interpret and are therefore useful as a first approach to determining the applicability of an assay. The zona-free hamster oocyte sperm penetration assay (SPA) has been demonstrated to predict the functional activity of sperm reasonably well, although exceptions occur. The percentage of swelling in the HOS test correlates highly ($r = 0.90$) with the percentage of penetration obtained in the HOS if ejaculates with normal sperm parameters are used (8). However, when ejaculates from infertility patients are tested, such a high correlation is not present (9–11).

This is not surprising, because these ejaculates frequently suffer from more than one abnormality, or a different parameter is abnormal than in the HOS test. For instance, sperm may have an intact plasma membrane, possess normal motility, and give a positive reaction in the HOS test, but lack the acrosome, possess low acrosin levels, and be unable to penetrate zona-free hamster oocytes (12).

Some investigators have criticized the HOS test because of the rather low correlation of the percentage of swelling with the percentage of penetration of zona-free hamster oocytes when abnormal ejaculates are used. Such criticism is unjustified. If a high correlation between test values and percentage of penetration is required, no sperm test would be valid, since none of the presently employed sperm parameters correlate well with the percentage of penetration (13, 14). Therefore, when one is using patient ejaculates, ranges should be selected for normal and abnormal. When a test is in the abnormal range, the SPA should usually also be abnormal. However, if a single test gives normal results, the SPA may give normal or abnormal results, depending on whether the other sperm parameters are normal or abnormal.

Ejaculates are classified as normal in the HOS test when ≥60% of the sperm swell, and abnormal when <50% of the sperm react. Between 50% and 59% reactive sperm is taken as a gray area, where no definitive diagnosis can be reached. Using these values, the HOS test is 75% to 85% predictive of the outcome (normal/abnormal) of the SPA when patient ejaculates are tested using the data from Chan (9) as recalculated by Jeyendran and Zaneveld (15), Collins (16), Langenbucher (17), and Bastias (11). An abnormal HOS test is more predictive of the outcome of the SPA than a normal HOS test.

Human in vitro fertilization (IVF) can also be used to assess the validity of an assay. Ejaculates can be classified as fertile if the sperm fertilize one or more oocytes and as infertile if no oocytes become fertilized. Error is present in this evaluation, since lack of fertilization may be due to other factors than those associated with sperm; e.g., the oocyte may be abnormal. Overall, a distinct difference should be present in the mean and range of assay values between those sperm populations that fertilize eggs and those that do not. In order to trace these values to the original ejaculates, no swim-up or other sperm selection procedures can be used for IVF. The values of the standard semen parameters for the fertile and infertile ejaculates overlapped almost completely (18). By contrast, all the semen samples that fertilized oocytes showed ≥60% reaction in the HOS test, whereas the majority of the infertile semen samples showed <60% swelling (18).

Correlation of the in vitro fertilizing capacity of the sperm with the HOS test was higher ($r = 0.56$) than that with the other semen parameters ($r = -0.04$ to 0.25). Since that publication, additional ejaculates have been evaluated, so that the total number is now 121. Using the HOS test as the independent variable and IVF outcome (fertile/infertile) as the dependent variable in a forward logistic regression analysis, it can be calculated that the HOS test correctly predicts IVF outcome 88.4% of the time, with 12.0% false positives and 7.7% false negatives. As shown by Vantman (19) and Basuray (20), differentiation of the various types of swelling may further aid in eliminating the false-positive results.

The above data were obtained in the absence of sperm selection procedures, e.g., by swim-up. Selection of spermatozoa before IVF alters the sperm population so that the normal and abnormal values for the ejaculates may not apply, and the relationship with IVF outcome may be different. The sperm populations obtained after a swim-up or sperm-rise procedure usually produce a significantly higher percentage of swollen sperm in the HOS test than the original ejaculate (21–24).

In vivo studies also support the usefulness of the HOS test, although the data are somewhat limited. If fertility is associated with a normal HOS test, the majority of the ejaculates from presumably fertile men should give a positive HOS test. It can be assumed that men who have fathered children are still fertile, although exceptions occur. For this reason the HOS test was applied to 1890 men who requested a vasectomy (25). The large majority (96%) of the ejaculates produced a positive HOS test ($\geq$60% swollen spermatozoa), averaging 83% swelling. Similarly, studies by Kolodziej (26) and Van Kooij (10) showed that all the ejaculates obtained from presumably fertile men produced, respectively, >65% ($n = 38$) and 55% ($n = 16$) swollen sperm in the HOS test, with average values of 77% and 71%, respectively. In contrast, Spittaler and Tyler (21) reported an average of 58% swollen sperm with a range of 25% to 91% ($n = 45$) in the ejaculates of presumably fertile men. However, weighting the data by removing the dead sperm resulted in an average of 72%, with a range of 46% to 100%. Langenbucher (17) found that pregnancies occurred only with ejaculates that had $\geq$60% swollen sperm in the HOS test (the number of pregnancies was not stated). These data indicate that fertility is generally associated with a positive HOS test.

Infertility may be due to an abnormal HOS test, to other sperm abnormalities, or to female factors. Therefore, large differences in mean assay values between fertile and infertile men may not be present. However, a larger percentage of infertile men than fertile men should produce an abnormal HOS test, if the test is valid. This is indeed the case. Kolodziej (26) and Katzorke (27) reported that about 40% of the ejaculates obtained from male partners of infertile couples produced <60% swelling, i.e., in the suspect or abnormal range. The data by Van Kooij (10) also indicate that about half of patients with abnormal spermiograms had an HOS test that was suspect or abnormal. This is in contrast to the studies with fertile men, in which the large majority of the ejaculates produced a normal HOS test. Nachtigall (28) and Perez-Pelaez (29) reported that tamoxifen treatment of subfertile men can improve the ejaculates from <60% sperm swelling in the HOS test to a normal percentage of swelling, with concomitant fertility.

The HOS test is simple, economical, and can readily be performed in laboratories with limited resources and equipment. After being subjected to hypo-osmotic conditions, the spermatozoa may be fixed for later observation, which is of advantage under field or other conditions. Most of the in vitro and in vivo data obtained so far indicate that the HOS test correlates well with the outcome of fertility, if abnormal and normal ranges are used. The HOS test values cannot be predicted from the values obtained with the more standard semen parameters. Therefore, it is recommended that the HOS test be used as an additional fertility indicator.

Relationship between Male Fertility and HOS: the Tygerberg Experience

Over the past 2 decades, it has become clear that the functional competence of human sperm is not necessarily reflected in the conventional semen profile (30), thus yielding an uncertain prognosis for the infertile couple. Many functional assays have been developed, the most popular being the SPA (30, 31); these assays, however, are time-consuming and complex.

In contrast, the HOS test is comparatively simple, able to assess the integrity and functional ability of the sperm membrane (8). The sperm membrane system is important not only for cell protection and energy metabolism; it is also imperative for normal fertilization (capacitation, acrosome reaction, and receptor-mediated functions). When exposed to hypo-osmotic conditions, only viable sperm can maintain osmotic equilibrium. This results in the inflow of water, causing the plasma membrane to bulge. The sperm tail appears to be particularly susceptible: it curls under these conditions.

The assay was first developed for human sperm by Jeyendran (8), who found the test to be extremely accurate ($r = 0.94$) and reproducible. A strong correlation ($r = 0.90$) was also found between sperm fertilizing capacity, as measured by the SPA, and sperm swelling. Lower correlations were observed between the HOS test and sperm morphology ($r = 0.30$), motility ($r = 0.61$), and viability ($r = 0.52$).

The HOS test was performed in our study as described by Jeyendran (8). Two hundred sperm were evaluated for swollen tails, and the percentage of swollen sperm was calculated for each semen sample. Samples with >60% swollen sperm were considered normal, 50% to 60% doubtful, and <50% abnormal. The correlation of the HOS test to the percentages of normal sperm and living sperm, and to SPA and human IVF, as well as the relationship between HOS test ranges and the above factors, was investigated in a study at the Tygerberg infertility clinic.

The strongest correlation ($r = 0.76$) of the study was obtained between the percentage of living cells and the percentage of swollen sperm. Van Kooij (10) also obtained a good correlation, an understandable outcome, as there should be a relationship between the percentage of living cells and membrane function. A linear regression analysis, however, indicated that, on average, 30% of all "dead" sperm were still able to swell. (Explanations for this outcome could be that the HOS test measures only a subset of all membrane functions, supravital stain exclusion is not absolute, and an intermediate state of death exists.) This fact must be kept in mind when one is determining the true ranges of fertility for the HOS test.

Normal sperm morphology has been shown to be a good predictor of male fertility (32, 33), if evaluated using our strict criteria. A strong correlation with this parameter would thus suggest that the HOS test may have a role in male fertility diagnosis. Only a moderately strong correlation ($r = 0.50$) was obtained in our study; similar low-positive correlations were obtained by other groups (8–10). Three major fertility groups have been identified (33) with the help of normal sperm morphology: one fertile (>14%) and two subfertile groups (<4% and 5% to 14%). The fertilization rates of these groups are 85% to 88%, 7.6%, and 63.9%, respectively. Assessing the predictability of the HOS test according to these groups, we verified the relatively low correlation (Table 5.13). However, there was a distinct association between an abnormal HOS test (<50%) and a normal morphology of <5%. Of the 13 patients with a normal morphology of <5%, eight (61.5%) had an HOS test of <60%, and 75% of these (6 of 8) had an abnormal HOS test (<50%). An abnormal HOS test may therefore indicate that the fertilizing potential of a patient may be severely reduced.

Unlike Jeyendran (8), we found only low-positive correlations between the HOS test and the SPA ($r = 0.42$) and between the HOS test and human IVF ($r = 0.24$); 97.4% (38 of 39) and 94% (46 of 49) of all patients able respectively to penetrate (SPA) or fertilize (IVF) at least one oocyte had a normal HOS test (>60%) (Tables 5.14 and 5.15). Similarly, a high proportion of patients unable to penetrate (81.2%; 13 of 16) or fertilize (78.6%; 11 of 14) an oocyte had a normal HOS test. The test thus seems to be

Table 5.13.
Percentage of Swollen Sperm as Predictor of Normal Morphology

| HOS | Normal Morphology | | |
	<5% (n = 13)	5–14% (n = 37)	>14% (n = 61)
<60%	8 (61.5%)	6 (16.2%)	3 (4.9%)
≥60%	5 (38.5%)	31 (83.8%)	58 (95.1%)

subject to a high level of false-positive results. A low rate of false negatives was evident, however, for no patients with <50% swollen sperm were able to penetrate or fertilize an oocyte.

An abnormal HOS test (<50%) may thus be of significant diagnostic value, as it may be a sure indication of a low-normal morphology and reduced fertilizing potential. Further investigation is needed, however, to confirm the predictive value of an abnormal HOS, because of the low number of such results encountered in our study. However, a normal HOS test should be used in conjunction with all available parameters and assays in the fertility assessment of a patient.

Table 5.14.
Association between the HOS Test and the SPA

| HOS | SPA (per Patient) | | |
	0% (n = 16)	>0%–10% (n = 10)	>10% (n = 29)
<60%	3 (18.8%)	0 (0%)	1 (3.5%)
≥60%	13 (81.2%)	10 (100%)	28 (96.5%)

References

1. Glass E, Ericsson R: Spontaneous cure of male infertility. Fertil Steril 31:305, 1979
2. Collins J, Wrixon W, Janes L, Wilson E: Treatment-independent pregnancy among infertile couples. N Engl J Med 309:1201, 1983
3. Steinberger E, Smith KD, Rodriguez-Rigau LJ: Relationship between the results of semen analysis and the fertility potential of the couple. In Schirren C, Holstein AF (eds): Diagnostic Aspects in Andrology, vol 8. Berlin: Grosse Verlag, 1983, p 10
4. Blasco L: Clinical tests of sperm fertilizing ability. Fertil Steril 41:177, 1984
5. Bostofte E, Serup J, Rebbe H: Interrelations among the characteristics of human semen and a new system for classification of male fertility. Fertil Steril 41:95, 1984
6. Zaneveld LJD, Jeyendran RS: Modern assessment of semen for diagnostic purposes. Semin Reprod Endocrinol 6:323, 1988
7. Rogers BJ, Bentwood BJ: Capacitation, acrosome reaction and fertilization. In Zaneveld LJD, Chatterton RT (eds): Biochemistry of Mammalian Reproduction. New York: John Wiley & Sons, 1982, p 203
8. Jeyendran RS, Van der Ven HH, Perez-Pelaez M, Crabo BG, Zaneveld LJD: Development of an assay to assess the functional integrity of the human sperm membrane and its relationship to other semen characteristics. J Reprod Fertil 70:219, 1984
9. Chan SYW, Fox EJ, Chan MMC, Tsoi W, Tang LCM, Tang GWK, Ho P: The relationship between the human sperm hypoosmotic swelling test, routine semen analysis, and the human zona-free hamster ovum penetration test. Fertil Steril 44:668, 1985

Table 5.15.
Association between the HOS Test and Human Fertilization

	Human IVF (per Patient)		
HOS	0% (*n* = 14)	>0% to <100% (*n* = 34)	100% (*n* = 15)
<60%	3 (21.4%)	1 (2.9%)	2 (13.3%)
≥60%	11 (78.6%)	33 (97.1%)	13 (86.7%)

10. Van Kooij RJ, Balerna M, Roatti A, Campana A: Oocyte penetration and acrosome reactions of human sperm. II. Correlation with other seminal parameters. Andrologia 18:503, 1986

11. Bastias C, Thompson T, Buck A, Hinson M, Rogers BJ: Relationship between the hypoosmotic swelling (HOS) test and the sperm penetration assay (SPA). J Androl 8:20P, 1987

12. Jeyendran RS, Van der Ven HH, Kennedy WP, Heath E, Perez-Pelaez M, Sobrero AJ, Zaneveld LJD: Acrosomeless sperm: a cause of primary male infertility. Andrologia 17:31, 1985

13. Hall J: Relationship between semen quality and human sperm penetration of zona-free hamster ova. Fertil Steril 35:457, 1981

14. Stenchever M, Sadoni L, Smith W, Karp L, Shy K, Moore D, Berger R: Benefits of the sperm (hamster ova) penetration assay in the evaluation of the infertile couple. Am J Obstet Gynecol 143:91, 1982

15. Jeyendran RS, Zaneveld LJD: Human sperm hypoosmotic test. Fertil Steril 46:151, 1986

16. Collins JA: Diagnostic assessment of the infertile male partner. In Kistner RW, Barbieri R (eds): Current Problems in Obstetrics, Gynecology and Fertility, vol 10. Chicago: Year Book, 1987, p 203

17. Langenbucher H, Buck S, Riedel HH, Mettler L: The importance of various in vitro sperm tests for the evaluation of ejaculate quality. Presented at the 12th World Congress on Fertility and Sterility, Singapore, 1986

18. Van der Ven HH, Jeyendran RS, Al-Hasani S, Perez-Pelaez M, Diedrich K, Zaneveld LJD: Correlation between human sperm swelling in hypoosmotic medium (hypoosmotic swelling test) and in vitro fertilization. J Androl 7:190, 1986

19. Vantman D, Zinaman M, Sherins R: Dissociation of hypo-osmotic tail swelling patterns in sperm from fertile and infertile men. J Androl 8:24P, 1987

20. Basuray R, Tarchala S, Van der Ven H, Perez-Pelaez M, Jeyendran R: Differential evaluation of HOS test minimizes false positive results. J Androl 8:25P, 1987

21. Spittaler PJ, Tyler JPP: Further evaluation of a simple test for determining the integrity of spermatozoal membranes. Clin Reprod Fertil 3:187, 1985

22. Garrison CP, Snoey D, Ford RB, Nezhat C: Methods for semen munipulation to improve the hypoosmotic sperm swelling test (HOS): possibility of increasing the fertilizing ability of individual semen samples (Abstract). In: Proceedings of the 42d Annual Meeting, American Fertility Society, and 18th Annual Meeting, Canadian Fertility and Andrology Society, Toronto, 1986

23. Huszar G, Parikh F, Corrales M: HOS and supravital staining in the initial and migrated sperm fractions of normospermic and oligospermic specimens. J Androl 9:45P, 1988

24. Centola GM, Emilson LBV: Sperm washing for intrauterine insemination: a technical and qualitative improvement. Presented at the Vth World Congress on In Vitro Fertilization and Embryo Transfer, Norfolk, VA, 1987

25. Zaneveld LJD, Jeyendran RS, de Castro MPP, Silveira PJM: Analysis of prevasectomy ejaculates by the hypoosmotic swelling (HOS) test. J Androl 8:19P, 1987

26. Kolodziej FB, Katzorke TT, Propping D: Der schwelltest als funktionstest der spermatozoen und seine wertigkeit in der andrologischen diagnostik. In Semm K, Ahn J, Rohof D (eds): Physiologie und Pathologie der Fortpflanzung: X Veterinaer-Humanmedizinische Gemeinschaftung. Berlin, 1985, p. 36

27. Katzorke TT, Kolodziej FB, Propping D: The hypo-osmotic swelling test and its significance. Presented at the 12th World Congress on Fertility and Sterility, Singapore, 1986

28. Nachtigall M, Viehberger G, Lunglmayer G, Van der Ven HH, Szalay S, Aigner H: The effect of tamoxifen on the sperm swell test. Helv Chir Acta 53:279, 1986

29. Perez-Pelaez M, Jeyendran RS, Tarchala SM, Damirayakhion M: Possible role of tamoxifen citrate in the therapy of oligozoospermic men. J Androl 9:P36, 1988

30. Yanagimachi R: Zona-free hamster eggs: their use in assessing fertilizing capacity and examining chromosomes of human spermatozoa. Gamete Res 10:187, 1984
31. Rogers BJ: The sperm penetration assay: its usefulness reevaluated. Fertil Steril 43:821, 1985
32. Kruger TF, Menkveld R, Stander FSH, Lombard CJ, Van der Merwe JP, van Zyl JA, Smith K: Sperm morphologic features as a prognostic factor in in vitro fertilization. Fertil Steril 46:1118, 1986
33. Kruger TF, Acosta AA, Simmons KF, Swanson RS, Matta JF, Oehninger S: Predictive value of abnormal sperm morphology in in vitro fertilization. Fertil Steril 49:112, 1988

Section G:

HAMSTER ZONA-FREE OOCYTE HUMAN SPERMATOZOA PENETRATION ASSAY

R. JAMES SWANSON, R.N., PH.D., ANIBAL A. ACOSTA, M.D., SERGIO OEHNINGER, M.D., KEVIN COETZEE, M.S., AND THINUS F. KRUGER, M.D.

The Norfolk Protocol

The sperm penetration assay (SPA), a somewhat complicated animal assay, requires the sophisticated orchestration of a large number of sequential events. Although each technician tends to develop his/her own unique interpretation of any assay, it is imperative to follow well-established procedures when one initiates this assay. The following protocol may seem at times to be tediously detailed and pedantic, but we hope that it will provide insight into troubleshooting the SPA in established programs when the procedure fails, as well as give understanding and confidence to the novice learning the SPA.

ANIMALS AND OVA HARVEST

Technicians in our laboratory have retrieved a reasonable number of ova (25 to 60) from hamsters varying in age from 5 weeks to 14 months. However, for routine usage we prefer mature (8- to 26-week-old) female Syrian outbred hamsters housed in a light- and temperature-controlled room with 14 hours of light and 10 hours of darkness. (This timing maintains the hamsters in consistent 4-day cyclicity at 21° to 25°C.) Water and food (Purina RMH 3000) are available ad libitum, and the cages are changed twice a week. The animals are housed four per $38 \times 30 \times 16$-cm cage; overcrowding can cause reduced or absent ovulation. After they are uncrated, they are allowed to acclimate for at least 1 week before use.

Two hamsters per semen specimen are injected intraperitoneally (IP) with pregnant mare's serum gonadotropin (PMSG, Sigma) at approximately 21 IU/100 g of body weight on the day of estrus (a viscous, stringy—5 to 20 cm—vaginal discharge), followed 58 to 60 hours later by IP injection of human chorionic gonadotropin (hCG, Sigma), approximately 20 IU/100 g of body weight. (Eggs can be recovered from non-estrus-injected, naturally cycling females, but with much more variability in the number of ova. We retrieve an average of 5 to 10 ova on the morning of estrus when eggs are needed on an emergency basis.) The hCG injection is timed to occur 15 to 18 hours before sacrifice. Between 25 and 60 ova are collected from each yielding hamster; 60% to 100% of the animals can be expected to give eggs. For each specimen 30 to 50 ova are used, with the higher number preferred.

The hamsters are sacrificed by cervical dislocation or by CO_2 or N_2 asphyxiation, depending on the preference of the technician; no differences have been observed in the quality of ova collected. Oviducts are dissected out, along with a small portion of the uterus, after the abdomen is skinned and the peritoneal cavity is opened. Although the procedure is not scrupulously sterile, all tools are heat-sterilized, culture medium is filter-sterilized, and all cultureware is sterile. No attempt is made to maintain an absolutely sterile field. The oviducts are placed in a 60×15-mm petri dish (on a cold pack) containing enough Biggers, Whitten, and Whittingham (BWW) 0.3% bovine serum albumin (BSA)—the medium used for all ova processing—to cover the ducts.

The oviducts are flushed with a 26-gauge needle on a 3-cc syringe filled with BWW 0.3% BSA. The dissecting scope is fitted with a fiberoptic light source above and a base light beneath, with the base at ambient temperature. A long cumulus mass is extruded after flushing with a strong, steady flow from the fimbriated end. The cumulus is picked up with a 100-μl pipette and transferred to a 35×10-mm petri dish, which has been placed on the cold pack beforehand. After all the ducts are flushed and the cumulus masses are collected into the 35×10-mm petri dish, the dish is removed from the cold pack. An equal volume of 460 units/ml hyaluronidase (Sigma) is added, approximately 0.1% solution. After the cumuli are broken down, in approximately 5 minutes, the ova are removed with a mouth pipette (a Pasteur pipette drawn fine over a bunsen burner with the tip broken off at a diameter slightly larger than an ovum) and washed three times sequentially in three 100-μl dots of medium. A 100-μl dot of fresh BWW 0.3% BSA is placed in the middle of a 35×10-mm petri dish, and the washed ova are delivered to this dish, which is then replaced on the cold pack.

Four 100-μl dots of medium are placed in the lid of a 60×15-mm petri dish. To one dot, 25 μl of trypsin-EDTA (Sigma) are added (300 units/ml), approximately 0.1% solution. The other three dots are used for washing the ova after trypsinizing. Twenty to 50 ova, depending on the technician's expertise, are picked up via mouth pipette from the 35×10-mm petri dish on the cold pack and are placed in the trypsin solution. Ova must be watched carefully, as in 2 to 5 minutes the zona should expand and the ova appear to be somewhat distorted. The ova should be picked up individually as they reach this stage and moved with the pipette to the first washing dot, in groups of 5 to 10, until all the ova are recovered from the trypsin. They should then be washed with some force through the other two dots. It is important to ensure that the zona is removed from each ovum and that all the polar bodies are removed.

The trypsinized ova should then be placed in a fresh 100-μl dot in a 35×15 mm petri dish on the cold pack. This procedure should be followed as many times as necessary to obtain the required number of ova. The same trypsin solution should not be used more than three times. Additional ova are processed to allow for loss during the trypsinizing step. Ova held too long in the pipette may stick to the glass walls.

SPERM PREPARATION

Patients should be screened before the superovulation protocol is started to determine the presence of a sufficient number of motile sperm. A minimum total of 10^6 motile sperm must be recovered to perform the SPA properly. A donor specimen needs to be run simultaneously as a control. Specimens should be collected by masturbation after 3 to 5 days of abstinence and should be allowed to liquefy for 30 minutes. If the specimen is not liquefied by that time, it may be placed in a 37°C incubator for up to a total of 60 minutes. An initial count and motility are then performed, and the volume and pH are measured.

Four 15-ml centrifuge tubes are labeled with the specimen number. If the specimen has $\leq 20 \times 10^6$ motile sperm in the total ejaculate, the total specimen must be used. If the specimen is viscous, the entire specimen should also be used. The semen is added and mixed thoroughly with a pipette. At this time any macroglobules present will have settled to the bottom of the tube and should be removed before centrifugation. The mixture is then divided evenly among the four tubes. If the total is <2 ml, only two tubes are used. If the specimen is viscous, the volume of BWW 0.3% BSA should be doubled.

The four tubes are then centrifuged for 10 minutes at $270 \times$ g; the supernatant is removed and discarded. The remaining pellets are resuspended in 500 μl of BWW 0.3% BSA per tube. If the pellets are very small, it is best to reduce to two tubes at one time, making 1.0 ml per tube. Tubes are centrifuged a second time for 10 minutes; the supernatant is carefully removed with a Pasteur pipette and discarded. The remaining pellets are carefully overlaid with 500 μl of BWW 0.3% BSA per tube. The tubes are placed in a humidified 5% CO_2-in-air, 37°C incubator for 1 hour with the caps loosened.

At the end of the hour, the tubes are removed from the incubator and the supernatants are removed without disrupting the pellet. The supernatant is saved; count, motility, and volume are measured again. The motility of the separation should be >80%. If 2×10^6 motile sperm are not recovered, the supernatant should be mixed with the pellets; count and motility should be measured again. The specimens are then replaced in the humidified 5% CO_2-in-air, 37°C incubator with the caps loosened, until the pre-incubation is complete and the hamster ova are prepared and ready to be inseminated. Pre-incubation is approximately 3 to 4 more hours (total of 6 hours) for short-term SPA and 16 to 20 hours for long-term SPA.

INSEMINATION

The sperm concentration should be adjusted to 10×10^6 motile sperm per milliliter, or 10^6 motile sperm per 100 μl. If the concentration is too high, as is commonly seen, dilution is necessary. The recovery volume is divided by the total number of motile sperm recovered; this yields the volume containing 10^6 motile sperm. For example, (2.0 ml recovery)/(50×10^6 total motile sperm) = 0.040 ml/10^6 motile sperm. Therefore, 40 μl of sperm solution with 60 μl of BWW 0.3% BSA is used to produce the 100-μl dot. Two 100-μl dots are used for insemination, each containing 10^6 motile sperm. Two such dots are placed in one dish, and one dish is used per specimen. Mineral oil is then placed around—but not completely over—the dots.

If the concentration is too low, 10-minute centrifugation should be repeated; then only enough supernatant should be removed to establish the proper concentration. For example, if the recovery volume is 2.0 ml, the total number of recovered motile sperm is 5×10^6; 1.5 ml of supernatant is removed after centrifugation, leaving 500 μl. The pellet is then resuspended in the remaining volume. Two aliquots of 100 μl of this solution are used to form the insemination dots.

After all the specimens are set up in this manner, the ova are added; 25 are pipetted into each dot. Enough mineral oil is now added to the dish to cover each dot completely. The dishes are then placed in a humidified 5% CO_2-in-air, 37°C incubator for 2.5 to 3.5 hours. The remaining medium should be kept in the incubator.

MOUNTING EGGS ON SLIDES

Two slides per specimen are labeled; they must be dust-free. For each slide, a 22×22-mm coverslip is prepared by placing a small dot of petroleum jelly-paraffin (15:1) mixture on each of the four corners. These are placed upside down on the edge of the table until used. The mouth pipette is loaded with approximately 50 μl of fresh BWW 0.3% BSA, with care taken to rinse out any debris. It is important that the pipette tip be clean and free of debris to avoid destroying the ova. At this time, dishes are removed from the incubator. Beginning with the donor, one group of ova are pipetted out of one of the dots and washed twice in 100-μl dots of fresh BWW 0.3% BSA in a 60×15-mm petri dish. Approximately 25 μl of BWW are pipetted onto the middle of a labeled slide with 15 to 25 ova. A prepared coverslip is placed over the drop and pressed down rapidly until the drop is contacted; this prevents the ova from moving. Air bubbles which occur at this point are of no concern.

The slide is set aside until the same procedure is completed with the remaining ova for that patient. The first slide is then pressed down on the corners of the coverslip with a pair of forceps. If air bubbles are present around the ova, the coverslip is gently pressed until the bubbles move away from the ova. As the coverslip is pressed, the petroleum jelly/paraffin drops in the corners should rebound; all four corners should be thus checked. This technique should yield an even and proper squash of the ova and should be repeated for each slide. All excess solution should be sucked away with bibulous paper tissue. Removing solution helps to flatten the ova, but care must be taken—too much flattening can result in exploding ova. With a phase microscope, no staining should be necessary, and the slides can be read immediately.

SCORING RESULTS

Under oil immersion on a phase microscope, each ovum is observed for penetration. Penetration has occurred when a decondensed sperm head is noted with an attached tail (Fig. 5.13). If a tail is not seen, one may be observing the pronucleus of the ovum. The decondensed head appears as a large round or oval clearing or distortion in the egg cytoplasm. The number of penetrations per ovum is recorded. After all ova are scored, the percentage of ova with one or more penetrations is calculated. The donor should have a minimum of 20% of the ova penetrated to consider the SPA valid for the day.

CLINICAL RESULTS

Most researchers report a good correlation, 80% to 90%, between the SPA and IVF results. In our results with the technique, IVF showed a correlation in 82% of cases when the SPA was >10%. On the other hand, IVF was successful in 65.8% of cases when the SPA indicated <10% of the oocytes penetrated. Even when the SPA showed 0% penetration, IVF still showed good results in 66.7% of cases. Therefore, with the technique we are using, the SPA seems to have a good prediction potential when it is normal.

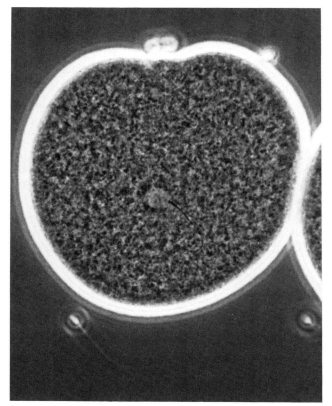

Figure 5.13. Zona-free hamster ovum with one decondensed human sperm head and detached tail in proximity. The wide white band is the oolemma, with several human sperm attached. (Oil immersion)

Section H:

FLUOROCHROME ACRIDINE ORANGE TEST

ELIZE PRETORIUS, M.S., AND THINUS F. KRUGER, M.D.

Although there are standard laboratory procedures to classify a semen sample as fertile or infertile, additional information on the DNA content of a sample seems to be theoretically important. The fluorochrome acridine orange (AO) test was described by Tejada (1), after an original version by Evenson (2). This test is based on the principle that *AO binding to double-stranded normal DNA results in green fluorescence*, while AO binding to denatured, single-stranded DNA results in red fluorescence. An abnormally high percentage of denatured sperm heads (red) can thus be associated with decreased male fertility, while a high percentage of green sperm cells indicates a normal semen sample.

The work of Evenson (2) was based on boiling semen samples from infertile patients, after which the red and green cells were counted by flow cytometry. He demonstrated that staining sperm cells with AO enabled him to estimate the fertility status of the patient. However, the equipment he used was expensive and specialized.

Tejada (1) introduced the idea of an "effective sperm count" (ESC), which is obtained by multiplying the percentage of green-fluorescing sperm by the sperm count. He showed that an ESC of ≥ 50 10^6/ml can be used as a cut-off value to classify a patient as fertile or infertile. During the Fifth World Congress on In Vitro Fertilization in 1987, Botes (3) presented the results of his research on AO staining of sperm cells. The percentage of preovulatory oocyte cleavage 44 hours after insemination was compared with the ESC of the husband, which revealed a significant difference between the division of oocytes with an ESC >50 and an ESC of <50.

Methods

The Tejada method for AO staining (1) begins with a routine semen analysis of each semen sample. After liquefaction, the semen is divided into two portions, one for semen analysis and one for AO staining. A drop of liquefied semen is pipetted onto a glass slide and covered with a coverslip. Motility and forward progression rate of the sperm cells are judged by phase contrast microscopy (Nikon, 400×). A sperm count is performed by Neubauer hemocytometer (improved double lining) and phase contrast microscopy (Zeiss, 400×). (The performance of the semen analysis is discussed in Chapter 4.)

The preparation of the semen for AO staining requires the following:

1. 1.0 ml of semen is added to 3.0 ml of sterile TC-Tyrode's solution (NaCl 8.0 g; KCl 0.2 g; $CaCl_2$ 0.2 g; $MgCl_2 \cdot 6H_2O$ 0.1 g; $NaH_2PO_4 \cdot 2H_2O$ 0.064 g; glucose 1.0 g; $NaHCO_3$ 3.0 g; bovine serum albumin 2.5 g; natrium pyruvate 0.011 g; Novopen (Novo Industries, Johannesburg, South Africa) 0.075 g—in 1 liter of water). The suspension is thoroughly mixed and centrifuged at 1300 × g for 5 minutes (Sorvall GLC-1).
2. The washing procedure is repeated once.
3. The final pellet is resuspended in 1.0 ml of TC-Tyrode's solution.
4. Two microscope slides are prepared for each patient. Medium-thick smears are made and allowed to airdry for 20 minutes.
5. The slides are fixed in Carnoy's solution (150 ml methanol + 50 ml acetic acid) overnight. (The Carnoy's solution is prepared daily.)
6. After fixation, slides are removed and left to airdry for a few minutes.
7. The AO stain is now prepared. The AO stock solution consists of 1.0 g AO (Sigma No. A-6014) in 1000 ml of distilled water. This must be stored in the dark at 4°C. To prepare the working solution, 10.0 ml stock solution is added to 40.0 ml of 0.1-M citric acid and 2.5 ml of 0.3-M $Na_2HPO_4 \cdot 2H_2O$. All solutions must be at room temperature. The pH of the working solution is 2.5.
8. Three to four milliliters of working solution are pipetted onto the fixed glass slides and left for 10 minutes.
9. The slides are gently rinsed with distilled water, and each slide is covered with a coverslip.

10. The excess water is removed by gently pushing each coverslip. Nail polish is applied to prevent each slide from drying.
11. The slides are kept in a moist Petri dish for microscopic examination.
12. A fluorescence microscope with an excitation filter of 490 nm and a 530-nm barrier filter is used to evaluate the slides. The magnification consists of a $100 \times$ oil immersion objective lens and $15 \times$ eyepieces. Evaluation time should not exceed 40 seconds per field.

Evaluation of Slides

Normal sperm heads reveal a definite green fluorescence. As described by Tejada (1), most of the red sperm cells do not stain clearly red, but a wide range of yellow, orange, and red can be observed. These cells are all classified as red, since denaturation which has already started is considered abnormal. The ribonucleic acid (RNA) content of the cytoplasmic droplet at the neck region shows a definite red color, while the rest of the sperm head fluoresces green. These cells are considered normal, since the RNA content of the cytoplasmic area normally stains red (4).

A total 300 cells are counted on each glass slide, and the average of the two slides prepared for each patient is reported. The results are expressed as a percentage of green cells, since these cells consist of normal double-stranded DNA which is supposed to have a fertilizing potential. For example:

$$\frac{150 \ (\text{green cells})}{300 \ (\text{total cells})} = 50\% \text{ green cells}$$

Fresh Semen Versus Frozen Semen

Tejada (1) mentioned that the semen samples were studied in either a fresh or frozen state. It is not clear, however, whether any of these test samples were frozen and rethawed; one must assume that the fresh or frozen state of the semen did not influence the test results.

A study was conducted by the Reproductive Biology Unit of Tygerberg Hospital to investigate the AO results of a freshly prepared semen sample versus a frozen semen of the same patient. The slides were prepared as described above. After resuspension of the final semen pellet in 1.0 ml of Tyrode's solution, 0.5 ml of resuspended solution was frozen. Two medium-thick smears were made of the freshly washed portion and fixed overnight in Carnoy's solution; 3 to 5 days later, the frozen portion was thawed and smears were made.

The study included 20 male patients who visited the Andrology Unit for routine fertility investigations. The results are represented in Table 5.16. Unfortunately, 14 (70%) of the 20 test samples did not show good correlation between the percentage of green cells found in the fresh and frozen portions. Although the study was small, it became clear that freezing the semen samples clearly modified the results. Swollen green sperm heads were observed in some semen samples after thawing, while other samples revealed only bright red sperm heads. Only 6 (30%) of the 20 test samples showed a difference of ≤5% between the percentage of green cells. It is also clear from Table 5.16 that 7 of the 14 cases where no correlation between fresh and frozen portions was noted, an increase in the percentage of green cells occurred after thawing.

Table 5.16.
AO Results of Freshly Washed Semen Portions versus Thawed Portions of Each Test Sample

Sample No.	Freshly Washed Portion (% green cells)	Thawed Semen Portion (% green cells)
1	38	23
2	41	39
3	23	76
4	37	36
5	57	91
6	31	80
7	59	52
8	58	21
9	67	58
10	56	70
11	45	72
12	80	65
13	52	14
14	55	60
15	56	54
16	77	83
17	70	65
18	39	93
19	63	29
20	55	87

AO Test Results Compared to Fertility Potential

Forty-eight couples undergoing in vitro fertilization (IVF) at Tygerberg Hospital were included in a preliminary study. On the day of oocyte aspiration, the husband provided a semen sample, a portion of which was prepared for AO staining. Ovulation induction was performed as described in Chapter 6, and the same laboratory procedures were followed for all 48 couples. The small number of patients could be attributed to the following:

1. Insufficient semen volumes did not allow AO preparation in addition to fertilization of the oocytes.
2. More than two oocytes had to be aspirated.
3. Patients in whom non-fertilization was attributed to an infection or cell damage were omitted.

Test results in these couples were evaluated. To determine the cutoff value for the normal percentage of green cells, box plots of the data were analyzed. If one looks at the box plots given *by the 25th percentile* of the total data set, one finds that 47% green cells gave a good discrimination for fertilization of the oocytes. The cutoff was not tested statistically, however, because of the small number of patients ($n = 7$) in the non-fertilization group. Because of the agreement in results, we selected 45% as a technical cut-off value for laboratory convenience. Group 1 consisted of patients with ≤45% green cells; group 2 consisted of those with >45% green cells.

In group 1, a total of 42 oocytes were aspirated. Of these 42, 14 (33.3%) were successfully fertilized in the IVF laboratory. In group 2, 185 oocytes were aspirated, of which 125 (67.58%) were successfully fertilized. The results of Sokoloski (5) showed that, of the 72 patients tested with the AO method, 17 also underwent IVF procedures. Of these 17 patients, six had an abnormal AO result and fertilized only 13% (four of 30) of the oocytes, while with a normal AO result, the fertilization rate was 47% (39 of 83). In our study, the patients were grouped as follows:

0 = patients with no fertilization ($n = 7$);
1 = patients with partial fertilization: some oocytes fertilized while others remained unfertilized ($n = 26$);
2 = all oocytes fertilized ($n = 15$).

The mean values for AO in the 3 groups were compared by a multiple comparison test (Tukey's Studentized Range Test for variables: HSD). According to the results, patients with no fertilization showed an average of 34.6% green cells (SD = 17.95). This result was significantly different from the other groups: an average of 62.4% green cells (SD = 14.55) in the group with partial fertilization and 63% (SD = 13.17) average in the group with total fertilization. It can be concluded that if the percentage of green cells is <45%, the probability of oocyte fertilization is lower, while a percentage of >45% green cells indicates a higher possibility of fertilization.

Sperm Cell Morphology and Fertility Potential

Sperm cell morphology in the 48 couples who underwent IVF treatment and AO evaluation can be divided into three groups according to the criteria of Kruger (6). Group A consists of patients with ≤4% normal morphology, group B consists of those with 5% to 14%, and group C consists of those with >14%. In group A, 18 oocytes were harvested; none were fertilized in vitro.

In group B, 84 oocytes were harvested, of which 50 (59.5%) fertilized. If the oocytes in this group are divided according to their maturation status, 62 of the 84 were metaphase I, of which 30 (48%) were fertilized. Of the other 22, classified as metaphase II, 20 (90%) were fertilized in vitro.

In group C, 84 (72%) of 116 oocytes fertilized. When these 116 oocytes are divided according to their maturation status, 78 of the 116 were metaphase I; of these, 57 (73%) were fertilized. Of the other 38, classified as metaphase II, 27 (71%) were fertilized.

From these results it is clear that, although group A consisted of a small number of oocytes ($n = 18$), the prognosis for fertilization was poor when the normal sperm morphology was <4%. In group B, maturation of the oocytes played an important role, as detected by the difference in the fertilization rate between metaphase I and II oocytes (48% vs. 90%, respectively). In group C, oocyte maturation did not play any significant role: the fertilization rate was 71% and 73% in metaphase I and II oocytes respectively.

Table 5.17.
Comparison of Fertilization Rates and Sperm Cell Morphology/AO Testing

	Correlation[a]	Number of Samples	Probability
Fertilization and morphology	0.35	48	0.014
Fertilization and AO	0.37	48	0.0088
Fertilization (MI)[b] and morphology	0.29	45	0.056
Fertilization (MI) and AO	0.39	45	0.0075
Fertilization (MII) and morphology	0.27	26	0.1726
Fertilization (MII) and AO	0.06	26	0.74

[a]Spearman correlation test.
[b]MI, metaphase I; MII, metaphase II.

Conclusion

Thus, AO test results shed more light on sperm cell morphology. The relationship between fertilization rates and test results of sperm cell morphology and the AO test are shown in Table 5.17. The relationships between fertilization and morphology or AO are not strong but are in the same range. Therefore, AO test results show the importance of careful morphological evaluation of each semen sample. Although human male fertility can be judged by a semen analysis alone, the AO test provides additional information on the potential of male fertility and can be used as an additional test in IVF.

References

1. Tejada RI, Mitchell JC, Norman A, Marik JJ, Friedman S: A test for the practical evaluation of male fertility by acridine orange (AO) fluorescence. Fertil Steril 42:87, 1984.
2. Evenson DP, Darzynkiewicz Z, Melamed MR: Relation of mammalian sperm chromatin heterogeneity to fertility. Science 210:1131, 1980.
3. Botes ADE, Van der Merwe JV: The effective sperm count correlated with fertilization in vitro. Presented at the Vth World Congress on In Vitro Fertilization and Embryo Transfer, Norfolk, VA, 1987.
4. Ichimura S: Differences in red fluorescence of acridine orange bound to single stranded RNA and DNA. Biopolymers 14:1033, 1975.
5. Sokoloski JE, Quigley MM, Thomas AJ: Relationship of human sperm DNA stability and fertility potential. Presented at the 12th Annual Meeting of the American Society of Andrology, Denver, CO, 1987.
6. Kruger TF, Acosta AA, Simmons KF, Swanson RJ, Matta JF, Veeck LL, Morshedi M, Brugo S: New method of evaluating sperm morphology with predictive value for human in vitro fertilization. Urology 30:248, 1987.

Part Two—Methodology

Section A:

THE NORFOLK EXPERIENCE

LUCINDA L. VEECK, M.L.T., LISA J. BROTHMAN, B.S.,
CATHY H. AMUNDSON, B.S., AND SIMONETTA
SIMONETTI, M.S.

Initial Screening

The andrology laboratory in Norfolk completes a thorough screening of all husbands on their initial visit. This evaluation includes volume, pH, count, motility, morphology, and *Ureaplasma urealyticum* screening. If there appears to be a problem with the specimen, additional specimens may be required and further testing carried out: washed sperm recovery analysis, ATP, acrosin, antibodies, microbiology screening, and hamster penetration tests. Results of these tests are relayed to the in vitro fertilization (IVF) laboratory before the couple's first IVF attempt.

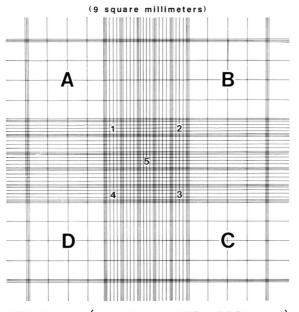

White blood area (counted in areas A,B,C, and D (4sq. mm.))
Red blood area (counted in areas 1,2,3,4, and 5 (80/400sq. mm.))

Figure 5.14.   Improved Neubauer ruling for one counting chamber area.

Semen Collection for IVF

The husband is directed by the embryology laboratory to collect a semen sample at a specific time, which might be anywhere from 30 minutes after oocyte retrieval to much later in the day, depending on oocyte maturity. A semen sample is collected in a sterile specimen container, and instructions are provided which detail the collection of a sterile specimen. The husband is instructed not to use a condom, cream, or lubricant because of the potential toxicity. Also provided is an information slip which asks for his name, birthdate, social security number, date and time of collection, date of previous ejaculation, and whether or not any of the specimen was spilled. The sample is then delivered to the desk in the hospital recovery room, and the lab is notified.

If a husband has difficulty collecting a specimen, he may go back to his hotel room or home to collect, have his wife's assistance, or use a special non-toxic condom obtained from a clinician. In more difficult cases the sample may be collected before oocyte retrieval by coitus interruptus. While a fresh specimen is desirable, a frozen specimen can also be used. A frozen back-up sample is requested of all husbands who anticipate any potential difficulty in collection.

Determination of Concentration, Motility, and Morphology in the Original Sample

MANUAL METHODS

Motility

Forty μl of semen sample are placed on a microscope slide with a coverslip. The percentage of motility is determined by counting motile and immotile sperm in five randomly selected fields containing at least 100 cells ($\times 400$) on an inverted microscope. Phase contrast microscopy is used.

Concentration

With distilled water, original samples are diluted 1:50. Both chambers of a Neubauer-ruled hemocytometer are loaded with diluted sample and scanned under low power to ensure even distribution of sperm and of obvious clumping. Five red blood cell (RBC) areas are counted using $400\times$ magnification (Fig. 5.14). If the specimen is poor, four white blood cell (WBC) areas are counted (Fig. 5.14), or a more concentrated dilution of the sample is used. The counts of both chambers are averaged, and the sperm concentration (in $10^6/\text{ml}$) is calculated using the following formulas:

RBC Area
1:100 dilution: Avg. no. of sperm counted $\times$ 5 = concentration (in $10^6/\text{ml}$);
1:50 dilution: Avg. no. of sperm counted $\times$ 2.5 = concentration (in $10^6/\text{ml}$);
1:10 dilution: Avg. no. of sperm counted $\times$ 0.5 = concentration (in $10^6/\text{ml}$);
1:5 dilution: Avg. no. of sperm counted $\times$ 0.25 = concentration (in $10^6/\text{ml}$);
1:2 dilution: Avg. no. of sperm counted $\times$ 0.1 = concentration (in $10^6/\text{ml}$).

WBC Area
1:100 dilution: Avg. no. of sperm counted $\times$ 0.25 = concentration (in $10^6/\text{ml}$);
1:50 dilution: Avg. no. of sperm counted $\times$ 0.125 = concentration (in $10^6/\text{ml}$);

1:10 dilution: Avg. no. of sperm counted $\times$ 0.025 = concentration (in 10^6/ml);
1:5 dilution: Avg. no. of sperm counted $\times$ 0.0125 = concentration (in 10^6/ml);
1:2 dilution: Avg. no. of sperm counted $\times$ 0.005 = concentration (in 10^6/ml).

Morphology

In the day-to-day preparation of sperm for IVF, it is not practical to stain and analyze slides for assessment of morphology. A critical morphological assessment is done, however, as part of the initial screening, and results of this evaluation are very important to the IVF lab in determining the concentration of sperm which will be used for insemination. Slides for morphology are made up from the IVF sample, but analyzed only if an unanticipated poor fertilization result occurs or as part of research studies.

COMPUTERIZED ANALYSIS

The CellSoft computer system consists of an IBM PC with disk drive, 256 K memory, monochrome monitor, keyboard, printer and digitizer, high-resolution video camera, recorder and monitor, Makler cell-counting chamber, and Olympus microscope with $10 \times$ objective. This system will simultaneously evaluate motility, concentration, velocity, and linearity.

To evaluate basic concentration and motility, 5 μl of undiluted sample are placed on the microscope stage. The threshold must be calibrated using the keyboard until the black images of the sperm heads on the digitizer are the same size as the white sperm heads on the video monitor. The threshold may be recalibrated during an analysis, if necessary.

To process an original specimen, three fields or 200 cells (whichever comes last) must be counted. A print-out will specify the number of cells counted, number and percentage of motile and immotile cells, concentration (in 10^6/ml) of the sample, and average velocity and linearity.

Sperm-Washing Procedures

RATIONALE FOR SPERM-WASHING AND INCUBATION PROCEDURES

Norfolk protocols for IVF sperm preparation involve washing and incubation of the sperm specimen or motile sperm migration out of whole seminal plasma. These steps are necessary for the following reasons:

1. Many sexually transmitted organisms are found in semen, including aerobic and anaerobic bacteria, genital mycoplasma, and *Chlamydia trachomatis*. Washing and/or incubating sperm in media containing antibiotics removes or retards the growth of these microbes from the preparation used for insemination.
2. The swim-up or motile migration portion of the sample improves motility and morphology over the original semen specimen.
3. Seminal plasma contains inhibitors to fertilization which must be separated from sperm cells. The washing and migration steps mimic a natural situation wherein sperm are separated from seminal plasma by transversing uterine and tubal fluids before reaching the oocyte. In addition, washed sperm may undergo or initiate capacitation during the incubation phase of the preparation procedure. Though poorly understood, capacitation involves changes in the spermatozoal membrane and serves as a precursor to the spermatozoon acrosome reaction.

TECHNIQUE

For our purposes, a normal semen specimen has the following parameters: count of $>20 \times 10^6$/ml, motility of $>30\%$, and morphology with $>14\%$ normal forms.

Normospermic Samples (Sperm Swim-up or Rise Technique)

1. Volume, viscosity, color of the specimen, and time analysis began are all recorded.
2. After liquefaction, 5 µl of sample are loaded onto the Makler chamber for analysis. A morphology slide is prepared for the andrology laboratory with another 5 µl.
3. One-fourth milliliter of semen is aliquoted into each of four 15-ml centrifuge tubes. An additional 0.5 milliliter of insemination medium (Ham's F-10 + 7.5% human fetal cord serum) is added to each and mixed. Tubes are centrifuged for 10 minutes at 427 × g.
4. Supernatants are removed with a 9-inch sterile Pasteur pipette, and pellets are resuspended.
5. One-half milliliter of insemination medium is added to the pellets, mixed, and recentrifuged. Supernatants are again removed.
6. Without disturbing the pellets, 0.5 milliliter of insemination medium is gently layered over the pellets. Tubes are placed slightly slanted in a specimen container, and caps loosened on the tubes.
7. Tubes are incubated at 37°C in 5% CO_2 in air for 1 hour.
8. Supernatants are removed and placed in a small Falcon #2003 culture tube. This is the motile fraction which will be used for insemination.
9. Five microliters of this motile fraction are loaded onto the Makler chamber for analysis of count and motility.

Subnormal Samples (Sperm Swim-up or Rise Technique)

Oligospermic, asthenospermic, and teratospermic samples are generally handled in the same manner as normospermic samples, with the following changes:

1. The entire sample is used and divided up into 8 to 16 centrifuge tubes.
2. A greater amount of the sample is aliquotted (up to 0.5 ml) into each tube if volume is sufficient; otherwise, smaller volumes are used.
3. A small amount of medium is layered over pellets to contain the motile fraction, as little as 0.1 ml.
4. One must be prepared to spin down the final volume and/or to use microtiter dishes to reach a desirable concentration for insemination.
5. Pellets may be relayered to obtain another rise specimen.
6. In extreme cases the motile fraction may be remixed with the pellet and used for insemination in this form.

Cryopreserved Samples

1. At least two cryovials are thawed for use.
2. Samples are allowed to thaw at room temperature for 40 minutes with the laminar hood shut off. Insemination medium should be at room temperature.
3. The thawed specimen is pipetted into a centrifuge tube, and the volume is noted.
4. Double the volume of insemination medium is added to the sample by drops. This should be done slowly so that the sperm are not damaged by sudden changes in osmolarity.
5. This final volume is divided among four centrifuge tubes and centrifuged.
6. Supernatants are removed and pellets resuspended in 0.5 ml of insemination medium. At this time 5 µl of the sample are loaded onto a Makler chamber for determination of concentration and motility. A lower motility may be expected in a cryopreserved specimen.
7. The sample is washed and centrifuged once more, as for a normal specimen.
8. Pellets are layered with 0.1 to 0.5 ml of medium and incubated for 1 hour, as for a normal specimen.

9. Supernatants (motile fraction) are removed and reassayed before insemination, as for a normal specimen.

Extremely Viscous or Agglutinated Samples

If a sample does not liquefy in approximately 20 minutes after collection, one or more of the following steps may be necessary:

1. Vigorous pipetting with a 10-ml pipette may be done to break up the viscous mass.
2. A larger amount of medium may be added to the original specimen and mixed vigorously. This may also be done after the first wash.
3. A third wash may be required.
4. Placing the sample at 37°C for 30 minutes may assist in reducing viscosity.

Sperm Migration Technique

1. Insemination medium is mixed with an inert, high-molecular-weight polysaccharide such as Sperm Select (Pharmacia Laboratories, Sweden).
2. Sperm are allowed to incubate for 1 hour in the viscous solution at 37°C in order for motile sperm to swim or migrate out of the viscous portion.
3. Motile sperm recovery is excellent without centrifugation and washing procedures.
4. This technique is suitable for normospermic, subnormal, cryopreserved, and viscous samples.

Determination of Concentration and Motility in the Washed Sample

After washing twice (optional) and incubating (1 hour) the sperm, the motile fraction that will be used for insemination is analyzed by manual or computerized methods. For manual methods a 1:2 or 1:5 dilution is typically used. In computerized analysis, 10 fields or 100 cells must be analyzed. Care must be taken to select random fields outside the chamber grid.

The final volume of washed specimen to add to an oocyte is calculated as follows:

$$\text{Volume to be added} = \frac{\text{Total number of motile sperm desired}}{\text{Number of motile sperm per milliliter recovered}}$$

In the Norfolk program, the number of sperm desired for insemination is 5×10^4/ml of insemination medium (normal males); 3 ml of medium are used in an organ culture dish. Therefore, a total of 0.15×10^6 motile sperm are required for insemination (5×10^4/ml $\times$ 3 ml = $15 \times 10^4 = 0.15 \times 10^6$ total sperm). One would divide this number (0.15×10^6) by the actual number of recovered sperm per milliliter (for example, 10×10^6/ml) to achieve the appropriate volume to be used for insemination (0.015 ml or 15 µl).

Sperm concentrations used for insemination are generally as follows:

1. Normal samples: 50,000 motile sperm (m) per milliliter of medium;
2. Cryopreserved samples: at least 100,000 m/ml of medium;
3. Subnormal samples: 200,000 to 1×10^6 m/ml of medium, depending upon the severity of the problem;
4. Poor hamster penetration assay: 500,000 m/ml of medium;
5. Antisperm antibodies: up to 500,000 m/ml of medium, depending upon the severity of agglutination.

ALTERNATIVE ACTION WHEN THE FINAL SAMPLE IS EXTREMELY POOR (LOW CONCENTRATION, LOW MOTILITY, NON-PROGRESSIVE MOTILITY)

1. The final motile fraction may be gently centrifuged for 5 minutes and the resulting pellet added to a single organ culture dish, micro dish, or medium droplet under oil to maximize sperm concentration around the oocyte(s).
2. Oocytes may be combined in a single culture dish or micro dish or in a medium droplet under oil to make the best use of the few available sperm.
3. The observation of a very low concentration of sperm in the final supernatant may indicate very poor motility (failure to swim into supernatant) and/or very poor morphology, which affects normal motility. In some cases the collection of a fresh sample may result in improved quality. It has been our experience that often a second sample, collected as soon as 1 to 2 hours after the first, may show improved semen parameters in routinely normospermic men.
4. In cases involving known subfertile males, a donor backup sample may be desired by the couple undergoing IVF.

OVERNIGHT MAINTENANCE OF WASHED SPECIMENS

Washed specimens are stored overnight at room temperature under 5% CO_2 in air. These samples may be used on the following day to inseminate immature oocytes which have matured in vitro.

For reinsemination of an unfertilized oocyte, the original sample from the previous day is often used, if it appears normal and has succeeded in fertilizing other oocytes. If the original specimen was very poor or if fertilization failed to occur, a fresh sample is requested. In some cases, a donor sample is used if the original specimen was extremely poor and the patient demonstrated a history of fertilization failure.

Abnormal or Failed Fertilization

PATIENT FOLLOW-UP

The embryology laboratory must notify the primary physician of failed fertilization and must supply all pertinent sperm and oocyte information. The andrology laboratory may be contacted to complete a further workup on the patient. With the additional information, causes and possible remedies for fertilization failure may be discovered and overcome.

INCIDENCE AND CAUSES

1. Pre-zygotes displaying one pronucleus are generally thought to be caused by oocyte activation without sperm penetration or with penetration but without sperm head decondensation. The problem may be related to trauma in oocyte collection and is often associated with aged oocytes.
2. Pre-zygotes displaying three pronuclei (tripoloidy) may be the result of:
   a. Failure of the block to polyspermy;
   b. Penetration by a binucleate spermatozoon;
   c. Retention of the first or second polar body of the oocyte;
   d. Penetration of a binucleate oocyte;
   e. Poor culture conditions, causing *a* or *c*.

Oocyte immaturity, especially post-maturity, is often associated with the development of ≥3 pronuclei after insemination.

Table 5.18.
Fertilization Success v. Oocyte Maturation at Collection (Norfolk Series 18–29)

Oocyte Maturation at collection	No. of Oocytes	Fertilization per Oocyte (%)	Pregnancy per "Pure Transfer"[a] (%)
Metaphase II	2980	92	27 (388 transfers)
Metaphase I (reached MII in less than 15 hr)	1568	86	20 (86 transfers)
Metaphase I (required more than 15 hr to reach MII)	392	69[b]	50 (6 transfers)
Prophase I	2347	52[b]	3 (38 transfers)

[a]"Pure transfers": Only pre-embryos developed from one maturational status transferred in transfer cycle (as opposed to a "mixed" transfer, where MII and MI oocytes transferred together). (MI, metaphase I; MII, metaphase II.)
[b]Semen sample 24 hours old by insemination, resulting in reduced fertilization success.

Correlation of Semen Factors with IVF Success

Which factors of the basic semen analysis give us an estimate of the fertilizing ability of sperm collected for IVF? What is the result in terms of pregnancy with male factor populations? Tables 5.18 to 5.22 demonstrate the Norfolk experience in regard to parameters of male partner assessment and the relationship to clinical success.

OOCYTE MATURITY AT COLLECTION

Rates of fertilization may be correlated to the degree of oocyte maturity at the time of IVF collection. Those oocytes collected at a fully mature state (metaphase II) exhibit a high fertilizing potential. Oocytes of intermediate maturity (metaphase I) exhibit a slightly lowered fertilization success, and fully immature oocytes (prophase I) demonstrate the lowest potential (Table 5.18). The significance of the age of the semen sample is not overlooked in these results; reduction of fertilization rates is directly related to the age of the washed sperm at the time of insemination. Oocytes collected at earlier stages of maturity, and therefore inseminated with sperm of longer capacitation time, demonstrate a reduced fertilization rate. Pregnancy rates are significantly lower only for oocytes which are collected in a fully immature state.

VOLUME AND VISCOSITY

Not surprisingly, neither semen volume nor viscosity demonstrates any particular relationship to fertilization, pregnancy, or ongoing pregnancy rates (Table 5.19). Semen volumes in the hypospermic (<1.0 ml) and hyperspermic (>8.0 ml) ranges fail to demonstrate any reduction of reproductive performance, even with volumes as low as 0.2 ml and as great as 11.0 ml. The presence of viscous seminal fluid, while sometimes technically difficult to deal with, poses no detriment to IVF treatment.

SPERM CONCENTRATION

Sperm concentration in the range of 20 to 400×10^6/ml shows very little effect on fertilization and pregnancy rates. Below the level of 20×10^6/ml, one begins to notice a

Table 5.19.
Fertilization and Pregnancy Success vs. Semen Volume and Viscosity (Norfolk Series 1–30)

Volume	No. of Cycles	Fertilization per Oocyte (%)	Pregnancy per Transfer (%)
0–1 ml	329	83	27
1.5–5.0 ml	1916	86	28
5–8.0 ml	136	85	27
8.5+ ml	15	89	40
Viscosity			
Viscous	731	87	30
Not viscous	1665	85	27

reduction in fertilizing ability, a reduction far more apparent at concentrations below 10 $\times$ 10^6/ml. Transfer rates per patient drop as a result of this diminished fertility, but it appears that the chances of pregnancy are not significantly lower if the patient reaches the transfer stage (Table 5.20). Taken as a single parameter, sperm number alone is a poor indicator of fertilizing capacity, as some males with concentrations well below normal possess the ability to fertilize all oocytes, while others in this range fail to fertilize even one.

MOTILITY

The percentage of motile sperm in the original ejaculate plays a role similar to that of sperm concentration in terms of fertilization. A slight reduction in fertilization is noticed below the 30% level, with a resulting decrease in transfer rate (Table 5.21). However, the pregnancy rate after transfer is not greatly affected. It is possible that the practice of increasing the number of sperm for insemination in cases of low motility has reduced the risk of fertilization failure.

MORPHOLOGY

Table 5.22 indicates that the percentage of sperm with normal morphology is the most significant parameter in IVF success. A strict method of morphology determination has been used for the Norfolk patients included in the data shown in this table. (Details of

Table 5.20.
Fertilization and Pregnancy Success vs. Sperm Concentration in Original Ejaculate (Norfolk Series 1–30)

Concentration (10^6/ml)	No. of Cycles	Fertilization per Oocyte (%)	Pregnancy per Transfer (%)
<20 $\times$ 10^6	111	62	28
20–49 $\times$ 10^6	436	80	29
50–99 $\times$ 10^6	857	88	29
100–199 $\times$ 10^6	697	90	27
200–399 $\times$ 10^6	213	90	26
>400 $\times$ 10^6	11	87	10

Table 5.21.
Fertilization and Pregnancy Success vs. Sperm Motility in Original Ejaculate (Norfolk Series 1–30)

Motility (%)	No. of Cycles	Fertilization per Oocyte (%)	Pregnancy per Transfer (%)
<20	63	62	33
<30	140	69	33
≥30	2255	87	27
>80	279	90	26

the techniques and criteria are elsewhere in this book.) In general, fertilization rates, pregnancy rates per transfer, and ongoing pregnancy rates per transfer and per cycle are all reduced in patients with severe teratozoospermia. Male subfertility is likely to involve a combination of sperm deficiencies which affect the functional ability of most or all of the sperm in a sample. The ability of a single parameter to serve as a prognostic tool is limited by this multifactorial association. While it is sometimes difficult to assess clinical findings and relate them to reproductive potential, prognostic value can be best placed on morphology when assessment is done by the strict criteria of evaluation.

Table 5.22.
Fertilization and Pregnancy Success vs. Sperm Morphology in the Original Ejaculate (Norfolk Series 25–28)[a]

Morphology Pattern	No. of Cycles	Avg. Normal Forms (%)	Fertilization per Oocyte (%)	Pregnancy per Transfer (%)	Ongoing Pregnancy per Transfer (%)
>14% normal forms (control group)	41	18.4±3.5	94	44	32
4–14% normal forms (G pattern)	144	7.3±2.8	86	44	25
<4% normal forms (P pattern)	47	1.4±1.2	45	14	7

[a]Data taken from Oehninger S, Acosta AA, Morshedi M, Veeck L, Swanson RJ, Simmons K, Rosenwaks Z: Corrective measures and pregnancy outcome in in vitro fertilization in patients with severe sperm morphology abnormalities. Fertil Steril 50:283, 1988.

Section B:

THE TYGERBERG EXPERIENCE

THINUS F. KRUGER, M.D., AND FRIK S. H. STANDER, CHIEF CLINICAL TECHNOLOGIST

In vitro fertilization (IVF) and embryo transfer have become an integral part of infertility management. Certain types of infertility previously regarded as incurable can now be treated successfully. However, comprehensive endocrine and ultrasonographic resources, high laboratory standards, and meticulous clinical techniques are prerequisites for the successful application of the procedure. Many years of experimentation by pioneering units were required to perfect the methods being used today (1–9). The IVF clinic at Tygerberg Hospital established its protocol after a critical comparison of the methods and results reported by seven of the foremost clinics in the world: three in Australia, two in the United States, one in England, and one in Austria.

Comparison of Laboratory Procedures

CULTURE MEDIA

The seven groups use Ham's F-10, Whittingham's T6, Earle's, or B-2 Menezo culture medium. Trounson (10) conducted a randomized trial of four different culture media and found no significant difference in pregnancy rates when embryos were cultured in Ham's F-10, Whittingham's T6, Earle's, and modified Witten's media. Earle's solution has been advocated because of its relatively simple chemical composition (11). Feichtinger (12) compared Menezo B-2, B-2 supplemented with bovine serum albumin (BSA), and Ham's F-10. The fertilization rates were similar in these three media, but the cleavage rate was lowest in B-2 contining BSA.

The effect of a higher potassium ion concentration in Ham's F-10 was evaluated by the group at Royal Women's Hospital, Victoria, Australia. Their conclusion was that doubling the concentration of potassium ions in the culture medium produces better results (13, 14). Human tubal fluid has a unique elemental composition characterized by high concentrations of potassium and chlorine but low concentrations of calcium relative to the range of normal human serum values. Sodium and magnesium concentrations in oviductal fluid are similar to serum levels (15, 16).

An important principle is that the culture medium must contain few chemical components in order to facilitate quality control and must be easy to prepare in the laboratory (17). Once the patient's serum or (non) pooled human fetal cord serum is added, the solution is no longer a fully defined medium. It would appear from the literature that there is no statistically significant difference between results obtained with the various media. According to Trounson (10), ''None of the culture media tested show any distinct improvement in implantation rate of embryos, and further refinements to existing media or completely new media may be necessary to increase pregnancy rates.''

Table 5.23.
Properties of Different Grades of Water

Test	Grade I	Grade II
Conductance (μS/cm)	0.1–0.055	2–1
Resistivity (mohm/cm)	10–18	0.5–1
Total dissolved solids (ppm)	Limit of detection	<0.05
Organic solutes (ppm)	Limit of detection	<0.1
pH range	6.5–7.0	6.5–7.0
Bacterial count (colonies/100 ml)	Nil	Nil
Silica, SiO_2 (ppm)	<0.005	<0.005
Trace dissolved metals (ppm)	<0.005	<0.005

Because of the simplicity of Ham's F-10, the unit at Tygerberg Hospital chose this medium for IVF and gamete intrafallopian transfer (GIFT) procedures.

WATER

Intensively purified water for washing culture equipment and preparing media is essential for good results in IVF. The types of purified water in use range from twice-distilled water (18), and pure "Analar" water from British pharmacies, to the six-times distilled rain water used in Adelaide, Australia, because of the poor results achieved with purified city water (19). Improvement in water purity was one of the factors that increased the fertilization rate in Norfolk (20).

Water distilled in glass may contain particulate and volatile organic impurities which can decrease fertilization and cleavage rates, despite rigorous redistillation. For this reason, Laufer (21) recommends the use of ultrapure high-pressure liquid chromatography-grade water.

In a study performed at the Infertility Clinic of Tygerberg Hospital (22), grade 1 and grade 2 water were compared using the mouse oocyte system. Grade 1 water (18 mohm/cm resistivity) was obtained by single-stage reverse osmosis (RO). A Rogers prefilter and a cellulose acetate RO membrane were used. Deionization took place within a two-bed weak-base anion system (water obtained from Sabax Laboratories, Johannesburg, South Africa). Grade 2 water was also obtained from Sabax (AFF 7114 sterile Baxter water for irrigation) (Table 5.23). Mouse embryos were cultured in Ham's F-10 medium prepared with grade 1 and grade 2 water; grade 1 water was used in the test group and grade 2 water in the control group. The two-cell embryos were randomly divided into test and control groups; 92% cleaved to the blastocyst stage in the test group (grade 1 water), and 91.8% cleaved to the blastocyst stage in the control group (grade 2 water). Cleavage was the same in both groups.

Because grade 2 water is easily obtainable and commercially available in South Africa, we decided to use it in the human IVF program launched in 1983 at Tygerberg Hospital. The first pregnancy followed soon after (23) and led to the birth of the first IVF baby in South Africa on April 29, 1984. Our fertilization rate of 77.7% per oocyte has been satisfactory since May 1984 (24) and compares favorably with that of the leading IVF clinics as does our pregnancy rate of 23% per transfer; to date, 170 babies have been born. (To establish our own water purification system to produce grade 1 water would have meant a capital outlay of at least $5000, whereas the average cost of obtaining grade 2 water is 60¢ per liter.)

SERUM

Either patient serum (18, 19, 25–28) or human fetal cord serum (20, 29) is used with good results among the different groups. (For practical considerations, patient serum supplementation is used in our program.)

The metabolism of the early-stage embryo is believed to be unaffected by the absence of serum macromolecules, but at the later stages of development the omission of such substances may lead to unfavorable results. Therefore, when the embryo is cultured in the absence of the macromolecules present in the serum, its metabolism could be suboptimal (30).

In Vienna, Feichtinger (12) observed that the cleavage rate in Menezo B-2 medium containing BSA was significantly lower than that in B-2 containing serum and in Ham's F-10 containing serum. We feel that the low cleavage rate could be due to the lack of serum in the medium. After observing pronuclei, we believe that the addition of serum to B-2 with BSA probably prevented this low cleavage rate.

Leung (31) recently reported a controlled trial comparing fetal cord serum with maternal serum. In the maternal serum group, the pregnancy rate was 23%, compared with 38% in the fetal cord serum group ($P<0.05$). The conclusion was that, for human IVF and embryo development, fetal cord serum is a better supplement than maternal serum in Ham's F-10 medium.

If embryos are cultured in a simple medium—without serum, for example—cleavage occurs, but embryonic metabolism declines with time (30). In a study performed at the Reproductive Biology Unit of Tygerberg Hospital (32), the cleavage rate in a simple medium with no serum supplementation was 66.7%; with 10% serum added to the growth medium, 83.3%. As there was a statistically significant difference between the cleavage performance of the two groups, the authors questioned the advisability of serum omission. The preparation of serum by immediate centrifugation may also improve the results (33).

INSEMINATION MEDIUM

The insemination medium consists of 90% Ham's F-10 and 10% heat-inactivated maternal serum. The serum is prepared as described by Leung (31). The oocytes are incubated in a 3037 Falcon culture dish for 5 to 6 hours before insemination (17). The central well of the culture dish is filled with 1.5 cc of insemination medium, and 5 cc of Ham's F-10 are placed in the surrounding well to keep the osmolarity constant (34).

Ham's F-10 medium is freshly prepared weekly; the osmolarity is adjusted to 280 with a pH of 7.9 to 8.0 after preparation. After gassing the medium in a 5% CO_2-in-air incubator (Forma Scientific 3157) for 24 hours, the pH is 7.4 (pH meter, Autocal PHM 83). The medium is tested weekly in the two-cell mouse embryo system (90% must reach the blastocyst stage for acceptability). If this standard is not reached, new medium is prepared and tested.

To maintain quality control, the following routines are carried out daily (35):

1. The percentage of CO_2 in the incubator is tested with a Fyrite gas analyzer.
2. The pH of the medium is measured in a 3037 Falcon petri dish, simulating the conditions in which the oocytes and spermatozoa are kept.

3. The osmolarity in a 3037 Falcon petri dish is recorded after 24 hours (Vapor Pressure Osmometer, model no. 5100 c; Wescor, Inc., Logan, Utah).
4. The temperature in the incubator is maintained at 37°C.
5. The humidity is tested to keep it at 95 to 98%.

GROWTH MEDIUM

The growth medium consists of 20% maternal serum plus 80% Ham's F-10. The oocytes are transferred 17 to 20 hours after insemination. The oocytes are dissected with a number 30 needle, and fertilization is documented (36). The next morning (±40 hours after insemination), the embryos are inspected for cleavage.

GAS MIXTURES

Most culture media rely on 5% CO_2 in the surrounding atmosphere to establish and maintain pH, usually ranging from 7.3 to 7.4. A humidified atmosphere is also required to stabilize osmolarity (10). Two gas mixtures are generally used: the 5% CO_2, 5% oxygen, and 90% nitrogen system (7, 9), and the 5% CO_2-in-air system (12, 20, 37). Pregnancies have been obtained from embryos cultured under 5%, 10%, and 20% oxygen concentrations, suggesting that oxygen at these levels does not have a major effect on human embryo viability (10, 20). Feichtinger and Kemeter (25) consider that the 5% CO_2-in-air has superseded previous gas mixtures through its simplicity. They did not find a significant difference between the fertilization rates in the two systems (12). In the different groups, the pH ranged between 7.3 and 7.4, with most groups preferring 7.4. The Norfolk group (20, 38) states that an adjustment of the pH to 7.4 in the medium, as well as improvement in the purity of the water, increased the fertilization rate in their program (20, 38). Because of the simplicity of the 5% CO_2-in-air system, we use it at the clinic at Tygerberg Hospital.

CULTURE VESSELS

It would appear that the 5-ml tissue culture tube (Falcon 2058) is the most popular method for culturing embryos (11, 17, 19). Others, including the Tygerberg clinic, use a welled organ-culture dish (Falcon 3037) (20) or NUNC multidish (12).

The Bourn Hall group prefers to culture embryos in droplets of medium beneath liquid paraffin. Although good results are obtained, the danger of toxicity exists. Feichtinger and Kemeter (25) state that the effectiveness of using tubes is compromised by the danger of losing the egg or embryo during routine manipulations. These problems do not arise using a multidish. This system of the 3037 Falcon dish is simpler, easier for observation and manipulation of the egg or embryo, and hence may be regarded as the safest, most efficient procedure.

If culture conditions without oil are used, the volume of the medium must be increased, and better control of the humidity in the incubator is mandatory (4). To achieve this, an additional incubator is often necessary because a large number of oocytes in one incubator means that the internal environment is frequently disturbed by opening and closing the doors (31).

PREPARATION OF SPERMATOZOA

Most groups use two washes of a small sample of semen to prepare a suspension of spermatozoa for insemination (27, 39). All groups preincubate the spermatozoa at 37°C except the Bourn Hall group, who maintain sperm at room temperature (4).

With group variations, 10,000 to 100,000 motile spermatozoa per milliliter of culture medium are commonly used (17, 27, 40). Fertilization may be achieved by relatively low numbers of spermatozoa. The reduction of the concentration to 10,000 to 50,000 sperm per milliliter does not affect the high rate of fertilization and can be considered a benefit in the IVF system because it decreases the chance of polyspermy. Since polyspermy cannot be predicted, it is advisable to remove the corona cells 15 to 18 hours after insemination to exclude the condition; at 40 hours, cleavage of polyspermic eggs may appear entirely within normal limits (36).

When human spermatozoa prepared by washing (which removes nearly all seminal plasma components) are compared with those collected by an overlay technique (which provides a highly motile sperm preparation but retains some seminal plasma components), there is a noticeable difference in their ability to penetrate zona-free hamster ova. The washed spermatozoa achieve their maximal fertilizing capacity after 6 hours of incubation with ova, whereas the spermatozoa collected by the overlay technique reach a comparable value only after 22 hours of incubation (41, 42).

Semen samples at Tygerberg Hospital are obtained 1 to 3 hours before insemination. The semen is allowed to liquefy at room temperature; 1 cc of semen is mixed with 2 cc of insemination medium. Centrifugation is performed at 200 × g for 10 minutes, and the supernatant fluid is discarded. The procedure is repeated. One cubic centimeter of insemination medium is used for the final step, and the semen is placed in the incubator in 5% CO_2-in-air for 30 to 45 minutes (17). The final count is performed, and 100,000 motile spermatozoa are added per milliliter of insemination medium.

FERTILIZATION

Most groups delay insemination for at least 5 to 6 hours, with some individual variations. Trounson (17) achieved a marked improvement in fertilization rate when insemination was delayed for 5 to 6 hours. This delay also achieved improvement at the Royal Women's Hospital (43). After fertilization, the rate of cleavage is the same whether insemination is delayed or not (43).

There was no significant difference in the fertilization rate for eggs from leading follicles, irrespective of whether insemination was immediate or delayed. However, when eggs obtained from secondary follicles were compared, it became evident that incubation before insemination significantly increased the fertilization rate. Lopata (43) noted that the pre-incubated eggs had a greater capacity to produce embryos which progressed to implanting blastocysts. The delayed insemination technique also improved the results in Norfolk (38). This was also the experience of Testart (44) with mature + + and less mature + oocytes, where the incidence of fertilization was increased by 28%.

Feichtinger (12) inseminated 38 to 42 hours after the human chorionic gonadotropin (hCG) injection, irrespective of the time of laparoscopy. His group matured oocytes in medium containing 75% follicular fluid (45). The Bourn Hall group did not find any improvement in the fertilization rate in cases of delayed insemination if the oocyte was mature (46). However, at present most groups use the delayed insemination technique.

Lately, the fertilization principles used in Tygerberg Hospital are those followed by the Norfolk group. We did use the principles outlined by Trounson (delayed insemination) but feel that it is more logical to wait for the polar body to appear before insemination is attempted.

EXAMINATION OF OOCYTES AND EMBRYOS

Most groups remove corona and cumulus cells 12 to 18 hours after insemination to examine the oocytes. Denudation is achieved by fine-gauge needles or drawn Pasteur pipettes. It is of value to detect polyspermic fertilization (36); the criterion for normal fertilization is cleavage of pronuclear oocytes (see Part 1, Section A of this chapter: Basic Semen Analysis).

The fertilized oocytes are placed in fresh culture medium; some groups increase the concentration of serum, while others do not. The Monash, Australia, group uses 10% serum in the embryo growth medium, while other groups use 15% or 20% serum as a routine, with no apparent differences in pregnancy rates among the major groups. The first cleavage of the oocyte occurs 22 to 30 hours after insemination; thereafter, divisions occur at 10- to 12-hour intervals (10, 19).

Regular cleavage and uniform blastomeres are important elements of normal embryonic development. Fragmentation and uneven cleavage may be indicative of abnormal development or suboptimal culture conditions.

EMBRYO TRANSFER

The embryo or embryos at the 4- to 8-cell stage are transferred 45 to 48 hours after insemination. No medication is given to patients before the transfer, but they have been examined in a previous cycle, are well prepared, and know exactly what to expect (35).

Patients are placed in the lithotomy position for the transfer procedure. The gynecologist scrubs as for a routine operation but does not wear gloves. The patient is positioned and draped with sterile towels, and the cervix is cleaned with Ham's F-10. The embryos are then brought to the gynecologist for transfer (35).

The embryologist uses a transfer medium consisting of 75% serum plus 25% Ham's F-10 (12). In Tygerberg Hospital, up to four embryos are transferred at each procedure. The rest of the technique is as outlined by Kerin (47, 48). A Tomcat catheter (Mondject, St. Louis, Mo.) is used. After 6.5-cm of the catheter is inserted into the uterus, 15 to 25 units of transfer medium are carefully injected in the uterus. The Tomcat catheter is turned 180° and removed after 30 seconds.

Of more than 1,000 cases treated in the Reproductive Biology Unit of Tygerberg Hospital, only two ectopic pregnancies have occurred.

References

1. Steptoe PC, Edwards RG, Purdy JM: Human blastocysts grown in culture. Nature 229:132, 1971
2. Edwards RG: Studies on human conception. Am J Obstet Gynecol 117:587, 1973
3. Steptoe PC, Edwards RG: Birth after the reimplantation of a human embryo. Lancet 2:336, 1973
4. Edwards RG, Steptoe PC, Purdy JM: Establishing fullterm human pregnancies using cleaving embryos grown in vitro. Br J Obstet Gynaecol 87:737, 1980
5. Steptoe PC, Edwards RG, Purdy JM: Clinical aspects of pregnancies established with cleaving embryos grown in vitro. Br J Obstet Gynaecol 87:757, 1980
6. Steptoe PC, Edwards RG: Reimplantation of a human embryo with subsequent pregnancy. Lancet 1:880, 1976
7. Lopata A, Brown JB, Leeton JF, McTalbot J, Wood C: In vitro fertilization of preovulatory oocytes and embryo transfer in infertile patients treated with clomiphene and human chorionic gonadotropin. Fertil Steril 30:27, 1978
8. Lopata A, Johnston WIH, Hoult KJ, Speirs AL: Pregnancy following intrauterine implantation of an embryo obtained by in vitro fertilization of a preovulatory egg. Fertil Steril 33:117, 1980
9. Lopata A: Successes and failures in human in vitro fertilization. Nature 288:642, 1980

10. Trounson A: Factors controlling normal embryo development and implantation of human oocytes fertilized in vitro. In Beier HM, Lindner HR (eds): Fertilization of the Human Egg in Vitro. Berlin: Springer-Verlag, 1983, p 236

11. Purdy JM: Fertilization and preimplantation growth in vitro. In Edwards RG, Purdy JM, (eds): Human Conception in Vitro. London: Academic Press, 1982, p 135

12. Feichtinger W, Kemeter P, Szalay S: The Vienna program of in vitro fertilization and embryo transfer—a successful clinical treatment. Eur J Obstet Gynecol Reprod Biol 15:63, 1983

13. Johnson I, Lopata A, Speirs A, Martin M, Olivia K: Current status of an in vitro fertilization programme and early pregnancy diagnosis. In Beier HM, Lindner HR (eds): Fertilization of the Human Egg in Vitro. Berlin: Springer-Verlag, 1983, p 271

14. Lopata A: Factors influencing the growth of human preimplantation embryos in vitro. In Edwards RG, Purdy JM (eds): Human Conception in Vitro. London: Academic Press, 1982, p 207

15. Borland RM, Biggers JP, Lechene CP, Taymor ML: Elemental composition of fluid in the human fallopian tube. J Reprod Fertil 58:479, 1980

16. Lippes J, Enders RG, Pragay DA, Bartholomew WR: The collection and analysis of human fallopian tubal fluid. Contraception 5:85, 1972

17. Trounson AO, Mohr LR, Wood C, Leeton JF: Effect of delayed insemination on in vitro fertilization culture and transfer of human embryos. J Reprod Fertil 64:285, 1982

18. Marrs RP, Vargyas JM, Gibbons E, Saito H, Mishell DR: A modified technique of human in vitro fertilization and embryo transfer. Am J Obstet Gynecol 147:318, 1983

19. Quinn P, Warnes GM, Kerin JF, Kirby C: Culture factors in relation to the success of human in vitro fertilization and embryo transfer. Fertil Steril 41:202, 1984

20. Wortham JWE, Veeck LL, Witmyer J, Sandow BA, Jones HW: Vital initiation of pregnancy (V.I.P.) using human menopausal gonadotropin and human chorionic gonadotropin ovulation induction: phase II—1981. Fertil Steril 40:170, 1983

21. Laufer N, De Cherney AH, Haseltine RP: The use of high-dose human menopausal gonadotropin in an in vitro fertilization program. Fertil Steril 40:734, 1983

22. Kruger TF, Van Wyk H, Stander FSH, Smith K, Menkveld R, Van der Merwe JP: A comparative analysis of grade 1 and grade 2 water in the Tygerberg Hospital in vitro fertilization programme. S Afr Med J 71:162, 1987

23. Kruger TF, Van Schouwenburg JAM, Stander FSH, Van den Heever AD, van Zyl JA, Menkveld R, Kopper K, De Villiers A, Conradie E, Odendaal HJ, De Villiers JN: Results of phase I of the in vitro fertilization and embryo transfer programme at Tygerberg Hospital. S Afr Med J 67:751, 1985

24. Kruger TF, Van der Merwe JP, Stander FSH, Menkveld R, Van den Heever AD, Kopper K, Odendaal HJ, van Zyl JA, De Villiers JN: Results of the in vitro fertilization programme at Tygerberg Hospital, phases II and III. S Afr Med J 69:297, 1986

25. Feichtinger W, Kemeter P: A simplified technique for fertilization and culture of human preimplantation embryos in vitro. Acta Eur Fertil 14:125, 1983

26. Edwards RG, Steptoe PC: Current status of in vitro fertilization and implantation of human embryos. Lancet 2:1265, 1983

27. Mahadevan MM, Trounson AO, Leeton JF: Successful use of human semen cryobanking for in vitro fertilization. Fertil Steril 40:340, 1983

28. Edwards RG, Fishel SB, Purdy JM: In vitro fertilization of human eggs: analysis of follicular growth, ovulation and fertilization. In Beier HM, Lindner HR (eds): Fertilization of the Human Egg in Vitro. Berlin: Springer-Verlag, 1983, p 169

29. Nayudu PK, Lopata A, Leung PCS, Johnston WIH: Current problems in human in vitro fertilization and embryo implantation. J Exp Zool 228:203, 1983

30. Fishel SB, Edwards RG, Purdy JM: In vitro fertilization of human oocytes: factors associated with embryonic development in vitro; replacement of embryos and pregnancy. In Beier HM, Lindner HR (eds): Fertilization of the Human Egg in Vitro. Berlin: Springer-Verlag, 1983, p 251

31. Leung PCS, Gronow MJ, Kellow GN: Serum supplement in human in vitro fertilization and embryo development. Fertil Steril 41:36, 1984

32. Kruger TF, Stander FSH, Smith K, Van der Merwe JP, Lombard CJ: The effect of serum supplementation on the cleavage of human embryos. J In Vitro Fertil Embryo Trans 4:10, 1987

33. New DAT, Coppola PT, Cockroft DL: Improved development of head-fold rat embryos in culture resulting from low oxygen and modifications of the culture serum. J Reprod Fertil 48:219, 1976

34. Kruger TF, Stander FSH, Menkveld R, Lombard CJ: Osmolarity studies with different containers and volumes in a human in vitro fertilization programme. S Afr Med J 68:651, 1985

35. Kruger TF, Lopata A, Rosich HME, De Villiers JN, Stander FSH, Van der Merwe JP, Smith K, Menkveld R, van Zyl JA: Comparative analysis of in vitro fertilization methods for establishing successful embryo transfer clinics. Acta Eur Fertil 16:317, 1985

36. Wentz AC, Repp JE, Maxson WS, Pittaway DE, Torbit CA: The problem of polyspermy in in vitro fertilization. Fertil Steril 40:748, 1983

37. Wortham JWE, Veeck LL, Witmyer J, Jones HW: Vital initiation of pregnancy (V.I.P.) using human menopausal gonadotropin and human chorionic gonadotropin ovulation induction: phase I—1981. Fertil Steril 39:785, 1983

38. Jones HW, Jones GS, Andrews MC, Acosta A, Bundren C, Garcia J, Sandow B, Veeck L, Wilkes C, Witmyer J, Wortham JE, Wright G: The program for in vitro fertilization at Norfolk. Fertil Steril 38:14, 1982

39. Mahadevan MM, Trounson AO, Leeton JF: The relationship of tubal blockage, infertility of unknown cause, suspected male infertility, and endometriosis to success of in vitro fertilization and embryo transfer. Fertil Steril 40:755, 1983

40. Trounson A, Conti A: Research in human in vitro fertilization and embryo transfer. Br Med J 285:244, 1982

41. Quinn P, Whittingham DG: Albumin seminal plasma and mammalian fertilization. In Hafez ESE, Semm K (eds): In Vitro Fertilization and Embryo Transfer. Lancaster, England: MTP Press, 1982, p 31

42. Quinn P, Whittingham DG, Stanger JD: Interaction of semen with ova in vitro. Arch Androl 8:189, 1982

43. Lopata A: Concepts in human in vitro fertilization and embryo transfer. Fertil Steril 40:289, 1983

44. Testart J, Lassalle B, Frydman R, Belaisch JC: A study of factors affecting the success of human fertilization in vitro: influence of semen quality and oocyte maturity on fertilization and cleavage. Biol Reprod 28:425, 1983

45. Feichtinger W, Kemeter P, Szalay S, Janisch H: Early hormone parameters and embryo transfer. In Beier HM, Lindner HR (eds): Fertilization of the Human Egg in Vitro. Berlin: Springer-Verlag, 1983, p 229

46. Edwards RG, Fishel SB, Cohen J: Factors influencing the success of in vitro fertilization of alleviating human infertility. J In Vitro Fertil Embryo Trans 1:3, 1984

47. Kerin JF, Warnes GM, Quinn P: In vitro fertilization and embryo transfer program, Department of Obstetrics and Gynecology, University of Adelaide at the Queen Elizabeth Hospital, Woodville, South Australia. J In Vitro Fertil Embryo Trans 1:63, 1984

48. Kerin JF, Warnes GM, Jeffrey R, Cox LW, Broom TJ: A simple technique for human embryo transfer into the uterus. Lancet 2:726, 1981

CHAPTER 6

Evaluation and Preparation of Spermatozoa for Gamete Intrafallopian Transfer

JACOBUS P. VAN DER MERWE, M.D., THINUS F. KRUGER, M.D., GREG M. GROBLER, M.D., VICTOR HULME, M.D., MARIE-LENA WINDT, M.S., FRIK S. H. STANDER, CHIEF CLINICAL TECHNOLOGIST, KEVIN COETZEE, M.S., AND EVELYN ERASMUS, M.S.

Successful new techniques such as in vitro fertilization (IVF) and embryo transfer for the treatment of infertility have been developed in recent years (1, 2). An alternate technique for the treatment of infertile couples, when the wife has at least one patent fallopian tube, was described by Asch (3): gamete intrafallopian transfer (GIFT). This technique involves the placement of both sperm and oocytes into the fallopian tube, the normal site of human fertilization. It is done by means of laparoscopy or a mini-laparotomy (4).

Criteria for Patient Selection

A married couple is considered for infertility workup after failure to achieve a pregnancy in 2 years of unprotected intercourse. Those who have at least one patent fallopian tube on hysterosalpingogram and laparoscopy are considered for GIFT when more conventional and simpler treatments have failed.

Patients accepted into our GIFT program had the following diagnoses:

1. Unexplained infertility;
2. Male factor (teratozoospermia);
3. Mild or moderate endometriosis;
4. Cervical factor;
5. Immunological factor;
6. Pelvic adhesions that interfered with oocyte retrieval; and

256

7. Hyperstimulation during routine ovulation induction.

Materials and Methods

INDUCTION OF FOLLICULAR DEVELOPMENT

To maximize the recovery of fertilizable oocytes, a combination of clomiphene citrate and human menopausal gonadotropin (hMG) was given (5, 6). Treatment was inititated on day 3 to 6, depending on cycle length. The first day of treatment was determined by a formula based on the work of McIntosh (7).

Patients received 100 mg of clomiphene daily for 5 days. Two ampules (150 IU) of hMG were administered on day 2 of clomiphene treatment; this dosage was repeated twice on alternate days. On the day after the last hMG administration, the graafian follicles were measured by transabdominal ultrasonography, using a full bladder. If the leading follicle had not reached a mean diameter of 14 mm (measured in two planes), two more ampules of hMG were given daily until the follicle reached that diameter. From this stage on, the patient was followed by sonograph and by four blood samples per day to detect a possible luteinizing hormone (LH) surge. The first blood was taken at 8 A.M. and the last at 10 P.M. The final sample was taken just before human chorionic gonadotropin (hCG) administration. hCG was administered as soon as the leading follicle reached 18 mm in diameter, with two additional follicles of at least 16 mm in diameter. Follicle aspiration was done 36 hours after hCG administration. An LH surge was diagnosed by a doubling of the baseline level (8, 9). If a surge occurred, an estimate was made of the time of onset, and follicular aspiration was done by laparoscopy approximately 30 to 34 hours thereafter.

SEMEN PREPARATION

The husband was required to produce a semen sample 1 hour before laparoscopy was performed. The semen was prepared as described in Chapter 5 (10, 11).

LAPAROSCOPY AND FOLLICULAR ASPIRATION

Laparoscopy was performed as for IVF (12), using 100% CO_2 for pneumoperitoneum.

OOCYTE HANDLING

Aspirated oocytes were placed in individual culture dishes containing Ham's F-10 medium with 50% maternal serum in a CO_2-in-air incubator (Forma Scientific 3157).

OOCYTE EVALUATION

During phase I of our GIFT program, aspirated oocytes were evaluated for maturity by an embryologist using the criteria of the Tygerberg Hospital (13). A score was obtained for each oocyte by assessing the spinnbarkheit of the cumulus oophorus, the halo around the oocyte, the homogeneity of the cumulus cells, and the volume of follicular fluid. An oocyte was considered to be mature if the total score was >six of eight (13). On completion of evaluation, the four best oocytes were selected for transfer. During phase II of our GIFT program, we changed the methodology according to the criteria of Veeck (14).

The catheter used for transfer was loaded as follows (4): first, 25 μl of medium containing 100,000 sperm for normal semen parameters or 500,000 sperm for <14% normal morphology (10), as indicated by IVF studies (15); next, 5 μl of air; then two oocytes in 25 μl of medium; and finally 10 μl of medium. The loaded catheter was threaded through the cannula used for aspiration, and the tip was inserted for 2 cm through the fimbrial opening of the fallopian tube. There the contents of the catheter were deposited.

Patients were discharged on the day of the procedure or the following day, depending on their recovery from the general anesthesia.

Results

The outcome of GIFT in 312 consecutive cycles was analyzed, with patients classified according to the etiology of their infertility. The overall ongoing pregnancy rate was 19.6%, with a rate of 17.8% in the idiopathic group and 25.8% in the endometriosis group (Table 6.1).

MALE FACTOR: TERATOZOOSPERMIA

Patients were classified as having teratozoospermia when the sperm morphology was <14% normal forms, with a count of 20 × 10⁶, motility of >30%, and forward progression of 2+ arbitrary units, according to the parameters of Tygerberg Hospital (10). During phase I, only one pregnancy occurred in 16 cycles (6.25%) (Table 6.2); all these patients were in the G-pattern male factor group (see Chapter 5) with normal morphology of 5% to 14%. The husband of one woman who achieved a pregnancy had a morphology of 10% normal forms; at 32 weeks she delivered a normal baby.

In phase II, 102 cycles were analyzed and classified (Table 6.3). The ongoing pregnancy rate was 15 (19.2%) of 78 in the G-pattern group and one (4.2%) of 24 in the P-pattern group (≤4% normal morphology).

These figures are small, and some of the pregnancies are still in the early stages. Therefore, an accurate abortion rate cannot be given. However, early indications are that GIFT may be a means of treating infertile couples in whom the main cause of infertility is teratozoospermia in the husband, especially in the group with 5% to 14% normal forms. The increased pregnancy rate in this group since the implementation of phase II may be attributed to two things: first, increased concentration of spermatozoa to 500,000; second, better quality and more mature oocytes, selected according to the criteria of Veeck (14). This latter assumption is based on two observations:

1. In an unpublished study, Stander found no correlation between oocytes scored as mature according to the system of Testart (16) and oocytes classified as metaphase I and II according to Veeck.
2. Kruger (Chapter 5) pointed out that the fertilization rate in metaphase I oocytes was only 43.8% compared to a rate of 58.04% in metaphase II oocytes in patients with teratozoospermia.

IMMUNOLOGICAL FACTOR

The presence of antisperm antibodies is accepted as a possible cause of infertility (17). All males are screened by a mixed antiglobulin reaction (MAR) test (18).

In this series there were 16 couples with male immunological problems; the duration of infertility was from 2 to 12 years. A sperm-cervical mucus compatibility (SCMC)

Table 6.1.
Results of Phase I and II for GIFT (%Pregnancies)

Total number of cycles	312	
Pregnancies	95	(30.4%)
Ongoing pregnancies	61	(19.55%)
Idiopathic		
Total cycles	129	
Pregnancies	37	(28.6%)
Ongoing pregnancies	23	(17.8%)
Endometriosis (mild to moderate)		
Total cycles	24	
Pregnancies	7	(29.16%)
Ongoing pregnancies	6	(25.8%)
Hyperstimulation (anovulatory patients who hyperstimulated on hMG)		
Total cycles	5	
Pregnancies (ongoing)	4	
Male factor (teratozoospermia)		
Total cycles	118	
Pregnancies	30	(25.4%)
Ongoing pregnancies	17	(14.4%)
Immunological		
Total cycles	22	
Pregnancies	11	(50%)
Ongoing pregnancies	6	(27.2%)
Adhesions only		
Total cycles	14	
Pregnancies	6	(42.8%)
Ongoing pregnancies	5	(35.7%)

test with normal donor cervical mucus was done in 14 of 16 patients to confirm the presence of antibodies. The specific antibody type on the surface of the sperm was determined by the immunobead test (19) for immunoglobulin G (IgG), immunoglobulin A (IgA), and immunoglobulin M (IgM) antibodies. Results are summarized in Table 6.4.

The traditional treatment for antisperm antibodies in the woman is the use of a condom at every coitus for 6 to 12 months (20, 21). For men with antisperm antibodies, success has been reported with insemination of washed sperm (17). Very high doses of

Table 6.2.
Pregnancies in Patients with Teratozoospermia (<14% Normal Forms): Phase I

		Percentage of Normal Forms	
		0–4%	5–14%
Number of cycles	16	0	16
Pregnancies (%)	1 (6.25)	0	1 (6.25)
Ongoing pregnancies (%)	1 (6.25)	0	1 (6.25)

Table 6.3.
Pregnancies in Patients with Teratozoospermia (<14% Normal Forms): Phase II

		Percentage of Normal Forms	
		0–4%	5–14%
Number of cycles	102	24	78
Pregnancies (%)	29 (28.4)	4 (16.7)	25 (32.1)
Ongoing pregnancies (%)	16 (15.7)	1 (4.2)	15 (19.2)

Table 6.4.
Types of Antibodies on Spermatozoa of Different Patients as Detected by Direct Immunobead Test

Patient	SCMC (% positive)	IgA (%)	IgG (%)	IgM (%)
AduP	95	95–100	95–100	<10
LduP	98	80–90	10	—
JCduT	68	80–100	100	—
CAL	21	40–50	99	<10
KAM	—	100	90	—
JZ	—	70	70	—
IHJ	70–96	20–50	95	<10
BS	66	80	90–99	<10
MMB	60	90	90	—
SP	25	20	100	<10
DN	91	99	100	0
LJR	98	100	100	0
BAH	100	80	90	0
TR	8	50	70	0
JAB	92	99	80	<10
MC	94	100	95	0

steroids have also been used, with pregnancies reported (17, 22, 23); the side effects of such high doses, however, are well known.

Pregnancies have also resulted from IVF treatment of patients with immunological infertility (24). In Tygerberg we have treated this problem by using GIFT. Sixteen patients were treated in 22 cycles with 11 pregnancies, for an ongoing pregnancy rate of 27.2% (6 of 22). Although the numbers are small, they are encouraging (Table 6.1).

Windt (25) showed that the reason for success in the GIFT program is not a change in the antibodies on the sperm surface but perhaps an improvement in semen parameters, e.g., motility and forward progression. In addition, using GIFT eliminates the side effects associated with steroid treatment.

References

1. Steptoe PC, Edwards RG: Birth after reimplantation of a human embryo. Lancet 2:366, 1978

2. Buster JE, Bustillo M, Thorneycroft ZH, Boyer SP, Marshall JR, Seed RG, Louw JA: Nonsurgical transfer of an invitro fertilized donated ovum to an infertility patient. Lancet 1:816, 1983
3. Asch RH, Ellsworth LR, Balmaceda JP, Wang PC: Pregnancy following translaparoscopic gamete intrafallopian transfer (GIFT). Lancet 2:1034, 1984
4. Asch RH, Balmaceda JP, Ellsworth LR, Wong PC: Gamete intrafallopian transfer (GIFT): a new treatment for infertility. Int J Fertil 30:41, 1985
5. Kruger TF, Van der Merwe JP, Stander FSH, Menkveld R, Van Den Heever AD, Kopper K, Odendaal HJ, van Zyl JA, De Villiers JN: Results of the in vitro fertilization programme at Tygerberg Hospital: phases II and III. S Afr Med J 69:297, 1986
6. Van der Merwe JP, Kruger TF, Lombard CJ, Muller LM: Ovulation induction for in vitro fertilization in Tygerberg Hospital. S Afr Med J 71:515, 1987
7. McIntosh JEA, Matthews CD, Crocker JM, Broom TJ, Coa LW: Predicting the luteinizing hormone surge: relationship between the duration of the follicular and luteal phase and the length of the human menstrual cycle. Fertil Steril 34:125, 1980
8. Vargyas JM, Morente C, Shangold G, Marrs RP: The effect of different methods of ovarian stimulation for human in vitro fertilization and embryo replacement. Fertil Steril 42:745, 1984
9. Quigley MM, Schmidt CL, Beauchamp PJ, Maklad NF, Berkowitz AS, Wolf DP: Preliminary experience with a combination of clomiphene and variable dosages of menopausal gonadotropins for enhanced follicular recruitment. J In Vitro Fertil Embryo Trans 2:11, 1985
10. Kruger TF, Menkveld R, Stander FSH, Lombard CJ, Van der Merwe JP, van Zyl JA, Smith K: Sperm morphologic features as a prognostic factor in in vitro fertilization. Fertil Steril 46:1118, 1986
11. Kruger TF, Acosta AA, Simmons KF, Swanson RJ, Matta JR, Veeck LL, Morshedi M, Brugo S: New method of evaluating sperm morphology with predictive value for human in vitro fertilization. Urology 30:248, 1987
12. Kruger TF, Lopata A, Rosich HME, De Villiers JN, Stander FSH, Van der Merwe JP, Smith K, Menkveld R, van Zyl JA: Comparative analysis of in vitro fertilization methods for establishing successful embryo transfer clinics. Acta Eur Fertil 16:317, 1985
13. Kruger TF, Stander FSH, Smith K, Van der Merwe JP, Lombard CJ: The effect of serum supplementation on the cleavage of human embryos. J In Vitro Fertil Embryo Trans 4:10, 1987
14. Veeck LL, Maloney M: Insemination and fertilization. In Jones HW Jr, Jones GS, Hodgen GD, Rosenwaks Z (eds): In Vitro Fertilization—Norfolk. Baltimore: Williams & Wilkins, 1986, p 168
15. Oehninger S, Acosta AA, Morshedi M, Veeck L, Swanson RJ, Simmons K, Rosenwaks Z: Corrective measures and pregnancy outcome in in vitro fertilization in patients with severe sperm morphology abnormalities. Fertil Steril 50:283, 1988
16. Testart J, Frydman R, De Mouzon J, Lassale B, Belaisch JC: A study of factors affecting the success of human fertilization in vitro. I. Influence of ovarian stimulation upon the number and condition of oocytes collected. Biol Reprod 28:415, 1983
17. Shulman S, Harlin B, Davis P, Reyniak JV: Immune infertility and new approaches to treatment. Fertil Steril 29:309, 1978
18. Hendry WF, Stredonska J, Lake RA: Mixed erythrocyte-spermatozoa antiglobulin reaction (MAR test) for IgA and sperm antibodies in subfertile males. Fertil Steril 37:108, 1982
19. Clark GN, Elliott PJ, Smaila C: Detection of sperm antibodies in semen using the immunobead test: a survey of 813 consecutive patients. Am J Reprod Immunol Microbiol 7:1123, 1982
20. Shulman S: Treatment of immunological infertility. In Shulman S (ed): Reproduction and Antibody Response. Cleveland, OH: CRC Press, 1975, p 93
21. Shulman S: Immunologic barriers to infertility. Obstet Gynecol Surv 27:553, 1972
22. Boettcher B, Kay DJ, Fitchett SB: Successful treatment of male infertility caused by antispermatozoal antibodies. Med J Aust 2:471, 1982
23. Franken DR, Slabber CF, Giesteira MVK: Corticosteroid therapy in a case of immunologic infertility: a preliminary report. Andrologia 14:256, 1982
24. Ackerman SB, Graff D, van Uem JFHM, Swanson RJ, Veeck LL, Acosta AA, Garcia JE: Immunological infertility. Fertil Steril 42:474, 1984
25. Windt M, Menkveld R, Kruger TF, van Zyl JA: Effect of sperm washing and swim-up on antibodies bound to sperm membrane: use of immunobead sperm cervical mucus contact tests. Arch Androl 22:55, 1989

CHAPTER 7

Evaluation and Preparation of Spermatozoa for Intrauterine Insemination

Part One—The Norfolk Experience

Section A:

METHODOLOGY

NANCY J. ALEXANDER, PH.D., AND STEVEN B. ACKERMAN, PH.D.

Therapeutic intrauterine insemination (TII) has been increasingly used in the last 5 years. Indications have included oligozoospermia, asthenozoospermia, pyospermia, hostile or absent cervical mucus, cervical stenosis, and immunological infertility (Table 7.1).

TII by husband is most frequently applied for cases of poor sperm quality, especially oligozoospermia or asthenozoospermia (1). The decision to use TII by husband for patients with these conditions must be based on a thorough clinical evaluation. The husband's spermiogram should be consistently poor for at least three evaluations without an indication that aggressive therapy (such as varicocelectomy or endocrine treatment) would be useful. Although poor success rates of TII by husband can be expected when sperm concentrations are very low, pregnancies have been achieved with as few as 10^6 motile sperm. Generally speaking, however, pregnancy rates are very low when $<10 \times 10^6$ motile sperm can be harvested from the ejaculate (2).

To remove prostaglandins and prepare the sperm for TII, various approaches have been developed. All methods result in a sperm loss compared to the untreated ejaculate. The characteristics of the sample must be taken into consideration when selecting a preparation method.

262

Table 7.1.

Possible Indications for Therapeutic Insemination by Husband

Female factors
    Anatomic defect of the vagina or cervix
    Hostile cervical mucus
    Immunological infertility
    Sexual dysfunction
Male factors
    Anatomic defect of the penis
    Retrograde ejaculation
    Sexual/ejaculatory dysfunction
    Semen volume deficit or excess
    Semen liquefaction defects
    Immunological infertility
    Oligozoospermia
    Asthenozoospermia
Other factors
    Idiopathic poor postcoital test
    Use of husband's semen following sterilization or death

Sperm Washing

Washing is the most straightforward method of removing seminal plasma and concentrating sperm cells, and affords the greatest sperm recovery. Culture medium plus serum or albumin is used to maintain sperm motility (3% to 5% albumin or 7% human serum). Because of possible transmission of the virus for acquired immune deficiency syndrome (AIDS), the wife's serum is collected and added to the sample to maintain motility. Usually midcycle serum is used, although our studies suggest that the serum collected in the follicular phase best maintains sperm motility. The semen specimen is collected in a clean cup, and about 8 ml of sterile medium, such as Ham's F-10, are added. Since high centrifugation can damage sperm membranes, the speed of $300 \times g$ for 10 minutes is used. There are many variations of the sperm-washing procedure. For example, Perrone (3) and Testart (4) suggest two washes, followed by an incubation that allows the sperm to swim down into a layer with a higher percentage of albumin. The sample is centrifuged again and resuspended in 0.5 ml of medium for insemination.

Swim-Up

To perform a swim-up, the semen sample is layered under 1 to 2 ml of protein-supplemented buffer and incubated for 90 minutes at 37°C. Some groups allow the sperm to migrate into a diluent layer from a centrifuged pellet of washed semen. The medium is centrifuged (speeds not greater than $300 \times g$) and the pellet resuspended in 0.5 ml of medium for insemination.

When low sperm count is a problem, an enhancement, although small, can be achieved by dividing the semen specimen into smaller samples, increasing the surface area by turning the test tube almost horizontally, and incubating in 5% CO_2 in air. All the overlaying buffer layers are collected and concentrated by centrifugation (5).

Sperm that migrate into the overlying buffer have an increased number of morphologically normal forms, increased motility, and even a better fertilizing potential, as evidenced by hamster egg penetration results (6), although the total number of sperm is markedly reduced. If a semen sample is contaminated with large amounts of debris or white blood cells, allowing sperm to swim away from these components may be useful for subsequent fertilization.

Percoll Separation

Percoll, a suspension of colloidal silica particles conjugated to the inert substance povidone, exploits weight differences to filter debris or white blood cells from sperm cells. Either continuous or discontinuous Percoll gradients can be used to accomplish the separation. A layer of liquefied semen is placed over the top of the Percoll and centrifuged at 700 $\times$ g for 45 to 60 minutes. The layer of sperm is aspirated, rediluted in buffer, centrifuged, and resuspended in 0.3 to 0.5 ml of culture medium for insemination. This procedure provides better sperm return than the swim-up method. Many laboratories report enhanced motility, velocity, and longevity after such gradient separation procedures.

Filtration

Another way to remove seminal contaminants is to use glass wool, rayon, sterile cotton gauze, or albumin column filters. A potential disadvantage of this approach is that foreign material may be washed into the specimen ultimately used for insemination.

Removal of Bacteria

Seminal plasma is colonized by a wide variety of aerobic and anaerobic bacteria, as well as chlamydia and mycoplasma. Cervical mucus has always been considered an effective barrier, but when TII is performed, this barrier is bypassed. When peritoneal fluid is cultured after TII, positive cultures are found to the bacteria in the semen specimen (7). For this reason, penicillin (6000 IU/100 ml) and streptomycin (12,000 IU/100 ml) are added to the culture medium used for dilution of the specimen.

References

1. Beck WW: Artificial insemination and semen preservation. In Lipshultz LI, Howards SS (eds): Infertility in the Male. New York: Churchill Livingstone, 1983, p 381
2. DiMarzo SJ, Rakoff JS: Intrauterine insemination with husband's washed sperm. Fertil Steril 46:470, 1986
3. Perrone E, Testart J: Use of bovine serum albumin column to improve sperm selection for human in vitro fertilization. Fertil Steril 44:839, 1985
4. Testart J, Lassalle B, Frydman R, Belaisch JC: A study of factors affecting the success of human fertilization in vitro II. Influence of semen quality and oocyte maturity on fertilization and cleavage. Biol Reprod 28:425, 1983
5. Makler A, Fisher M, Murillo O, Laufer N, DeCherney A, Naftolin F: Factors affecting sperm motility. IX. Survival of spermatozoa in various biological media and under different gaseous compositions. Fertil Steril 41:428, 1984

6. Russell LD, Rogers JB: Improvement in the quality and fertilization potential of a human sperm population using the rise technique. J Androl 8:25, 1987
7. Stone SC, de la Maza LM, Peterson EM: Recovery of microorganisms from the pelvic cavity after intracervical or intrauterine artificial insemination. Fertil Steril 46:61, 1986

Section B:

CLINICAL ASPECTS

FRANCISCO IRIANNI, M.D., ANIBAL A. ACOSTA, M.D., SERGIO OEHNINGER, M.D., AND MARIA ROSA ACOSTA, B.S.

Since the pioneer work of Dickinson (1) in 1920 and Hanson and Rock (2) in 1951 established the possibility of therapeutic intrauterine insemination (TII), the method has been used extensively in many centers of reproductive endocrinology worldwide. In a first review, Mastroianni (3) recommended that, because of no positive results, the procedure should be abandoned until the technique could be improved.

The indications have been quite diverse (4–9), with variable degrees of success depending on the type of male or female problem for which the procedure was used. Several reviews (10–12) have tried to establish the indications, techniques, and results obtained in the different etiologies.

There are a number of variables besides patient selection and definition of the pathologies which increase the difficulty of assessing the value of this technique in the management of infertility. The variables include the method of sperm preparation (4–6, 9, 13–19), the timing and number of inseminations per cycle (4, 7, 13, 19–27), the techniques of insemination used, the varying manner of reporting results and the inherent pitfalls, and the frequent lack or inappropriateness of control groups.

The experience of the Norfolk program with TII is reviewed and reported in this chapter. This modality of treatment was started as a therapeutic procedure by one of us (A.A.A.) in 1979, with or without simultaneous ovulation stimulation or induction. During the initial 2 years, tentative attempts were made using different types of stimulation and different methods of sperm preparation. We present our experience from 1982 to May 1987, a period for which the best documentation and follow-up are available.

Materials and Methods

A total of 121 couples in 300 treatment cycles underwent 334 TII procedures. Each patient had an average of 2.47 cycles during which TII was carried out and a mean of 1.1 TIIs per cycle was performed. The mean age of the female population treated was 30.4 years, the youngest being 24 and the oldest 42 years of age.

Table 7.2.
Norfolk Program—Therapeutic Intrauterine Insemination

Type of Stimulation	Number of Cycles (n = 300)	
Natural cycle	163	(54.3%)
Natural cycle and progesterone	11	(3.6%)
Natural cycle and hCG	7	(2.33%)
Clomiphene and hCG	55	(18.3%)
Gonadotropins	64	(21.3%) { 55 hMG-hCG 9 FSH-hMG-hCG

Eighty couples were diagnosed as having primary infertility, with an average of 4.19 years' duration (shortest, 1 year; longest, 15 years). Forty-one couples were seen for secondary infertility with a mean of 2.4 years' duration (shortest, 6 months; longest, 10 years).

In almost every case, the husband's semen was used, except for two patients in whom donor insemination was used because of an irreversible male factor and a noncorrectable cervical factor.

In 163 cycles (54.3%), natural ovulation was used; in 11 (3.6%) the natural cycle was supplemented with progesterone (vaginal suppositories or intramuscular injections) during the second part of the cycle because of a confirmed or suspected luteal phase defect. In seven (2.33%) a midcycle injection of 10,000 IU of human chorionic gonadotropin (hCG) was given to trigger ovulation, to improve the timing of TII, and to further stimulate corpus luteum function. In 55 cycles (19.3%) a clomiphene citrate stimulation plus hCG was used, and in 64 cycles (21.3%) gonadotropin stimulation was carried out (Table 7.2).

Since the indications for TII were ill-defined when the procedure was incorporated into the therapeutic armamentarium, various categories of patients were treated in Norfolk by this technique (Table 7.3). In 40 cases (103 cycles) the indication was a pure male factor; in 11 cases (33 cycles) it was a male factor combined with a partial tubal factor; and in 22 cases (62 cycles) the indication was a male factor combined with

Table 7.3.
Norfolk Program—Therapeutic Intrauterine Insemination

Indications	No. of Patients	No. of Cycles
Pure male factor	40	103
Male factor and partial tubal factor	11	33
Male factor and ovulatory dysfunction	22	62
Pure ovulatory dysfunction	23	45
Endometriosis with mechanical tubal factor	7	21
Pure partial tubal factor	2	5
Unexplained	11	19
Pure cervical factor	5	12
Total	121	300

ovulatory dysfunction. As this work evolved over more than 5 years, the definition of a male factor has changed. Patients included had a sperm density $<20 \times 10^6$ (the majority $<10 \times 10^6$); an initial motility $<40\%$; and/or a morphology $<40\%$ by the classic criteria or $<14\%$ with the new, strict criteria, and/or $<10\%$ by the hamster sperm penetration assay. Whenever a male factor was involved, we followed a protocol outlined at the beginning of the program: three or four attempts at TII if the male had $>10 \times 10^6$ sperm with rapid progressive motility recovered in the swim-up procedure and the wife was suitable for this therapy. If the number of sperm recovered was 5 to 10×10^6, the couple was offered the option of entering the in vitro fertilization (IVF) program if they wished. If the number of sperm was $<5 \times 10^6$, the couple were advised to undergo IVF as a primary procedure.

Within the category of partial tubal factor, there were patients with unilateral adhesive disease, unilateral tubal occlusion, or a history of pelvic inflammatory disease with no demonstrable sequelae or bilateral tubal patency.

Ovulatory dysfunction was defined as oligoovulation, abnormal sequence of events at monitoring during midcycle using hormone determinations and ultrasound scanning, or luteinized unruptured follicles that were treated with hCG. In 23 cases (45 cycles) the diagnosis was pure ovulatory dysfunction; in seven couples (21 cycles) TII was done because of endometriosis generating some mechanical partial tubal factor. In two cases (five cycles) a pure partial tubal factor was present, and in 11 couples (19 cycles) unexplained infertility was diagnosed. In five cases (12 cycles) TII was performed because of a pure cervical factor, either anatomical (post-conization) or functional (postcoital test negative or <3 motile sperm per high-power field and abnormal cross-match test). In several other cases a pure cervical factor was present with other etiological problems. Those cases were grouped under the other factor(s), since the cervical abnormality was bypassed by TII. Five women had had exposure to diethylstilbestrol (DES). One had a coexistent male factor, one had mild endometriosis, one had ovulatory dysfunction, one had unexplained infertility, and one had a cervical factor. One man who had had DES exposure had a severe sperm problem.

Monitoring the menstrual cycle varied according to the type of treatment. With natural cycles, monitoring was done by using the basal body temperature chart (BBT), cervical mucus index, and daily ultrasound examinations; later a urinary luteinizing hormone (LH) immunoassay was added to the protocol (28). In 27 cases progesterone (25-mg vaginal suppositories twice a day or 25 mg intramuscularly four times a day) was used to supplement the luteal phase whenever an inadequate phase was diagnosed or suspected.

Similar monitoring was used with clomiphene stimulation. In most of these cycles, 10,000 IU of hCG were injected when the leading follicle was 18 to 20 mm in diameter; insemination was performed 34 to 36 hours later.

When gonadotropins were used for stimulation, most cycles were done with the two human menopausal gonadotropin (hMG) protocol (29), and the monitoring was done by the same methods recommended for our IVF program (29). In nine cases, a combination of hMG, hCG, and follicle-stimulating hormone (FSH) was used (30). In all of these, insemination was carried out 34 to 36 hours after hCG injection.

The semen preparation technique has changed since the beginning, when Tyrode's solution was used; in the newer method, Ham's F-10 supplemented with 7.5% human fetal cord serum is used. The compositions of the solutions we used are listed in Table 7.4. The specimen was collected in the laboratory according to the

Table 7.4.
Formulas for Solutions

1. Baker's saline:
    15.0 g D-glucose;
    1.0 g sodium chloride;
    2.3 g sodium phosphate, dibasic, heptahydrate;
    0.05 g potassium phosphate, monobasic, anhydrous.
    Add distilled water to 500 ml. Adjust pH to 7.3. Filter-sterilize and store at 4°C.
2. Diluting fluid for sperm counts:
    50.0 g sodium bicarbonate;
    10.0 ml formalin (35%).
    Dilute to 1000 ml with distilled water and store at 4°C.
3. Ham's F-10 medium: Dissolve one package of Ham's F-10 culture medium (Cat. no. 430-1200, GIBCO, Grand Island, N.Y.) in 1 liter of distilled water. Dissolve the following in 250 ml of dissolved Ham's F-10:
    0.0625 g calcium lactate;
    0.015 g penicillin G, sodium salt (1670 units/mg);
    0.034 g streptomycin sulfate (735 units/mg).
    Filter-sterilize and store at 4°C. Immediately prior to use, warm required volume to room temperature. Add sterile, heat-inactivated (56°C for 30–45 minutes) human fetal cord serum to 7.5% solution (v/v). Adjust pH to 7.3 and filter-sterilize.
4. Tyrode's medium: Dissolve one package of Tyrode's Salt Solution (Cat. no. 460-1116, GIBCO, Grand Island, N.Y.) in 1 liter of distilled water. Dissolve the following in 250 ml of the dissolved Tyrode's salts:
    0.25 g sodium bicarbonate;
    0.075 g fructose (beta-D);
    0.011 g penicillin G, sodium salt (1670 units/mg);
    0.028 g streptomycin sulfate (735 units/mg);
    0.073 g glutamine;
    0.028 g sodium pyruvate.
    Adjust pH to 7.3. Filter-sterilize, aliquot into 15-ml sterile tubes, and store at 4°C.

specifications of the World Health Organization (WHO) (31). Volume, sperm density, and motility were determined in small aliquots. The remaining semen specimen was diluted 1:1 with Ham's F-10. The specimen was then aliquotted into 4-, 6-, 8-, or 15-ml centrifuge tubes according to volume, and the tubes were centrifuged at 290 × g for 10 minutes. The supernatant was discarded without disturbing the pellet, which was resuspended in 4 ml of Ham's F-10, and the number of centrifuge tubes was reduced to half. Centrifugation was performed again at 290 × g for 10 minutes, and the supernatant was again discarded without disturbing the pellet. The pellets were resuspended in 2 ml of Ham's F-10, pooled in one tube, and centrifuged again at the same speed for another 10 minutes. The supernatant was discarded; the pellet was resuspended in 250 µl of Ham's F-10 and was sent at body temperature to the physician who would perform the insemination.

When cryopreserved sperm were used for TII, the specimen was taken out of the liquid nitrogen and allowed to thaw at room temperature for 30 minutes. It was then placed in 15-ml centrifuge tubes; 2 ml of Ham's F-10 without serum supplementation were mixed well with the specimen and centrifuged at 290 × g for 10 minutes. The supernatant was discarded, and the specimen was resuspended in 250 μl of Ham's F-10 and sent to the physician.

When the sperm swim-up method was used, the technique was similar to the one performed in the IVF embryology laboratory. A basic semen analysis was performed on the specimen. Within 20 to 45 minutes post-emission, according to liquefaction, the semen was diluted 1:1 with separation medium (Ham's F-10 plus 7.5% human fetal cord serum). The specimen was then aliquotted into 4-, 6-, 8-, or 15-ml tubes and centrifuged at 290 × g for 10 minutes at room temperature. The supernatant was discarded, and 0.5 ml of separation medium was added to each tube, taking care not to disturb the pellet. Incubation was done for 1 hour at 37°C in a 5% carbon dioxide environment. The supernatants were collected from the tubes and pooled; motility and count were performed on the supernatant. The specimen was then sent to the physician for TII.

Collection and preparation of sperm in patients with retrograde ejaculation was as follows. An abstinence period of 4 to 7 days was advised, urine was neutralized for 3 days before the test with sodium bicarbonate by mouth, and avoidance of alcohol and other drugs was recommended. The patient urinated 1 hour before semen collection, collected the semen specimen, then produced another urine specimen within 5 minutes of ejaculation or as soon as possible. The pH, volume, and osmolality were checked in both urine specimens. The urine was centrifuged at 280 × g for 10 minutes. The pellet was resuspended in Tyrode's with 4% human serum albumin or in Ham's F-10 plus 15% fetal cord serum. The specimen was recentrifuged and the pellet resuspended in a minimal volume and overlaid with 0.2 ml of Tyrode's with 4% human serum albumin. It was then incubated for 2 hours at 37°C in 5% CO_2. The supernatant was collected, a sperm count and motility evaluation were performed, and the specimen was sent for TII.

The insemination technique used the same instruments used for embryo transfer (32), with the patient in the dorsal lithotomy or knee-chest position. The amount inseminated was usually 250 μl and was always less than 500 μl to avoid backflow.

There were difficulties during insemination, such as problems negotiating the cervix, bleeding, or backflow. The patient was left to rest for 30 minutes after the procedure in the supine position and was free to have intercourse afterward.

Monitoring was continued after TII until ovulation was documented by disappearance of the follicle, presence of cul-de-sac fluid by ultrasound, and/or a drop in estradiol values and an increase in progesterone values.

If the menstrual period did not occur 2 weeks after TII, blood was drawn for a β-hCG radioimmunoassay. In patients who had been stimulated with gonadotropins, the procedure was not repeated until one or two normal cycles had subsequently occurred.

Statistical evaluation was done using Student's T test, the chi square approximation (Kruskall-Wallis) test, and the Wilcoxon 2 sample test.

Results

A total of 21 pregnancies were obtained in 300 cycles (7.0% total pregnancy rate per cycle) in 121 patients (17.3% total pregnancy rate per patient). Eight pregnancies occurred during the first cycle, five during the second, five during the third, and three during the fourth. No pregnancies occurred after four inseminations (12 cases).

Twelve pregnancies were established in 80 patients with primary infertility: four in patients with 2 years or less of reproductive difficulties (33.3%), three in patients with 3

Table 7.5.
Results—21 Pregnancies in 17 Patients

13 Patients ———————— 1 pregnancy each	{	5 abortions 8 term pregnancies
4 Patients ———————— 2 pregnancies each	{	3 patients had 2 consecutive abortions 1 patient had 2 term pregnancies

Live births: 10 patients (47.6%), 3.33% per cycle.
Abortion: 11 patients (52.4%)

---

years of infertility (25%), three in patients with 4 years of infertility (25%), and two in patients with 5 years or more (16.6%). In 41 patients with secondary infertility, nine pregnancies resulted: three in patients with 2 years or less of infertility (33.3%), two in patients with 3 years of infertility (22.2%), two in patients with 4 years of infertility (22.2%), and two in patients with 5 or more years of infertility (22.2%). No significant differences in the results were found when duration of infertility was taken into account.

Twenty-one pregnancies were obtained in 17 patients (Table 7.5); 13 had one pregnancy each (eight term and five miscarriages), and four had two pregnancies each (three had two consecutive abortions, and one had two term pregnancies). Ten babies were born (47.6% of the pregnancies), giving an overall term pregnancy rate of 3.3% per cycle and 8.2% per patient. Eleven patients had miscarriages (52.4% of the pregnancies).

If we now consider the pregnancy results according to the type of cycle (Table 7.6), five were obtained with natural cycles, of which four ended in spontaneous abortion, and one was a term pregnancy (0.6% term pregnancy rate per cycle). No pregnancies were obtained in the natural cycle group when progesterone was used for supplementation, and one term delivery was achieved when the luteal phase was stimulated with hCG during a natural cycle.

Six pregnancies developed when clomiphene stimulation was used (10.9% per cycle); two ended in spontaneous abortions, and four were delivered, including one set of twins. When gonadotropin stimulation was used, nine pregnancies were established (14.0% per cycle); four ended in spontaneous abortion, and four were delivered or

Table 7.6.
Pregnancy Results According to Type of Cycle Used

Type of Cycle	No. of Cycles	Total Pregnancies	Term Pregnancies	Term Pregnancies Per Cycle (%)	Outcome
Natural cycle	163	5	1	0.6	
Natural cycle + progesterone	11	0			
Natural cycle + hCG	7	1	1	14.2	
Clomiphene	55	6	4	7.2	1 set of twins
Gonadotropin	64	9	4	6.2	1 unknown

Table 7.7.
Pregnancy Results According to Etiology

Etiology	No. of Patients	No. of Cycles	Total Pregnancies	Term Pregnancies	Term Pregnancies per Cycle (%)
Male factor	40	103	3	1	0.9
Male + tubal factors	11	33	0		
Male + ovulatory factors	22	62	8	3	4.8
Ovulatory factor	23	45	8	4	8.8
Endometriosis	7	21	0		
Pure tubal factor	2	5	0		
Unexplained infertility	11	19	1	1	5.2
Cervical factor	5	12	1	1	8.3
Total	121	300	21	10	3.3

ongoing (one set of twins) at the time of this review. In one patient the pregnancy outcome was unknown.

When term pregnancies are considered according to the type of cycle, natural cycles rendered a total of two term pregnancies out of 181 cycles (1.1%); clomiphene produced four term pregnancies out of 55 cycles (7.2%), and gonadotropin stimulation induced four term pregnancies out of 64 cycles (6.25%). No statistically significant differences were found among these groups.

Results obtained in the etiological groups are shown in Table 7.7. No pregnancies were obtained in the combined male factor and tubal factor group, in the endometriosis group, or in the pure tubal factor group. No significant differences in the pregnancy rates were seen in the groups in which pregnancies were established.

When the groups are analyzed by both etiology and type of cycle (Tables 7.8–7.12), in the male factor group the only three pregnancies were achieved when clomiphene was used for stimulation; two ended in abortion, and one was a term pregnancy (in which donor semen had been used). Long-term follow-up of patients in the natural cycle group, in whom TII had failed, showed that two patients achieved pregnancy afterwards with natural intercourse, two became pregnant by IVF, and one had TII elsewhere but subsequently aborted. In the clomiphene-stimulated group, one patient achieved pregnancy with donor intracervical insemination. In the hMG- and hCG-stimulated group, one patient achieved pregnancy with natural intercourse and one with IVF.

In the male and tubal factor group, 11 patients had 33 cycles; no pregnancies were established. One patient achieved pregnancy later by IVF.

The results obtained in the male factor combined with ovulatory factor group are shown in Table 7.9. Among the patients with pregnancies, no significant differences were observed.

In patients with ovulatory factor (Table 7.10), no differences were shown between the groups. In the long-term follow-up, one patient in the natural cycle group became pregnant by the gamete intrafallopian transfer (GIFT) procedure. In the hMG-hCG

Table 7.8.
Pregnancy Results According to Etiology and Type of Cycle Used: Male Factor—40 Patients

Type of Cycle	No. of Cycles	Total Pregnancies	Term Pregnancies	Reproductive Performance after TII Failure
Natural cycle	76	0		2 pregnant with coitus
				2 pregnant with IVF
				1 pregnant with TII elsewhere
Natural cycle + progesterone	7	0		
Clomiphene	10	3	1	1 pregnant with ICI[a]-AID
hMG-hCG	9	0		1 pregnant with coitus
				1 pregnant with IVF
FSH-hMG-hCG	1	0		
Total	103	3	1	8

[a]Intracervical insemination.

group, one patient became pregnant with the same stimulation and natural intercourse; one became pregnant with gonadotropin-releasing hormone (GnRH) pump infusion and natural intercourse.

In the endometriosis group, seven patients had 21 cycles of treatment with no pregnancies established. Two patients achieved pregnancy with natural intercourse, and one became pregnant by IVF later. Of the partial tubal factor patients, two had five cycles of treatment and no pregnancies were obtained; follow-up also revealed no pregnancies.

In the unexplained infertility group (Table 7.11), only one pregnancy was obtained in the clomiphene-stimulated group.

In the cervical factor group (Table 7.12), the only pregnancy was in the natural cycle group with an hCG ovulatory dose.

The long-term follow-up in patients who failed to achieve pregnancy during treatment cycles, but achieved pregnancy in some other way afterwards, is summarized in Table 7.13.

Table 7.9.
Pregnancy Results According to Etiology and Type of Cycle Used: Male + Ovulatory—22 Patients

Type of Cycle	No. of Cycles	Total Pregnancies	Term Pregnancies
Natural cycle	20	4 (3 patients)	1
Natural cycle + progesterone	3	0	
Natural cycle + hCG	6	0	
Clomiphene	11	1	1
hMG-hCG	16	2 (1 patient)	
FSH-hMG-hCG	6	1	1
Total	62	8	3

Table 7.10.
Pregnancy Results According to Etiology and Type of Cycle Used: Ovulatory—23 Patients

Type of Cycle	No. of Cycles	Total Pregnancies	Term Pregnancies	Reproductive Performance after TII Failure
Natural cycle	15	1		1 with GIFT
Clomiphene	13	1	1	
hMG-hCG	16	5	2	1 with hMG + hCG + coitus 1 GnRH[a] + coitus
FSH-hMG-hCG	1	1	1	
Total	45	8	4	

[a]Gonadotropin-releasing hormone.

Discussion

Evaluation and discussion of TII as treatment for certain types of infertility using the available literature is an extremely difficult task, posing at times almost unsurmountable problems. In the first place, relatively few of the series report on a substantial number of patients (4, 14, 23, 24, 26, 33–36). The procedure has been used for many different indications; even for similar indications, definitions of the etiologies involved (male factor, unexplained infertility, cervical factor, ovulatory dysfunction) are so different that the populations are completely heterogeneous.

Since assisted reproduction methods such as IVF, GIFT, and direct intraperitoneal insemination (DIPI) have become available, different methods of sperm preparation have been developed and applied to TII. For the same reason, more sophisticated procedures for monitoring ovulation have been designed, and consequently the timing of insemination has become more accurate. Therefore, series reported earlier are impossible to compare with those reported more recently.

Another variable is the number of inseminations performed per cycle. Most of the reports, including our own, involve retrospective reviews, and therefore control groups were either lacking or inadequate. Very few have been designed as prospective studies (37).

The type of cycle used for TII—a natural cycle or a stimulated cycle using different combinations of ovulatory agents—introduces another important variable in evaluating results (16, 37).

Table 7.11.
Pregnancy Results According to Etiology and Type of Cycle Used: Unexplained Infertility—11 Patients

Type of Cycle	No. of Cycles	No. of Pregnancies	Outcome
Natural cycle	11	0	
Clomiphene	2	1	Birth
hMG-hCG	5	0	
FSH-hMG-hCG	1	0	

Table 7.12.
Pregnancy Results According to Etiology and Type of Cycle Used: Cervical Factor—5 Patients

Type of Cycle	No. of Cycles	Total Pregnancies	Term Pregnancies
Natural cycle	7	0	
Natural cycle + progesterone	1	1	1
Clomiphene	4	0	
Total	12	1	1

The way in which results are reported in most papers—pregnancy rate per patient—is perhaps not the best way to evaluate the results, efficiency, and cost-effectiveness of the method. Abortion rates and term pregnancy rates per patient and per cycle should be given routinely in order to determine the real value of this therapeutic approach.

The number of cycles to be performed before the procedure is abandoned should be about four, according to our experience. This coincides with most series already published (6–9, 13–14, 17, 21, 26–27, 33–39). If no pregnancy is achieved after four attempts, the situation should be reconsidered.

Table 7.13.
Reproductive Performance in Patients Who Did Not Achieve Pregnancy with TII in Norfolk

Etiology	No. of Patients	Cause of Eventual Pregnancy	Previous Stimulation
Male factor	8	Coitus: 3 patients (one with male on clomiphene)	2 on natural cycle 1 on gonadotropin
		IVF: 3 patients	2 on natural cycle 1 on gonadotropin
		TII elsewhere: 1 patient	Natural cycle
		ICI/AID:[a] 1 patient	Clomiphene
Male factor + tubal factor	1	IVF	Clomiphene
Ovulatory factor	4	GIFT: 1 patient	Natural cycle
		Ovulation induction with gonadotropin + coitus: 2 patients	Gonadotropins
		GnRH pump + coitus: 1 patient	Gonadotropins
Endometriosis	3	Coitus: 2 patients IVF: 1 patient	Natural cycle Gonadotropin

[a]ICI, intracervical insemination; AID, artificial insemination by donor.

In our series, patients with 2 years or less of reproductive difficulties had a 33.3% total pregnancy rate. Patients with 5 or more years had a 16.6% total pregnancy rate. Although the difference is not statistically significant, the trend seems to follow the rule in infertility cases that problems of more than 5 years' duration have a worse prognosis.

In the group of patients reported here, the term pregnancy rate per cycle was 3.3%. DiMarzo (38) reported 4.7% per cycle, Barwin (4) 6%, and Toffle (14) 3.6%. Cruz (26) in a prospective study had 6.2%, Confino (35) 5.8%, Belker (34) 3%, and Hoing (33) 4%. All found that large series gave similar results, and all pointed to a very low efficiency of treatment.

The total pregnancy rate per patient in our series (17.3%) was lower than those of some of the longer series in the literature, which fluctuated between 20% and 30% (21, 34–36, 38, 40–43), but is comparable to others that reported 10% and 20% success (6, 13, 14, 23, 26, 33, 44). Very few series exceeded the 30% total pregnancy rate per patient (4, 16, 19, 45).

The term/ongoing pregnancy rate per patient in our series was 8.2%. Most series in the literature had rates of 10% to 15% (6, 13, 14, 26, 33, 34, 38, 43). A few had 20% to 30% (35, 45). Unusually high results were reported by Barwin (4), 48%; White (19), 55.5%; and Gerris (16), 37.9%. Quagliarello (41) had results similar to ours, 8.8%.

The literature very rarely presents breakdowns of results by type of cycle. In our series the use of natural cycles seems to be extremely inefficient (1.1% term pregnancy rate per cycle); stimulated cycles, using clomiphene or gonadotropins, seem to improve the efficiency somewhat, although statistical analysis did not show any significance.

ANALYSIS OF RESULTS ACCORDING TO INDICATIONS

More detailed and critical evaluation of the results of the method in each of the indications may produce useful information to clarify the real value of the procedure.

Male Factor Infertility

In male factor infertility, the differences in threshold and parameters used to define the problem are staggering. Some authors simply mention the presence of a male factor without definition (36, 37, 46). Others use strict criteria and define oligoasthenoteratozoospermia as a concentration of $<10 \times 10^6$ sperm per milliliter, progressive motility of $<30\%$, and ideally shaped sperm $<20\%$ (16). A third group uses parameters that allow inclusion of specimens that can be considered normal by other researchers' standards. For instance, Kerin (21) defines oligoasthenoteratozoospermia as a concentration of $<40 \times 10^6$ sperm per milliliter, motility of $<45\%$, and normal morphology of $<40\%$ in three different specimens. Among the other authors writing on the use of TII in male factor patients (4, 5, 13, 14, 17, 26, 27, 33, 35, 44, 45, 47), the criteria are spread between these two extremes.

Most have used the natural female cycle for TII (4, 13, 14, 21, 35, 36, 40, 44–47), some have used stimulated cycles (5, 17, 26, 27), and others have used both (16, 33).

Monitoring the cycle and timing the insemination are quite variable, with some using only the day of the cycle and the cervical mucus index (13), and others using BBT chart only (4), ultrasound only (38), or a combination of the latter two (14, 35). Some groups measured LH surge and performed insemination 15 hours (44), 24 hours (21, 33), or 24 to 36 hours (36) thereafter. Others used hCG at midcycle and performed insemination 24 hours (16), 28 hours (26), 34 hours (40), or 36 hours (27) thereafter. Others performed TII after the LH surge or hCG with no other specifications (5, 17).

Regarding sperm preparation, most authors preferred a swim-up procedure (21, 26, 27, 33, 36, 40, 44), some used washing (5, 14, 35, 45), and others used both (38, 47). Barwin (4) used frozen whole semen, Harris (13) used a migration into a diluent, and Glass (46) used filtration.

Most authors reported total pregnancy rates per patient of 13% to 25% (13, 14, 21, 26, 27, 33, 36, 38, 40), which is higher than our 7.5%. Barwin (4) reported a very high figure (66.6%) in mild oligospermia and 37.5 in severe oligospermia. Gerris (16) reported 50% in his group. Hewitt (5) had a low, 8.3%, pregnancy rate per patient. Of the series reporting the total pregnancy rate per cycle, Barwin (4) had 6% success rate in severe oligospermia, Cruz (26) showed 7.0%, Hoing (33) 6.9%, and Hewitt (5) 4.6%. Our series showed only 2.9%. Rare exceptions were Kerin (21) and Barwin (4), with pregnancy rates per cycle of 20.5% and 22.2%, respectively, using higher thresholds for classifying male factors.

The term pregnancy rates per patient and per cycle were given by two authors: Cruz (26), 11% to 12%; and Hoing (33), 4% to 6%. Again, our corresponding figures are much lower: 2.5% and 0.9%, respectively. Only Gerris (16) reported a pregnancy rate per patient of 50% and per cycle of 12% with all term deliveries; the author indicated that the best results were obtained when >500,000 sperm with good progressive motility are used. Four series showed no pregnancies (35, 44, 46, 47).

Unexplained Infertility

In unexplained infertility, very few series reported a substantial number of patients (22, 36, 37). Two authors (22, 36) had used natural cycles exclusively. Hewitt (5) had stimulated cycles using clomiphene-hCG, and Sher (27) had exclusively used an hMG-hCG protocol. Gerris (16) used all three methods, and Perino (17) used FSH-hMG-hCG and clomiphene-hMG-hCG. Serhal (37) published the only prospective randomized series, using the natural cycle with LH determinations, hMG-hCG followed by natural intercourse, and hMG-hCG with TII. The sperm preparation was swim-up in most cases, with plain washing in two series (5, 22).

Two series showed no pregnancies (17, 22). The rest had pregnancy rates per patient between 11% and 25%. Only Sher (27), with very few cases, and Serhal (37), in his randomized trial, reported a 40% pregnancy rate per patient. Our own experience yielded a 9% pregnancy rate per patient, a 5.2% pregnancy rate per cycle, and identical figures for term pregnancy rates.

Cervical Factor Infertility

In cervical factor infertility, the definitions are equally different. Most authors categorize the etiology using the concept of a poor or negative postcoital test, with or without definition of the term (no forward progression; absent mucus; poor or negative postcoital test with a negative in vitro test and negative bacteriology and immunology; <3 or <5 motile sperm per high-power field, etc.).

Most investigators used the natural cycle or the natural cycle with hCG (14, 34–36, 38, 40, 41, 44). Barwin (4) used the natural cycle and Premarin IV at midcycle. Hewitt (5) used clomiphene-hCG. Sher (27) used hMG-hCG, and Gerris (16) used both of the latter stimulations. Timing was based on LH surge or hCG injection. Sperm preparation was equally divided between swim-up and washing techniques.

Using the natural cycle, pregnancy rates per patient in the largest series varied from 30% (41) to 72.2% (4). Two series in this group obtained much poorer results: 14.2% and 15.7%, respectively (14, 44).

One group using clomiphene with or without hCG had a pregnancy rate per patient of 6.6% (5); and Arny and Quagliarello (48) in a small group reported 33.3%. With hMG-hCG, Sher (27) reported a 60% total pregnancy rate per patient in a very small group. DeVilliers (42) reported a 47.3% pregnancy rate per couple in a group of patients with infertility due to cervical factor. In the few reports giving the number of cycles used, the total pregnancy rate per cycle was much lower.

In our very small series, the total pregnancy rate was 20% per patient and 8.3% per cycle; the term pregnancy rates per patient and per cycle were identical.

Ulstein (43) used whole semen for insemination in couples with cervical factor infertility and obtained a 28.5% pregnancy rate per couple, but six of 10 aborted, perhaps because of concomitant poor semen quality. Glezerman (18), also using only fresh semen, reported 13 pregnancies in 25 couples inseminated with the first ejaculatory spurt, for a pregnancy rate per couple of 52% and an abortion rate of 33%.

PROBLEMS WITH TII

Very few problems have resulted from the application of TII, according to the available literature. In regard to the amount of sperm used, Shelden (49) pointed out that, when gonadotropin stimulation and multiple ovulation are used as part of the insemination protocol, the rate of multiple gestations is related to the sperm concentration in the specimen. A ceiling of 20×10^6 has been proposed to reduce the number of multiple pregnancies without impairing the monthly probability of conception.

Although the theoretical risk of transporting bacteria with the insemination exists, and Stone (50) has demonstrated the recovery of microorganisms from the pelvic cavity after the procedure, the cases of pelvic infections reported are extremely rare, and in our experience there are no instances of this complication. Uterine cramps have been reported after TII, with apparently no further consequences.

References

1. Dickinson R: Artificial impregnation: essays in tubal insemination. Am J Obstet Gynecol 1:225, 1920
2. Hanson FM, Rock J: Artificial insemination with husband's sperm. Fertil Steril 2:162, 1951
3. Mastroianni L Jr, Laberge JL, Rock J: Appraisal of the efficacy of artificial insemination with husband's sperm and evaluation of insemination technic. Fertil Steril 8:260, 1957
4. Barwin BN: Intrauterine insemination of husband's semen. J Reprod Fertil 36:101, 1974
5. Hewitt J, Cohen J, Krishnaswama V, Fehilly C, Steptoe P, Walters D: Treatment of idiopathic infertility, cervical mucus hostility and male infertility: artificial insemination with husband's semen or in vitro fertilization? Fertil Steril 44:350, 1985
6. Dmowski WP, Gaynor L, Lawrence M, Rao R, Scommegna A: Artificial insemination homologous with oligospermic semen separated on albumin columns. Fertil Steril 31:58, 1979
7. Corson SL, Batzer FR, Alexander NJ, Schlaff S, Otis C: Sex selection by sperm separation and insemination. Fertil Steril 42:756, 1984
8. Kredentser JV, Pokrant C, McCoshen JA: Intrauterine insemination for infertility due to cystic fibrosis. Fertil Steril 45:425, 1986
9. Scammell GE, Stedronska J, Dempsey A: Successful pregnancies using human seroalbumin following retrograde ejaculation: a case report. Fertil Steril 37:277, 1982
10. Nachtigall R, Faure N, Glas RH: Artificial insemination of husband's sperm. Fertil Steril 32:141, 1979
11. Allen NC, Herbert CM III, Maxon WS, Rogers BJ, Diamond MP, Wentz AC: Intrauterine insemination, a critical review. Fertil Steril 44:569, 1985

12. Alexander NJ, Ackerman S: Therapeutic insemination. Obstet Gynecol Clin N Am 14:905, 1987
13. Harris SJ, Milligan MP, Masson GM, Dennis KS: Improved separation of motile sperm in asthenospermia and its application to artificial insemination homologous (AIH). Fertil Steril 36:219, 1981
14. Toffle RC, Nagel TC, Tagatz GE, Phansey SA, Okagaki T, Waurin C: Intrauterine insemination, the University of Minnesota experience. Fertil Steril 43:743, 1985
15. Cohen MR: Intrauterine insemination. Int J Fertil 7:235, 1962
16. Gerris JM, Delbeke LO, Punjabi U, Buytaert P: The value of intrauterine insemination with washed husband's sperm in the treatment of infertility. J Reprod 2:315, 1987
17. Perino A, Cimino C, Catinella E, Barba G, Cittadine E: In vitro sperm capacitation and intrauterine insemination: a sample technique for the treatment of refractory infertility unrelated to female organic pelvic disease. Clinical results and immunologic effects: a preliminary report. Acta Eur Fertil 17:325, 1986
18. Glezerman M, Bernstein D, Insler V: The cervical factor of infertility and intrauterine insemination. Int J Fertil 29:16, 1984
19. White RM, Glass RH: Intrauterine insemination with husband's semen. Obstet Gynecol 47:119, 1976
20. Kaskarelis E, Comninos A: A critical evaluation of homologous artificial insemination. Int J Fertil 4:38, 1959
21. Kerin JFP, Kirby C, Peek J, Jeffrey R, Warnes GM, Matthews CA, Cox LW: Improved conception rate after intrauterine insemination of washed spermatozoa from men with poor quality semen. Lancet 1:533, 1984
22. Irvine S, Aitken J, Lees M, Reid C: Failure of high intrauterine insemination of husband's semen. Lancet 2:972, 1986
23. Yovich J, Matson P: Pregnancy rates after high intrauterine insemination of husband's spermatozoa or gamete intrafallopian transfer. Lancet 2:1287, 1986
24. Davajan V, Vargyas JM, Kleitzky OA, March CM, Bernstein GS, Mishell DR, Marrs RP: Intrauterine insemination with washed sperm to treat infertility. Fertil Steril 40:419, 1983
25. Marrs RP, Vargyas JM, Saito H, Gibbons WE, Berger T, Mishell DR Jr: Clinical applications of techniques used in human in vitro fertilization research. Am J Obstet Gynecol 146:477, 1983
26. Cruz RI, Kemmann E, Brandeis VT, Becker KA, Beck M, Beardsley L, Shelden R: A prospective study of intrauterine insemination of processed sperm from men with oligoasthenospermia in superovulated women. Fertil Steril 46:673, 1986
27. Sher G, Knutzen VK, Stratton CJ, Montakhab MM, Allenson SG: In vitro sperm capacitation and trans-cervical intrauterine insemination for the treatment of refractory infertility: phase I. Fertil Steril 41:260, 1984
28. Knee GR, Feinman MA, Strauss JF, Blasco L, Goodman DBP: Detection of the ovulatory luteinizing hormone (LH) surge with a semiquantitative urinary LH assay. Fertil Steril 44:707, 1985
29. Garcia JE, Jones GS, Acosta AA, Wright G Jr: Human menopausal gonadotropin/human chorionic gonadotropin follicular maturation for oocyte aspiration: phase I, 1981. Fertil Steril 39:167, 1983
30. Muasher SJ, Garcia JE, Rosenwaks Z: The combination of follicle stimulating hormone and human menopausal gonadotropin for the induction of multiple follicular maturation for in vitro fertilization. Fertil Steril 42:62, 1985
31. World Health Organization: Laboratory Manual for the Examination of Human Semen and Semen-Cervical Mucus Interaction. Cambridge: Cambridge University Press, 1987
32. Jones HW, Acosta AA, Garcia JE, Sandow BD, Veeck L: On the transfer of conceptuses from oocytes fertilized in vitro. Fertil Steril 39:241, 1983
33. Hoing LM, Devroey P, Van Sterteghem AC: Treatment of infertility because of oligoasthenoteratospermia by transcervical intrauterine insemination of motile spermatozoa. Fertil Steril 45:338, 1986
34. Belker AM, Cook CL: Sperm processing and intrauterine insemination for oligospermia. Urol Clin N Am 14:597, 1987
35. Confino E, Friberg J, Dudkiewicz AB, Gleicher N: Intrauterine insemination with washed human spermatozoa. Fertil Steril 46:55, 1986
36. Sueldo C, Hovel L, Gocke S: Intrauterine insemination for the treatment of infertility. Infertility 9:217, 1986
37. Serhal PF, Katz M, Little V, Woronowski H: Unexplained infertility—the value of Pergonal superovulation combined with intrauterine insemination. Fertil Steril 49:602, 1988
38. DiMarzo SJ, Rakoff J: Intrauterine insemination with husband's washed sperm. Fertil Steril 46:470, 1986
39. Urry RL, Middleton RG, McGavin S: A simple and effective technique for increasing pregnancy rate in couples with retrograde ejaculation. Fertil Steril 14:1124, 1986

40. Serhal PF, Katz M: Intrauterine insemination. Lancet 1:52, 1987
41. Quagliarello J, Arny M: Intracervical versus intrauterine insemination: correlation of outcome with antecedent postcoital testing. Fertil Steril 46:870, 1986
42. DeVilliers TJ, Kruger TF, Van der Merwe JP, Menkveld R: Kunsmatige intrauteriene inseminasie met gewaste voorbereide eggenootsemen. S Afr Med J 72:488, 1987
43. Ulstein M: Fertility of husbands at homologous insemination. Acta Obstet Gynecol Scand 52:5, 1973
44. Hull ME, Magyar DM, Vasquez JM, Hayes MF, Moghissi KS: Experience with intrauterine insemination for cervical factor and oligospermia. Am J Obstet Gynecol 154:1333, 1986
45. Baerthlein WC, Muechler EK, Chaney K: Simplified sperm washing techniques and intrauterine insemination. Obstet Gynecol 71:277, 1988
46. Glass RH, Ericsson RJ: Intrauterine insemination of isolated motile sperm. Fertil Steril 29:535, 1978
47. Thomas EJ, McTighe L, King H, Lenton EA, Harper R, Cooke ID: Failure of high intrauterine insemination of husband's semen. Lancet 2:693, 1986
48. Arny M, Quagliarello J: Semen quality before and after processing by a swim-up method: relationship to outcome of intrauterine insemination. Fertil Steril 48:643, 1987
49. Shelden R, Kemmann E, Bohrer M, Pasquale S: Multiple gestation is associated with the use of high sperm numbers in the intrauterine insemination specimen in women undergoing gonadotropin stimulation. Fertil Steril 49:607, 1988
50. Stone SC, de la Maza LM, Peterson EM: Recovery of microorganisms from the pelvic cavity after intracervical or intrauterine artificial insemination. Fertil Steril 46:61, 1986

Part Two—The Tygerberg Experience

GREG M. GROBLER, M.D., TOBIE J. DE VILLIERS, M.D., THINUS F. KRUGER, M.D., JACOBUS P. VAN DER MERWE, M.D., AND ROELOF MENKVELD, PH.D.

Therapeutic insemination by husband has been practiced for 200 years. The first recorded insemination (1) was performed in London in the 1770s by Dr. John Hunter in a patient whose husband had hypospadias. Since then, many methods of insemination have been tried, with varying degrees of success—from caps of semen placed over the cervix to intravaginal, intracervical, or intrauterine insemination (2, 3). Until recently, raw, unprepared semen was used, with widely varying results and with reported pregnancy rates up to 55% (4). In a review of the literature, however, Nachtigall (5) found that the average pregnancy rate using unprepared semen was actually about 18%. The method was unsatisfactory and caused unpleasant side effects, most commonly severe cramping of the uterus. This was probably due to prostaglandins in the seminal plasma, which possibly resulted in the expulsion of the semen from the uterus (1). Other complications—more serious but fortunately less common—included intrauterine infection and severe anaphylactic reaction (6–9).

Indications for therapeutic intrauterine insemination (TII) have been numerous and often arbitrary. The most common indication is an abnormality in one or more of the semen parameters. TII has also been used in patients with hostile cervical mucus, immunological problems (such as antisperm antibodies in the cervical mucus), and anatomical defects causing defective deposition of semen in the vagina (as in retrograde ejaculation). However, TII with unprepared semen is not likely to increase significantly the prospects of pregnancy in a case of abnormal semen parameters (1).

With the advent of in vitro fertilization (IVF) and embryo transfer, a new method of preparing semen for TII was developed. This method involves washing the sperm in a special medium, followed by a swim-up. The washed sperm are thus separated from the seminal plasma, and sperm quality is improved. Improvement in sperm motility and forward progression is attained, as the sperm with greatest motility are selected by the swim-up procedure (10, 11). Because there is a positive correlation between sperm motility and morphology, the latter can also be improved during semen preparation (11).

Is Intrauterine Insemination a Therapeutic Option?

In the Tygerberg experience, the use of unwashed sperm for TII or intracervical insemination produced very poor results and was discontinued. With the advent of washed sperm for IVF, studies in the literature reported an increased conception rate with husband's semen prepared for TII (10, 12). These reports rekindled our interest in the procedure, and we decided to reinstitute TII by husband, using washed semen, as a treatment modality for certain abnormalities including poor cervical mucus and teratozoospermia.

We have a particular interest in abnormal sperm morphology; Kruger (13) reported its effects on the fertilization potential of ova in vitro. He showed that, with a sperm morphology <14% normal, the fertilizing capacity of the semen is severely compromised. We therefore decided to include patients with teratozoospermia in our study to establish whether the pregnancy rate in this group could be improved.

Patient Workup for Intrauterine Insemination

All patients seen at the Tygerberg infertility clinic receive a standard workup. Thus, all patients selected for TII have all of the following procedures before insemination.

After the initial consultation and physical examination, patients are asked to return on the day of maximum flow in the subsequent menstruation. Six specimens of menstrual fluid are withdrawn from the vagina by flushing it with 10 cc of normal saline and aspirating the fluid into a syringe. The specimens are taken at intervals of at least 1 hour and are sent for *Mycobacterium tuberculosis* culture. (Specimens may be taken over more than one cycle, if this is more convenient.) We consider this an important step in the infertility workup because turberculosis is still a commonly diagnosed condition at our institution. If the culture is positive, the patient is placed on anti-tuberculosis therapy for 6 months, after which she is recultured before the infertility investigation is continued.

The next step involves daily ultrasound examinations from day 10 of the cycle to document the growth of the dominant follicle. Daily serum estradiol (E_2) and luteinizing hormone (LH) assays are performed from day 10 to determine the time of ovulation. The cervical mucus is also examined daily, and a cervical index is assigned according to the modified Insler method (14). We evaluate the mucus quantity (volume), translucency, liquidity, spinnbarkheit, and fern pattern. A score of 1 to 3 is possible for each category, with a maximum total score of 18. The mucus is considered poor if the index is <14. Once the index is at least 16 to 18, a postcoital test is performed 4 hours after intercourse. If the results are poor, a screening test for antibodies is performed on the cervical mucus (sperm-cervical mucus compatibility test). If an antibody problem is found, the patient is referred for further investigations (see Chapters 4 and 5).

Between days 21 and 24, the patient is given a diagnostic laparoscopy, chromopertubation, hysterosalpingogram, and endometrial biopsy under general anesthesia. The endometrium obtained is sent for histological dating and *Mycobacterium tuberculosis* culture. On day 24, blood is taken for progesterone assay to confirm ovulation.

The husband is scheduled for four semen analyses, done after 2 to 3 days of abstinence from intercouse, at intervals of 4 to 6 weeks. Disorders in the male are referred to our Division of Andrology for further evaluation.

Method of Insemination

TII is performed as near the time of ovulation as possible, as determined by daily ultrasound examinations and serum E_2 and LH assays. Once the semen has been washed and the swim-up has taken place, the prepared sperm are drawn into a tuberculin syringe attached to a Tomcat catheter (Monoject, St. Louis, Mo.).

The patient is placed in the lithotomy position and the cervix is visualized by means of a speculum. The Tomcat catheter is introduced into the uterus, with care not to damage the endometrium and cause bleeding. The full amount of prepared specimen

Table 7.14.
Analysis of Cycles in Patients Undergoing Intrauterine Insemination

Total number of patients	68
Total number of cycles	162
Number of inseminations per patient	2.47
Number of inseminations per cycle	1.68
Spontaneous cycles	93
Ovulation induction cycles (total)	69
Clomiphene	34
hMG	33
Clomiphene + hMG	2

(usually 0.6 to 0.8 ml) is then injected slowly into the uterine cavity. The patient lies on her back for 10 minutes and then is allowed to get up, with no restrictions other than refraining from intercourse for 2 days.

The Tygerberg Experience

From January 1986 to November 1987, TII was performed on 68 patients in 162 cycles—an average of 2.47 inseminations per patient. In 1987 the average patient age was 29.6 years. All patients had been trying to become pregnant for at least 18 months. The average duration of infertility in the group was 4.94 years (range, 2 to 11 years). Each patient received an average of 1.68 (range, 1 to 3) inseminations per cycle. There were 93 spontaneous cycles and 69 cycles in which some form of ovulation induction was indicated. In 33 of these cycles, human menopausal gonadotropin (hMG) was used for ovulation induction; in 34 cycles clomiphene citrate was used. Two patients who had been selected for gamete intrafallopian transfer (GIFT) were placed on the routine combination of hMG and clomiphene (see Chapter 6). However, their response to stimulation was poor, and only one or two follicles developed. It was therefore decided to perform TII instead, since GIFT is seldom attempted if <3 follicles are formed in response to ovarian stimulation (see Table 7.14). In 26 patients there was a cervical factor (cervical index <14), in 24 patients teratozoospermia (normal sperm morphology <14%) (12), and in 15 patients a normal sperm morphology of 15% to 20%. The sperm concentration in these patients was >20 × 10^6/ml, and motility was >30% (12).

There were 27 pregnancies, of which 22 resulted from TII, giving a pregnancy rate of 32.35% per patient and 13.58% per cycle in the TII group. There were 5 spontaneous pregnancies occurring in non-TII cycles, giving a spontaneous pregnancy rate of 7.35%. Among those who became pregnant, the average number of cycles per pregnancy was 2.5 (Table 7.15).

In the group with a cervical factor as the probable cause of infertility, there were 14 pregnancies, 13 of these after TII (50% per patient). There was only one spontaneous pregnancy, giving a pregnancy rate per patient of 3.84% (Table 7.16).

In patients with teratozoospermia there were 13 pregnancies, nine of which followed TII (21.95% per patient). Four pregnancies occurred spontaneously in non-TII cycles, giving a pregnancy rate of 9.75% per patient (Table 7.17). Among 10 patients with <10% normal sperm morphology, there was only one pregnancy (10% per patient). In 16 patients with a

Table 7.15.
Confirmed Pregnancies

Total number of patients	68
Total number of pregnancies	27
Pregnancies following TII	22 (32.35%)
Spontaneous pregnancies	5 (7.35%)
Pregnancy rate per cycle	13.58%
Average number of cycles per pregnancy	2.5

normal morphology of 10% to 14%, there were three pregnancies after TII (18.75% per patient) and two spontaneous pregnancies (12.5% per patient). In the 15 patients with a morphology of 15% to 20%, there were seven pregnancies; five followed TII (33.3% per patient), and two occurred spontaneously (13.3% per patient) (Table 7.18).

In the TII group there were no serious complications. A few patients complained of mild, transient lower abdominal cramping, which required no specific therapy.

Can Intrauterine Insemination Be Justified in Modern Practice?

TII is a controversial issue in the field of infertility. Many authorities believe that it has no therapeutic value (9). In the past, when one of the chief indications for TII was poor semen quality, TII with unwashed sperm failed to improve the chances of pregnancy (1). However, the improvement in sperm quality achieved by washing and swim-up may well increase the chance of pregnancy in teratozoospermic patients. Although our numbers are small, we have observed a tendency which suggests a cause-and-effect relationship (21.95% pregnancy rate in the TII group compared to 9.75% in the group becoming pregnant spontaneously).

In our institution, GIFT has also been used with some success in patients with abnormal sperm morphology. In a recent study, Van der Merwe obtained a 25.4% pregnancy rate per cycle in 118 cycles treated for teratozoospermia (see Chapter 6). We are optimistic that in the future TII may be offered as a valid alternative to patients with infertility due to abnormal sperm morphology. Because we have a considerable waiting

Table 7.16.
Analysis of Pregnancies in Patients with Poor Cervical Mucus

Total number of patients	26
Total number of pregnancies	14
Number of pregnancies following TII	13 (50%)
Spontaneous pregnancies	1 (3.84%)
Type of cycle resulting in pregnancy in TII group	
hMG stimulation	6
Clomiphene stimulation	3
Spontaneous	4
Number of cycles per pregnancy	2.75

Table 7.17.
Analysis of Pregnancies in Patients with Teratozoospermia (<20% Normal Sperm Morphology)

Total number of patients	41
Total number of pregnancies	13
Pregnancies following TII	9 (21.95%)
Spontaneous pregnancies	4 (9.75%)
Average number of TII cycles per pregnancy	2.4

list for the GIFT procedure, we schedule our teratozoospermic patients for two or three cycles of TII in the hope that they will become pregnant before a more invasive and costly procedure becomes necessary. If both these modalities fail, then donor insemination remains an alternative.

In patients with hostile cervical mucus, we believe that TII may be regarded as a valid option. Confino (15) reported a 68% pregnancy rate and Kirsch (12) a 75% rate in patients with a cervical factor. We consider our pregnancy rate of 50% as adequate and recommend that women with a cervical mucus problem undergo TII. The method is safe, minimally invasive, and has an acceptable success rate in this group.

One may speculate upon the reason for the increased pregnancy rate in these two groups of patients. The reason is probably a combination of factors. TII is timed to coincide with ovulation. The in vitro preparation of the sperm may enhance capacitation, which may improve the motility and the cervical mucus-penetrating ability of the sperm (16). Balmaceda (17) achieved an overall improvement of sperm motility from 51.7% to 85% and a pregnancy rate of 50%. TII may also allow a greater concentration of sperm to reach the fallopian tubes. This was demonstrated by Weathersbee (18), who showed that TII led to a 25% increase in peritoneal recovery of sperm compared to intracervical insemination.

Conclusion

Our numbers are small at present and should be viewed with caution. There is need for a controlled study, which we plan to begin soon. However, in the light of our experience and that of other authorities, we believe that TII has a place in the treatment

Table 7.18.
Pregnancies in Various Morphology Groups

Normal Morphology (%)	No. of Patients	No. of Pregnancies
<10	10	1
10–14	16	3 (following TII) 2 (spontaneous)
15–20	15	5 (following TII) 2 (spontaneous)

of infertile couples, on the waiting list for GIFT, who have hostile cervical mucus or abnormal sperm morphology. We also advocate GIFT as a therapeutic alternative to be used in conjunction with TII. As our numbers increase, it will become apparent whether or not this opinion is justified.

References

1. Beck WW Jr: Two hundred years of artificial insemination. Fertil Steril 41:193, 1984
2. Mishell DR Jr, Davajan V: Reproductive endocrinology, infertility, and contraception. Philadelphia: FA Davis, 1979, p 371
3. Glezerman M: Artificial homologous insemination in treatment of male infertility. In Bain J, Schill WB, Schwarzenstein L (eds): Treatment of Male Infertility. Berlin: Springer-Verlag, 1982, p 295
4. Barwin BN: Intrauterine insemination with husband's sperm. J Reprod Fertil 36:101, 1974
5. Nachtigall RD, Faure N, Glass RH: Artificial insemination of husband's sperm. Fertil Steril 32:141, 1979
6. Russel JK: Artificial insemination (husband) in management of childlessness. Lancet 2:1223, 1960
7. Swensen CE, Toth A, Toth C, Wolfgruber L, O'Leary WM: Asymptomatic bacteriospermia in infertile men. Andrologia 12:7, 1980
8. Stone SC, de la Maza LM, Peterson EM: Recovery of microorganisms from the pelvic cavity after intracervical or intrauterine artificial insemination. Fertil Steril 46:61, 1986
9. Hull ME, Magyar DM, Vasquez JM, Hayes MF, Moghissi KS: Experience with intrauterine insemination for cervical factor and oligospermia. Am J Obstet Gynecol 154:1333, 1986
10. Kerin JFP, Peek J, Warnes GM, Kirby C, Jeffrey R, Mathews CD: Improved conception rate after intrauterine insemination of washed spermatozoa from men with poor quality semen. Lancet 1:533, 1984
11. Mortimer D, Leslie DD, Kelly RW, Templeton AA: Morphological selection of human spermatozoa in vivo and in vitro. J Reprod Fertil 64:391, 1982
12. Kirsch SP, Scholer J, Servy SJ: Intrauterine insemination in infertility practice (Abstract). In: Program supplement, 41st Annual Meeting of the American Fertility Society, 1985, p 47
13. Kruger TF, Menkveld R, Stander FSH, Lombard CJ, Van der Merwe JP, van Zyl JA, Smith K: Sperm morphologic features as a prognostic factor in in vitro fertilization. Fertil Steril 46:1118, 1986
14. van Zyl JA: The role of the spermiogram with reference to infertility. (Doctoral Thesis). University of Stellenbosch, South Africa, 1975.
15. Confino E, Friberg J, Dudkiewicz AB, Gleicher N: Intrauterine inseminations with washed human spermatozoa. Fertil Steril 46:55, 1986
16. Sher G, Knutzen VK, Stratton CJ, Montakhab MM, Allenson SG: In vitro sperm capacitation and trans-cervical intrauterine insemination for the treatment of refractory infertility: phase I. Fertil Steril 41:260, 1984
17. Balmaceda JP, Schenken RS, Ellsworth LR: Intrauterine insemination with washed sperm as treatment of infertility. Fertil Steril 42:322, 1984
18. Weathersbee PS, Werlin LB, Stone SC: Peritoneal recovery of sperm after intrauterine insemination. Fertil Steril 42:322, 1984

CHAPTER 8

Evaluation and Preparation of Spermatozoa for Artificial Insemination by Donor

LUIS J. RODRIGUEZ-RIGAU, M.D.

Artificial—or therapeutic—insemination by volunteer donor (AID) has become a frequently used treatment for certain types of infertility, particularly severe male factor infertility. Each year in the United States an estimated 6,000 to 10,000 children are born by AID (1, 2). This chapter will review the clinical and technical aspects of AID, with emphasis on factors which affect the outcome. The selection and screening of donors will be discussed, particularly in light of the possible transmission of the human immunodeficiency virus (HIV). The legal, ethical, and social aspects of AID have been discussed elsewhere (3–7).

Indications for AID

Indications for AID in clinical practice include the following: (*a*) irreversible azoospermia or obstructive azoospermia where microsurgical repair is unwanted or impossible; (*b*) severe oligoasthenozoospermia which is untreatable or has not responded to treatment; (*c*) sexual dysfunction with total inability to ejaculate; (*d*) genetic or hereditary disorders; (*e*) previous exposure to radiation, chemotherapy, or toxic chemicals with fear of genetic consequences; (*f*) Rh incompatibility (severe Rh-isoimmunization, Rh-negative wife and Rh-positive husband); and (*g*) insemination of a single woman (acceptable at some centers).

Patient Evaluation

Selection and screening of donors for AID (1, 6, 8–10) involves four main aspects: (*a*) genetic screening; (*b*) screening for sexually transmitted infectious diseases; (*c*) fertility screening; and (*d*) proper matching of donor and recipients.

286

GENETIC SCREENING

An exhaustive medical and family history, as well as a physical examination, is the basis of identifying donors who may carry a risk for genetically transmitted disorders. While karyotypes are the definitive laboratory test, they are usually not obtained in many laboratories; in the Norfolk program, karyotyping has been established as mandatory. Prospective donors with a personal or family history for any non-trivial condition of possible genetic transmission are rejected (1, 6). Donors with a family history of a multifactorial disease (hypertension, diabetes, cancer, etc.) should not be matched with recipients who have a similar family history (1). Donors of certain ethnic groups require testing for specific conditions (sickle cell disease in blacks, Tay-Sachs disease in Ashkenazi Jews, thalassemia in Mediterranean populations, etc.).

SCREENING FOR SEXUALLY TRANSMITTED INFECTIOUS DISEASES

The initial screening involves a thorough personal, sexual, and medical history of prospective donors. Those at risk for acquired immune deficiency syndrome (AIDS) (homosexuals, bisexuals, those with multiple sexual partners, intravenous drug users, etc.) or other sexually transmitted diseases are rejected. If the history is totally negative, laboratory tests for HIV, syphilis, gonorrhea, chlamydia, hepatitis B, and cytomegalovirus (CMV) are performed. (Whether semen from CMV-positive donors is acceptable for CMV-positive recipients is a matter of controversy.) Some centers also test for *Mycoplasma hominis* and *Trichomonas vaginalis*. Donors are usually not tested for the herpes simplex virus, since the available tests lack sensitivity and specificity. Donors with a history of genital herpes (or donors whose sex partners have such a history) are usually rejected, although transmission of genital herpes by AID has not been demonstrated.

It is recommended that donors be rescreened, with laboratory retesting, at least every 6 months (6).

Until recently, some centers performed AID with fresh semen. However, fear of transmitting the HIV virus has abolished this practice. The knowledge that a donor could transmit the HIV virus for 3 months or more before he became seropositive has prompted such organizations as the American Fertility Society, the American Association of Tissue Banks, and the Centers for Disease Control to recommend the abandonment of the use of fresh semen for AID (9, 10). Most centers now perform AID exclusively with cryopreserved specimens which have been quarantined for at least 6 months, after which period the donors have been retested and found to be HIV-seronegative. Other centers have entirely ceased to perform AID because of the HIV risk.

FERTILITY SCREENING

Ideally, only donors of proven fertility should be accepted. All semen samples should be tested for sperm concentration, motility, and morphology. It is generally agreed that only samples with a post-thaw concentration of 30 to 50 $\times$ 10^6 motile sperm per milliliter should be used. Although minimum values for other parameters are not yet standardized, recent developments in the analysis of sperm motility now permit objective evaluation of directional motility and sperm velocity, and will allow these parameters to be incorporated into the screening of specimens to be used for AID.

PROPER MATCHING OF DONOR AND RECIPIENTS

The physical characteristics (height, body build, eye color, hair color and texture, complexion, etc.) and ethnic background of the donor should approach those of the husband as nearly as possible. Many centers also match blood groups. If optimal matching is impossible, AID may still be performed with the couple's consent.

Evaluation of the Couple

All couples desiring AID should undergo a complete evaluation prior to the initiation of treatment. This evaluation has several important goals:

1. Confirmation that AID is indicated (confirmation of the husband's irreversible infertility, confirmation of the wife's Rh-isoimmunization, etc.).
2. Medical and reproductive evaluation of the recipient: Detection of medical problems that would contraindicate pregnancy, detection of a familial history for disorders of multifactorial genetic origin (important in the selection of the donor; see above), and detection of reproductive disorders (e.g., uterine or tubal disease, ovulatory dysfunction). The thoroughness of the investigation of the recipient prior to initiation of AID varies among centers and is guided by the history of the patient.
3. Screening for sexually transmitted infectious diseases: Many centers screen both members of the couple with the same tests administered to the donor (HIV, gonorrhea, syphilis, chlamydia, hepatitis B, CMV, etc.).
4. Psychological screening: Some centers require psychological evaluation and counseling of all couples prior to the initiation of AID.

Preparation of the Semen and Insemination Techniques

When a fresh semen sample is to be used, although this is not recommended when performing AID, insemination should be performed within 2 hours of collection. When cryopreserved samples are used, insemination should be performed within 30 to 45 minutes of thawing. (The techniques of cryopreservation are discussed in Chapter 10.) Immediately before use, all samples should be examined to confirm adequate count, motility, morphology, absence of abundant white blood cells, etc.

The preferred insemination technique varies among centers and depends upon the circumstances of the recipients. A common technique involves intracervical injection of a small amount (0.1 to 0.3 ml) of semen, with placement of the remaining specimen against the cervical os and mucus, using a cervical cup or the speculum. Some centers omit intracervical injection and perform only paracervical insemination, with similar results. Contact of semen and cervical mucus for 30 minutes is usually sufficient. A test for sperm survival in the cervical mucus should be performed 12 to 24 hours after insemination in a patient not achieving pregnancy after several AID attempts, and in all subsequent attempts, to rule out hostile or incompatible cervical mucus.

Recently developed techniques of sperm preparation for therapeutic intrauterine insemination (TII) (see Chapter 7) can also be used for AID. Although TII is the preferred technique in recipients with a cervical factor (absent or inadequate cervical mucus, cervical stenosis, etc.), there is no indication that TII using donor semen produces better results than other techniques in recipients without a cervical factor and with good post-insemination sperm survival. Therefore, routine use of TII for AID is not justified at present.

Donor semen is sometimes used for in vitro fertilization, gamete intrafallopian transfer, intraperitoneal insemination, etc. The preparation of specimens for these procedures is discussed in Chapters 5, 6, and 9.

Results of AID

Many factors influence the results of AID, with pregnancy rates varying from 40% to 80% (11–13). It is difficult to compare these reports because of differences in recipient populations and in techniques. Curie-Cohen (12), in a survey of physicians in the United States who perform AID, found a highly significant correlation ($P<0.001$) between success rate and the size of the physician's practice: larger practices had higher pregnancy rates. Experience thus seems to be an important factor. For this reason—and to avoid controversy—the rest of this chapter will present the results of AID from the experience of the author and his colleagues.

The Texas Institute for Reproductive Medicine and Endocrinology is one of the few centers that have performed AID for many years with both fresh and cryopreserved semen, permitting comparison between similar populations of recipients. We have periodically analyzed and published our results (14–18).

INFLUENCE OF THE MALE FACTOR ON THE SUCCESS OF AID

We have studied the possible relationship between sperm output of the husband and the success rate of AID. The crude pregnancy rate for recipients with azoospermic husbands was 73%, not significantly different from the 71% pregnancy when the husbands' sperm count was $<10 \times 10^6$/ml. However, recipients whose husbands had a sperm count $>10 \times 10^6$/ml had a significantly lower pregnancy rate (54%) with AID, a rate not significantly different from the 53% pregnancy rate observed in the author's practice when no AID was performed and the female was treated. Other authors have published similar findings (19, 20). These data suggest that a female factor should be suspected in cases of moderate or mild oligospermia. AID should not be performed until the woman has undergone a thorough evaluation and until any disturbances which could be influencing her fertility potential have been treated for a sufficient time.

INFLUENCE OF FEMALE FACTORS ON THE SUCCESS OF AID

We have detected a 7% incidence of bilateral tubal obstruction in women referred to us for AID, with a higher incidence of other pelvic disorders such as endometriosis, pelvic adhesions, and unilateral tubal disease. Ovulatory dysfunction is even more common. We use a strict definition for normal ovulatory function (follicular phase, 14 ± 2 days; luteal phase, 14 ± 1 day), and we treat any patient who deviates from this norm. Over 50% of our AID recipients are thus treated.

Ovulatory dysfunction has a significant influence on the results of AID (15, 17). In patients with normal ovulation, our pregnancy rate was 84%, and an average of 2.9 cycles was required for pregnancy to occur. In recipients treated for ovulatory dysfunction, the pregnancy rate was 62% in an average of 5.2 cycles. The overall pregnancy rate was 72% in an average of 4.1 cycles. With normal ovulation, over 70% of the pregnan-

Table 8.1.
Comparison of AID Results with Fresh and Cryopreserved Semen in Patients with Normal and Abnormal Ovulation

	Pregnancy Rate (%)	Average No. of Cycles
Normal ovulation		
Fresh semen	88	1.9
Frozen semen	69	3.4
Abnormal ovulation		
Fresh semen	81	4.2
Frozen semen	49	9.3

cies occurred within three cycles of insemination, while the rate was over 70% in an average of five cycles for recipients with ovulatory dysfunction.

Our management of ovulatory dysfunction seems to have improved over the years. Before 1971, the average time required to achieve pregnancy in AID cases with ovulatory dysfunction was 8.8 cycles for a 51% pregnancy rate. Since 1971, the average time for these cases has been 3.4 cycles for a rate of 70%. It appears that treatment of even minor ovulatory disturbances, which might be of little significance in non-AID patients, improves the success of AID patients.

COMPARISON OF AID RESULTS WITH FRESH AND CRYOPRESERVED SEMEN

In our experience, pregnancy rates are slightly higher when AID is performed with fresh semen (76% with fresh, 64% with frozen). In addition, the time required for pregnancy to occur with fresh semen (2.8 cycles) is less than half that required with frozen semen (6.3 cycles). This difference is magnified when the influence of ovulatory dysfunction is also analyzed (Table 8.1). Thus, the use of frozen semen for AID delays the occurence of pregnancy, particularly in recipients with ovulatory dysfunction. Since we performed the inseminations every other day (as opposed to daily) until ovulation, we were interested in analyzing whether the timing of the insemination could be responsible for the differences in results with fresh and frozen semen. A review of the timing of insemination in conception cycles demonstrated that with fresh semen, an insemination was performed on the presumed day of ovulation (day 0) in 43.5% and on the day before (day −1) in 37.0%. With frozen semen, an insemination was performed on day 0 in 66.7% and on day −1 in only 6.7%. Thus it seems plausible that there were significant differences in the survival of fresh and cryopreserved sperm in the female reproductive tract, and timing the inseminations may take on greater importance when cryopreserved semen is used for AID. In patients with ovulatory dysfunction, where precise timing of ovulation is more difficult, daily insemination may be necessary when cryopreserved semen is used.

OUTCOME OF AID PREGNANCIES

When we compared matched AID and non-AID populations of infertile patients in our practice, we found similar rates of spontaneous abortion and multiple pregnancies. The duration of the pregnancies and the infant birth weights were also similar. A slight but significant increase in the male:female ratio of AID offspring was noted. The inci-

dence of congenital abnormalities was extremely low, no higher than in the non-AID infertile group or in the general population. No differences in outcome were found in a comparison of pregnancies initiated with fresh and with cryopreserved semen. However, recipients with treated ovulatory dysfunction had higher incidences of spontaneous abortion and of twins. This is not surprising, since most of these patients received clomiphene citrate or gonadotropins for ovulation induction.

References

1. Timmons MC, Rao KW, Sloan CS, Kirkman HN, Talbot LM: Genetic screening of donors for artificial insemination. Fertil Steril 35:451, 1981
2. Stone SC: Complications and pitfalls of artificial insemination. Clin Obstet Gynecol 23:667, 1980
3. Beck WW: A critical look at the legal, ethical and technical aspects of artificial insemination. Fertil Steril 27:1, 1976
4. David G, Price WS (eds): Human Artificial Insemination and Semen Preservation. New York: Plenum, 1980
5. American Fertility Society: Ethical considerations of the new reproductive technologies. Fertil Steril 46 (Suppl 1), 1986
6. American Fertility Society: New guidelines for the use of semen-donor insemination: 1986. Fertil Steril 46 (Suppl 2), 1986
7. American Fertility Society: Ethical considerations of the new reproductive technologies. Fertil Steril 49 (Suppl 1), 1988
8. Mascola L, Guinan ME: Screening to reduce transmission of sexually transmitted diseases in semen used for artificial insemination. N Engl J Med 314:1354, 1986
9. American Fertility Society: Revised new guidelines for the use of semen-donor insemination. Fertil Steril 49:211, 1988
10. Centers for Disease Control, Atlanta: Semen banking, organ and tissue transplantation, and HIV antibody testing. JAMA 259:1301, 1988
11. Koren Z, Lieberman R: Fifteen years experience with artificial insemination. Int J Fertil 21:119, 1976
12. Curie-Cohen M, Luttrell L, Shapiro S: Current practice of artificial insemination by donor in the United States. New Engl J Med 300:585, 1979
13. Hammond MG, Jordan S, Sloan CS: Factors affecting pregnancy rates in a donor insemination program using frozen semen. Am J Obstet Gynecol 155:480, 1986
14. Steinberger E, Smith KD: Artificial insemination with fresh or frozen semen: a comparative study, JAMA 223:778, 1973
15. Steinberger E, Rodriguez-Rigau LJ, Smith KD: The female factor in AID. In David G, Price WS (eds): Human Artificial Insemination and Semen Preservation. New York: Plenum, 1980, p 301
16. Steinberger E, Rodriguez-Rigau LJ, Smith KD: Comparison of results of AID with fresh and frozen semen. In David G, Price WS (eds): Human Artificial Insemination and Semen Preservation. New York: Plenum, 1980, p 283
17. Smith KD, Rodriguez-Rigau LJ, Steinberger E: The influence of ovulatory dysfunction and timing of insemination on the success rate of artificial insemination donor (AID) with fresh or cryopreserved semen. Fertil Steril 36:496, 1981
18. Smith KD, Rodriguez-Rigau LJ: The infertile couple. J Androl 4:111, 1983
19. Formigli L, Formigli G, Gottardi L: Artificial insemination by donor results in relation to husband's semen. Arch Androl 14:209, 1985
20. Alfredson JH: Success of donor insemination and male diagnosis. Acta Obstet Gynecol Scand 66:43, 1987

CHAPTER 9

Evaluation and Preparation of Spermatozoa for Direct Intraperitoneal Insemination

AGNES MENARD, M.D., CHRISTIANE WITTEMER, PH.D., LAURENCE MOREAU, M.D., AND PIERRE DELLENBACH, M.D.

The complex and selective migration of sperm throughout the female reproductive tract constitutes a true odyssey. Motility of the sperm as well as cervical, uterine, and tubal secretions are involved in this process. Only a small number of sperm actually reach the area of fertilization. Indeed, the probability of pregnancy is very low in the case of oligospermia or cervical mucus abnormalities, or in certain instances of unexplained infertility. Motile sperm can be found in the peritoneal fluid (PF) of the pouch of Douglas (1, 2). This criterion enabled Templeton to evaluate the prognosis of certain cases of unexplained infertility (3, 4). The prognosis was considered positive if motile sperm were found in the tubal ampulla or in PF, which can be considered the physiological environment of the fallopian tube and the ovary during ovulation.

In 1986 our team suggested that the direct supply of capacitated sperm to PF during ovulation could bypass certain obstacles inhibiting fertilization and could thus provide a useful treatment for certain cases of infertility (5). We suggested that this technique be named direct intraperitoneal insemination (DIPI) (6). This terminology has since been widely adopted. DIPI can be defined as the direct insemination of prepared sperm in PF during ovulation (7). Those working on this technique have greatly benefited from the progress made during the last decade in the fields of sperm preparation and programmed and timed induction of ovulation. The difficult passage of the sperm throughout the female genital tract is avoided through insemination in the pouch of Douglas. Bringing together of the sperm and the oocyte is possible through the motility of the male gamete and the transport of PF from the pouch of Douglas toward the fallopian tube and the uterine cavity.

An experiment first done by Conill Serra (8) and later by Pauerstein (9) attests to the existence of these movements of PF. China ink or radioactive particles injected into the pouch of Douglas were found in the cervix. They had migrated from the fallopian tube toward the uterus and vaginal cavity. The existence of these fluid movements is one of the reasons why the use of DIPI is justified. If the fallopian tubes function properly, after fertilization the egg will be carried to the uterine cavity.

The present study outlines the basis of this new infertility treatment. In the first part, a short summary of up-to-date information on the physiological and physiopathological aspects of PF is given. The second part deals with an analysis of techniques. The third part focuses on the results obtained and includes a discussion of these results.

Physiology of Peritoneal Fluid and Its Role in Reproduction

Claude Bernard was the first person to be interested in the "inner environment" of the human body. As early as 1850, he made the hypothesis that this inner environment was necessary for the development of organic beings. In accordance with his supposition, he suggested inseminating dogs or rabbits by injecting sperm into the peritoneal cavity near the ovaries. Work done by Novak in 1922 (10) proved the existence of "physiological ascites" in the peritoneum of the female. Variations in the volume of PF during the menstrual cycle were pointed out by Bissel in 1932 (11) and Rizzuti in 1950 (12). At about the same time, other authors—Decker (13) and Doyle (14, 15)—described the peristaltic movements of the fallopian tube. According to them, these movements suck in the oocyte, which is released when the follicle ruptures. Rubenstein (16), Horne (17), Ahlgren (1), and Templeton (4) studied the presence of motile sperm in PF, pointing out that they are still present a few hours after natural intercourse. Clear indication of sperm migration from the pouch of Douglas to the fallopian tube was shown by Settlage in 1973 (18). Since the beginning of this decade, Belgian and Dutch teams—Maathuis (19, 20) and Koninckx (21)—have devoted much time and work to the study of PF biochemistry. Numerous authors have recently been interested in the physiopathological aspects of PF, especially in cases of endometriosis (22–30).

PHYSIOLOGY AND PHYSIOPATHOLOGY

Origin

Present theory describes PF as an exudate of the active ovary. However, its true origin is a much debated question (19, 31, 32).

Volume

The volume of PF fluctuates greatly throughout the menstrual cycle (20, 31, 33, 34). During the follicular phase it increases progressively and reaches its maximum (approximately 20 ml) during the post-ovulation period (Fig. 9.1). After maintaining a certain level for 10 days, it suddenly drops when menstruation begins. Ovarian function explains these cyclic variations, which are dependent upon follicular activity, vascularization of the corpus luteum, and hormonal production. The volume of PF is very low (approximately 2 ml) in women who do not ovulate, who take oral contraceptives, or who have gone through menopause (31). In the case of endometriosis and in spite of contradictory opinions—Syrop (35), Mudge (36), Rock (37), Olive (38), and Drake (39)—the volume generally seems higher during the entire cycle.

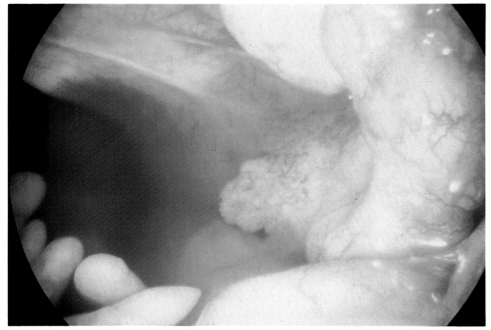

Figure 9.1. Laparoscopic view of the cul-de-sac at ovulation, documenting the presence of peritoneal fluid and a normal tube.

Biochemistry

The biochemistry of PF is complex, and the most recent experiments focus mainly on proteins and hormones. The distribution of proteins in PF is the same as in serum except that the percentage is lower (35% to 60%) (19–21). Identical variations are observed in PF and in uterine (40) and tubal secretions (41). These might be due to estrogens which influence vascular permeability (32). From a qualitative point of view, the most important proteins are the α- and β-globulins, antitrypsin, the C3 and C4 proteins, and albumin (5, 19, 42) which could play an important role in the phenomenon of capacitation (43).

The main hormones are present in PF. Results pertaining to follicle-stimulating hormone (FSH), luteinizing hormone (LH), and prolactin are still incomplete (21, 31, 44, 45). However, much work has been done on steroid hormones: 17β-estradiol (E$_2$) and progesterone (P) (21, 31, 44, 46). The amount of E$_2$ varies during the cycle. There is an equal amount in the serum and PF during the follicular phase. After ovulation and until the 26th day of the cycle, there is a significant increase of E$_2$ in PF (19, 20). The amount of P increases greatly in PF during the luteal phase, marking follicular rupture (34, 47–49). The amount is lower in the case of luteinized unruptured follicle syndrome. The same phenomenon can be observed in the case of extensive adhesions (34). In a mild case of endometriosis, the levels of steroid hormones E$_2$ and P are normal, but in the case of severe endometriosis the levels decrease (23, 48).

The concentrations of electrolytes found in PF are the same as those found in plasma and remain almost constant during the cycle (21). This is different from what happens in the uterine (40), tubal (41), and follicular (50) fluids. There the concentration of potassium increases during ovulation, thus favoring sperm capacitation (40).

Various other substances can be found in PF. In pelvic inflammatory disease, protein markers such as seromucoid a1, immunoglobulin M (28, 42), and prostaglandins (30, 51, 52) can be found. Thromboxane B2 and 6-ketoprostaglandin $F_{2-\alpha}$ and $F_{1-\alpha}$ are present in endometriosis (25, 39, 53).

Cytology

Numerous cells are found in PF (26, 35, 54): mesothelial cells, lymphocytes, histiocytes, monocytes, "menstrual detritus," and macrophages, the latter being predominant (85%) (55). Macrophages have multiple physiological functions which may be modified by pathological conditions (53, 56). They will phagocytize cellular debris, sperm, and red blood corpuscles (35, 57). They have a luteotropic function furthering the development of the corpus luteum and stimulating production of P by the oocyte cumulus complex (58, 59). When endometriosis is present, the phagocytic and cytotoxic potency of the macrophages in relation to the sperm is said to increase (53, 56). The production of fatty acids and prostaglandins which immobilize sperm is enhanced (39, 60). Antisperm antibodies activate the macrophages and, in doing so, facilitate sperm destruction (55, 61). An endometrial cellular reflux through the tubes is apparent not only in the physiological circumstances but also after uterine lavage (62, 63). There are few endometrial cells in the ase of tubal obstruction (64).

ROLE OF PERITONEAL FLUID IN REPRODUCTION

The complex role played by the peritoneal compartment during reproduction, whether it be in the transfer and survival of gametes or in fertilization, is for the most part misunderstood. The most recent studies have been devoted mainly to the analysis of pathological conditions and, in particular, to peritoneal endometriosis. Indeed, in the latter case, sperm are rapidly immobilized and phagocytized (57). In his experiments, Oak (65) shows that there is a significant immobilization of test sperm put into the PF of women with endometriosis. It can be hypothesized that the PF of these women contains a toxic immobilizing factor. According to Suginami (29), a peritoneal toxic factor present in endometriosis could inhibit the capture of the oocyte by the fimbria of the tube. Other experiments have led to results which contradict the aforementioned. In fact, the sperm penetration of hamster ova was not modified when macrophages extracted from the PF of women with endometriosis were added (58, 60). A negative aspect in the process of fertilization should also be considered, since the macrophages could secrete interleukin-1, which has a harmful effect on embryonic cleavage and development (66). In the mouse, cleavage of the two-blastomere embryo is inhibited by a factor also present in the PF of women with endometriosis (67). The ciliary and muscular activity of the tube could also be modified by prostaglandins in PF (30, 35). The increase in their concentration could thus affect the transport of sperm and the pickup of the oocyte (29, 30). These different experiments suggest that certain cases of subfertility or infertility, not due to any significant changes of pelvic anatomy, could be secondary to changes to the composition of the PF, thereby upsetting the balance in the complex interaction pertaining to fertilization.

Sperm-PF Interaction

The most advanced studies of the biochemistry of PF have certainly yielded extremely valuable information concerning some physiopathological aspects of infertility and have led to some positive conclusions.

These, however, belong to the field of research and cannot be applied to everyday medical practice. The previously mentioned Templeton test is, in fact, very difficult to carry out (4). With this in mind, we felt, as have other teams involved in this field (3, 4), that it would be useful to study the interactions between PF and sperm. This would enable us to decide which patients or couples would be eligible for DIPI. Before doing so, however, a simple way to collect a sample of PF from an outpatient had to be perfected. In most of the scientific work already done in the physiology and physiopathology of PF, it was aspirated at laparoscopy, directly under visual control, through a catheter or a long needle in the pouch of Douglas. The volume of PF can then be measured, and the aspect of the peritoneum can be assessed. It is also possible to determine whether the tubes are patent, whether there are any follicles in the ovaries, or if a stigma is present. Taking a sample of PF at laparoscopy is still a worthwhile procedure and may be done in an infertility patient if the procedure is performed during the periovulation period. The major inconvenience of this procedure is that it cannot be easily repeated. It would be most useful if, on a regular basis, a simple transvaginal puncture of the pouch of Douglas or culdocentesis could be done instead.

Actually, culdocentesis can be done by a simplified technique. It does not require any pre-medication or anesthetic and can be performed on an outpatient basis. Wiegerinck (68) proposed an interesting apparatus named ''Cupido System.'' Unfortunately, it is expensive and therefore not commonly used. In fact, culdocentesis can be performed very easily by using a thin Butterfly G19 needle, 22.2 mm in length and 1.1 mm in outer diamter (Venisystems, Abbott Ireland, Ltd., Sligo, Republic of Ireland), which is inserted with a forceps. The posterior vaginal fornix is punctured 1 cm behind the cervix, and the needle usually penetrates into the pouch of Douglas without any problem. PF flows back into the tube, and several milliliters can be collected in a sterile culture dish (Falcon 3001, Becton Dickinson Labware, Oxnard, Calif.) or can be withdrawn via gentle aspiration with a syringe. After being centrifuged, the sample of PF (3 to 20 ml) is put into 1.5-ml sterile micro-centrifuge test tubes (Treff, AG, Degersheim, Switzerland). The test tubes are then marked and frozen until needed for biological purposes. The sperm-PF interaction studies are usually done at a later date convenient for the spouse. Several studies accomplished by our team (5, 69) have provided the basis for a sperm-PF migration test (PFMT), which focuses on the interaction between sperm and PF. These studies are briefly summarized.

Survival of a Test Sperm in Different Peritoneal Fluids

Sampling of PF was done in this series at laparoscopy in 36 patients evaluated for infertility. Laparoscopy was performed as close as possible to the periovulation period. All important information about the etiological factors of infertility, the average number of days of the cycle, and the date of the patient's last menstrual cycle were recorded. Before surgery, the morphology of the ovary was determined by ultrasound. Ovarian activity was evaluated by measuring 17β-E_2 and LH plasma levels. The same determinations were done in the PF. Preparation of the sperm was done with the following protocol: Several ejaculates obtained from the same donor were used and verified as having the same characteristics. After liquefaction, adequate samples of sperm were divided in test tubes, and sperm were washed twice with 4 ml of Ham's F-10 (Gibco) added to each tube. Centrifugation was performed for 10 minutes at 500 × g and the supernatant discarded. One milliter of each sample of frozen PF was thawed until it reached room temperature and was added to each sample of sperm. One of the tubes was used as culture medium control: 1 ml of Ham's F-10 solution containing 20% calf serum.

After the addition of 1% of an antibiotic solution (10,000 IU of penicillin, 10 mg of streptomycin, and 25 mg of amphotericin B per milliliter; Gibco), the tubes were kept in an incubator (37°C, 5% CO_2 in air). Survival of sperm in PF was evaluated after 1, 24, 48, 72, 96, 120, and 144 hours in the incubator. The life span of the sperm varied by more than 144 hours in four samples; by more than 5 days in eight samples (21.6%); by more than 4 days in 11 samples (23.7%); by more than 48 hours in 22 samples (59.5%), and by more than 24 hours in 29 samples (78.4%). In one sample, all sperm were immotile after 1 hour. Results are given in Figure 9.2. This preliminary study shows that sperm may survive for several days in PF, whereas in the Ham's F-10 + serum test environment, there were hardly any motile sperm left after 48 hours. There is a close correlation between the moment when PF is collected and the survival of sperm. In fact, type 4 motility (direct transport and rapid sperm progression) is significantly more frequent in PF taken during ovulation than in PF withdrawn 48 hours later. The same experiment with the same results has been done on PF collected via culdocentesis when ovulation took place. This led us to propose the PFMT, which has now been standardized.

Sperm-Peritoneal Fluid Migration Test (PFMT)

Use of the PFMT is suggested in cases of unexplained infertility, as well as in cases where DIPI is being considered. The purpose of this test is to compare the survival and capacitation of sperm in PF and in a test environment (Menezo B2 now replaces Ham's F-10 + serum used in the first experiments). The procedure is as follows: a fresh ejaculate is obtained, using a proper receptacle (Prodimed, Neuilly-en-Thelle, France) and allowed to liquefy at room temperature. Two aliquots of 1 ml are taken and washed twice by centrifugation in 4 ml of Ham's F-10 (500 × g for 10 minutes). The supernatant is discarded, and the two pellets are respectively suspended in 1 ml of Menezo B2 medium (API-System S.A., La Balme les Grottes, Montalieu-Vercheu, France) and 1 ml of PF. The PF, previously obtained via culdocentesis, is kept frozen at −20°C after centrifugation. Before the experiment begins, the PF is thawed at room temperature. Both specimens are incubated in a 5% CO_2 environment at 37°C for 20 minutes. The motile sperm which have migrated into the PF and the culture medium are aspirated with a pipette in the supernatant and counted in a Makler chamber. In order to determine sperm survival in both environments, the following protocol has been adopted. Two samples of the supernatant (usually about 200 microliters) are aspirated with a pipette so that an average of 50,000 sperm can be placed in a droplet of PF or culture medium. These are placed in a sterile culture dish (Falcon 3001) covered with siliconate oil (200 fluid 50 CS; Dow-Corning, Belgium) and conserved in the incubator. Motility is repeatedly observed by microscope after 1, 3, 6, and 24 hours. When at least 5% of the sperm are motile (type 4 motility) after 24 hours of incubation, the test is considered positive. In most cases, survival is higher in PF than in the reference environment. If the test is negative, the same procedure is performed with a control sample of sperm so that the intrinsic quality of PF can be appreciated. The PFMT has been administered in 130

NUMBER OF PERITONEAL FLUIDS

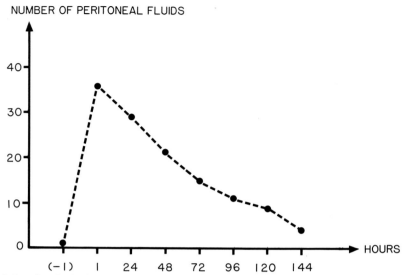

Figure 9.2.   Survival of sperm from one sample in 37 different peritoneal fluids. The number of motile sperm in peritoneal fluids after 1, 24, 48, 72, 96, 120, and 144 hours.

infertility cases (69). The volume of the PF sample collected each time during ovulation through culdocentesis was 1.5 to 30 ml (mean, 9 ml). Sperm survival and capacitation in PF was found in the majority of cases. The results are given in Figure 9.3. One hour after incubation, 10% or more of the sperm were observed with type 4 motility in 110 of 130 PF samples. A phenomenon of "late capacitation" was observed, and after 6 hours the figure changed to 124 of 130. A connection between the results obtained from this PFMT and the probability of pregnancy after DIPI can be made. This will be treated later in the discussion.

Direct Intraperitoneal Insemination (DIPI): Indications, Technique, and Results

DIPI as a new treatment of unexplained or cervical factor infertility was first proposed in April 1986 (6). Since that date, the main principles of the method have basically remained the same. First of all, a careful study of the etiology of the infertility is done, followed by a PFMT. The principle of DIPI having been accepted, the patient then undergoes a timed induction of ovulation. The prepared and capacitated sperm are inseminated 35 hours after human chorionic gonadotropin (hCG) has been administered. The stages of our present procedure are reported here.

INDICATIONS AND PRELIMINARY EXAMINATION

In order to best estimate the potential value of the method, our team enlarged the scope of indications during a set period of time. This helped distinguish which indications were optimal. In our present opinion, DIPI is not a first-line treatment of sterility and should therefore be proposed only in certain cases, such as cervical infertility, some cases of male subfertility and long-term unexplained infertility, and in cases of no success with traditional treatments. The criteria which determine whether a patient is eligible

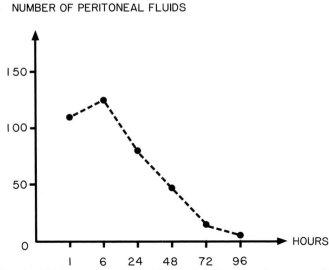

NUMBER OF PERITONEAL FLUIDS

Figure 9.3.   Results of 130 sperm-peritoneal fluid migration tests. Long-term (24-hour) survival of capacitated sperm was noted in 80 of 130 peritoneal fluids.

for DIPI are the same as for gamete intrafallopian transfer (GIFT) (70). DIPI is not done without first performing numerous and extensive tests which take into consideration the various etiologies of infertility. Before being accepted for treatment, the female patient must first undergo a pelvic examination and almost without exception must also have had laparoscopy and hysterosalpingography. Patients who have a documented history of pelvic infection or tubal pathology and/or surgery should be rejected. The cases of extrauterine pregnancy in our series are retrospectively explained by inadequate preliminary screening. All female patients and their spouses are subjected to extensive bacteriological tests (cervico-vaginal cultures, repeated sperm cultures) and tests to detect syphilis, *Chlamydia trachomatis*, or *Ureaplasma urealyticum* infection, or acquired immune deficiency syndrome (AIDS).

Diagnosis of cervical infertility was accepted after repeated examination of cervical mucus, based on the now accepted standards, with repeated poor or negative postcoital tests, even if the patient was treated with estrogen. Two types of defective cervical mucus are recognized: quantitative insufficiencies, which are characterized by a small volume; and qualitative insufficiencies, which are defined by an acid pH, inadequate penetration, and poor migration and survival of test sperm as well as husband's sperm.

The diagnosis of male subfertility is made according to the following criteria:

1. Oligozoospermia: sperm concentration per milliliter: $<20 \times 10^6$;
2. Asthenozoospermia: percentage of total sperm motility $<40\%$ after 1 hour;
3. Teratozoospermia: percentage of normal shapes $<40\%$.

The diagnosis of unexplained infertility is made when no pathology is detected after rigorous and complete examinations. Before trying DIPI, all couples were subjected to various medical treatments which included repeated traditional ovulation stimulation. A few patients who had had artificial insemination with a sperm donor were accepted. There was no positive result because the number of sperm in the pellets is usually small, and DIPI with donor sperm is no longer considered acceptable.

TECHNIQUE

Ovulation Induction Strategy

DIPI has never been attempted during a spontaneous cycle, and in all cases ovulation has been induced and timed using procedures improved for in vitro fertilization (71). The risk of multiple pregnancy is certainly one of the possible dangers inherent in the method, but several factors exist which favor this therapeutic strategy. Ovulation can be timed and insemination done at what appears to be the best time (inseminations in our experiments were done 35 to 36 hours after hCG).

Stimulation improves the peritoneal environment by increasing PF volume and its concentrations of E_2 and P. In the first attempts (72), traditional protocols with clomiphene and/or human menopausal gonadotropin (hMG) + hCG were used. These protocols have been perfected with better knowledge of ovarian response, and luteinizing hormone-releasing hormone (LH-RH) analogs are used when deemed necessary. Table 9.1 presents a summary of the nature and quality of stimulation methods used in a series of 124 cases analyzed in this paper.

Sperm Preparation

Sperm is collected in a graduated sterile receptacle (Prodimed) and allowed to liquefy for 30 minutes at room temperature. The following characteristics are then evaluated: volume, pH, number of round cells, total concentration of sperm (10^6/ml of semen), percentage of type 4 motile sperm, sperm with less motility, and immotile sperm. One milliliter of sperm is washed and centrifuged for 10 minutes at 500 $\times$ g with 4 ml of Ham's F-10, and the supernatant is discarded. Three milliliters of Menezo B2 (API-System) medium are then gently pipetted onto the pelleted sperm (while avoiding resuspension of the sperm) and incubated for 1 hour at 37°C (5% CO_2 in air). These manipulations are done with sterile graduated serologic pipettes in a laminar air-flow cabinet. The number of capacitated sperm in the supernatant are counted in a Makler chamber. Two hundred microliters are aspirated in a sterile dish (Falcon 3001), covered with siliconate oil (200 fluid 50 CS), and stored in the incubator for 24 hours (37°C; 5% CO_2 in air) so that sperm survival can be verified. The remaining part of the prepared specimen (approximately 3 ml; the capacitated sperm suspended in the Menezo B2 medium) is aspirated with a sterile syringe before insemination.

Insemination

DIPI can be performed on an outpatient basis. A speculum is inserted which exposes the posterior vaginal fornix. After careful disinfection, the pouch of Douglas is punctured with a thin, short needle (Butterfly G19; Venisystem, Abbott Ireland) held by a forceps. Puncture of the vaginal wall and the peritoneum is made by inserting the needle with a quick movement. Once it is in place, PF flows out spontaneously into the catheter. This reflux is a prerequisite to insemination. The culture medium containing the capacitated sperm is then injected. The patient may then return home as soon as the insemination has been completed. If on the following day an ultrasound examination reveals that follicular rupture has not taken place, a second sperm sample may be taken and inseminated. No other treatment is administered after DIPI. If the patient misses her period, pregnancy is diagnosed by determining β-hCG concentration in plasma and is later confirmed by ultrasound. The follow-up is of a traditional nature.

Table 9.1.
Number of Pregnancies in Response to Different Ovulation Induction Protocols

| | | Treatments | | |
| | | LHRH Analog | | |
	Clomiphene	Long Protocol	Short Protocol	hMG-hCG
Cycles[a]	176	29	11	5
Pregnancies	18	4	1	1

[a]221 cycle treatments for 124 couples.

RESULTS

The results presented here correspond to the total number of cases of infertility treated with DIPI between September 1985 and December 1987. Figure 9.4 summarizes the indications and the results. One hundred and twenty-four infertile couples were treated with one or several DIPIs. The etiological characteristics of the patients can be classified as follows: 19 cases of pure cervical infertility, 54 cases of cervical infertility associated with male subfertility, and 27 cases of infertility due predominantly to male subfertility. In three of the latter 27 cases, immunological infertility was also present. In the remaining 24 of 124 cases, the infertility was unexplained.

Overall Results: Pregnancies

Twenty-four pregnancies have been obtained with DIPI; five were miscarriages and two were extrauterine pregnancies. Among the pregnancies which lasted longer than 3 months, there were 13 single pregnancies, three twin pregnancies, and one triple pregnancy; 19.3% pregnancies per patient and 12% pregnancies per insemination cycle were obtained. These results should be analyzed in relation to the indications.

Analysis of the Results

Fourteen pregnancies were obtained in cases of associated cervical and male infertility, three pregnancies in cases of male subfertility (one of which was a case of immunological infertility), and two pregnancies in cases of unexplained infertility (Fig. 9.4). These results suggest that the best indication for DIPI is cervical infertility or cervical infertility associated with male subfertility.

DIPI and Sperm Quality

The important role played by the number and quality of inseminated sperm was assessed in a prospective series of cases treated in 1987. DIPI has been used on 71 couples who had a total of 123 inseminations. Figure 9.5 gives the main information about the number of inseminated sperm, which averaged 8×10^6. In 75% of the cases, $<30 \times 10^6$ sperm were deposited in the pouch of Douglas. No pregnancy ensued when $<1 \times 10^6$ sperm were used. The optimal number was about 10×10^6. Probability of pregnancy depended largely on the initial sperm motility (73). It varied considerably, from 10% to 80%. Figure 9.6 shows the qualitative categories of the sperm. In the majority of cases, initial motility was 30% or greater. If the motility was lower than 25% in fresh sperm, the patient did not become pregnant. Although these figures are too small, they nevertheless show that a high initial motility factor might be instrumental in obtaining a successful outcome. This study has proven that oligoasthenoteratozoospermia

NUMBER OF INSEMINATIONS

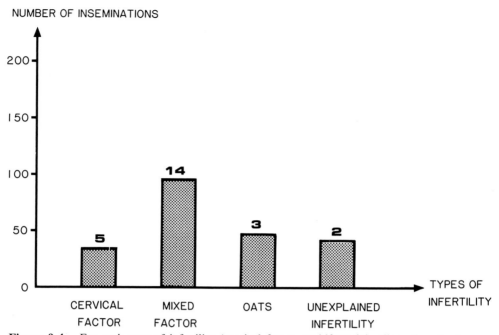

Figure 9.4. For each type of infertility (cervical factor, multifactorial, oligoasthenoteratozoo-spermia, and unexplained), the columns indicate the number of inseminations performed and the number of pregnancies obtained.

NUMBER OF INSEMINATIONS

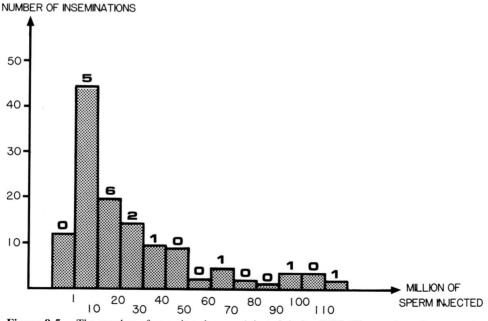

Figure 9.5. The number of capacitated sperm injected during DIPI. The number of pregnancies obtained in each class is at the top of the column. Results were obtained in 1987.

(OATS), a symptom of conjugal subfertility, should not be treated by intraperitoneal insemination.

Value of the Peritoneal Fluid Migration Test (PFMT) versus Sims-Hühner's Postcoital Test

The postcoital test is an essential part of any infertility check-up. The result of this test depends on two factors: the quality of cervical mucus and the quality of the sperm. This test is very valuable in predicting the patient's chances of becoming pregnant. If cervical mucus insufficiency exists without improvement after an estrogen treatment or ovulation stimulation, the test either cannot be done or loses it value. The PFMT can then be proposed. Our team also felt that it would be useful to study patients who had sufficient cervical mucus but who were infertile for apparently unexplained reasons. Results obtained from the Sims-Hühner test and from the PFMT (Table 9.2) were compared with the semen analysis, and correlations were poor. Sperm can be found in PF in some cases of severe OATS. PF can be of good quality in cases of qualitative or quantitative cervical mucus insufficiency. Inversely, in some cases the sperm and postcoital tests are good, but PFMT is negative. This hostility of the peritoneal environment could explain certain cases of unexplained infertility. No pregnancy ever resulted from DIPI in this situation. These patients probably need to be treated by in vitro fertilization, as Pampiglione (74) has shown that the results of DIPI may be correlated to the quality of PF. It is important to underline the fact that PFMT is a valuable means of determining whether DIPI will be successful or not. If the results of the PFMT are positive in the case of cervical mucus insufficiency (associated or not with a certain degree of OATS), the probability of DIPI being successful is high. If, on the other hand, the PFMT is negative and it seems impossible to collect even a small number of motile sperm, it would be better to consider in vitro fertilization.

Complications

Several types of complications may arise when treating infertility with DIPI. The risk of infection should be almost totally eliminated by thorough screening of the patients and their spouses. Adequate treatment is given in case of a vaginal infection or an infection in the sperm. (There were no infections in any of our patients.) Ectopic pregnancy is also one of the possible complications, and in our patient group there were two extrauterine pregnancies. Both are explained by preexisting tubal lesions not diagnosed because, for medical reasons, the patient had not had a laparoscopy beforehand. These two cases emphasize the absolute necessity of having a complete check-up, including hysterosalpingography and laparoscopy with normal results. Multiple pregnancies are a risk inherent in any hyperstimulation protocol. In spite of this fact, the majority of pregnancies were singletons, but there also were three twin pregnancies and one triple pregnancy.

Antisperm immunization seems to be more a theoretical than a real risk, but further studies should be done to evaluate that risk. Ahlgren (1, 2) showed that the presence of sperm in PF after natural intercourse or after artificial insemination did not lead to the formation of antibodies. Besides, the preparation of sperm by a washing technique decreases the number of antigenic proteins. In several patients from our group, antisperm antibodies in PF were looked for by the tray agglutination test (75). These patients had had several DIPIs in the past. The results of this research remain negative. One patient who had accomplished a full-term pregnancy resulting from DIPI conceived spontane-

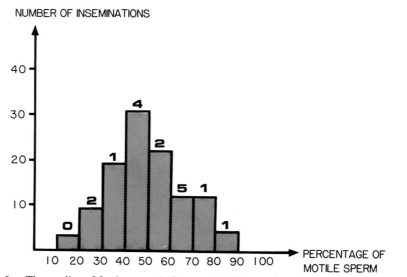

Figure 9.6.   The quality of fresh semen before each DIPI assay is estimated by the percentage of motile sperm. Each column indicates the number of inseminations performed with semen presenting the same rate of motile sperm. The number of pregnancies is indicated at the top of each column. These results were obtained in 1987.

ously 1 year later. This patient had a history of 6 years of primary infertility and had been unsuccessfully treated with various therapies, both traditional and more modern, such as intracervical or intrauterine inseminations. The fact that a spontaneous pregnancy occurred in this case leads one to believe that the treatment did not induce antisperm immunization. The problem nevertheless warrants systematic and more advanced studies.

Table 9.2.
Number of Pregnancies Obtained by DIPI Analyzed According to the Results of Three Tests

Spermogram[a]	Sims-Hühner Test	PFMT	Number of DIPI Procedures	Number of Pregnancies
−	−	+	24	6
−	−	−	11	1
+	−	+	14	5
+	+	+	10	1
−	+	+	7	1
−	+	+	4	1
+	−	−	3	0
+	+	−	1	0

[a]In all cases, + indicates normality. For spermogram, − indicates oligoasthenoteratozoospermia; for postcoital test, − indicates cervical insufficiency; for peritoneal fluid migration test, − indicates <5% of motile sperm after 24 hours of incubation.

Discussion

Fifteen percent of the couples who wish to have children have a problem of sterility or infertility. The etiological factors which concern the male or female partner or the couple are so numerous that many different treatments can be offered. Modern techniques such as in vitro fertilization are the most elaborate answers to the needs of these couples (76). However, they also represent a departure from the natural reproduction process, which, aside from the technical aspects, may bring to mind ethical or religious considerations.

Elaborate infertility treatment techniques are numerous and include intracervical insemination (77), in vitro fertilization (71, 77), intrauterine insemination (78, 79), and GIFT (70, 80). These techniques involve sperm preparation and a timed induction of ovulation. DIPI may well play an interesting role in this range of treatments. The relatively simple and innocuous nature of this technique justifies increasing the number of patients treated with it. In our patient group, DIPI has proven to be an answer to certain difficult cases of long-term infertility. This result is in itself an extremely satifactory one. We have also stressed that doing a laparoscopy to collect PF was not necessary, but much remains to be done in this field. We can foresee that in the near future biochemical studies and the discovery of specific markers will help focus on the etiological problems of certain infertilities, thus providing the best treatment in the best conditions.

What are the results obtained with DIPI, and how do they compare with those obtained with other sophisticated infertility treatments? The results obtained by our team in a large patient group resulted in a 19% pregnancy rate per couple and a 12% pregnancy rate per therapeutic cycle. These results must be compared to those obtained by other teams who published favorable statistics such as a 33.3% pregnancy rate per cycle or dubious results such as a 10% pregnancy rate per cycle (81–85). These results are presented in Table 9.3. Lack of randomization of patients makes it impossible to pinpoint the exact place of DIPI with respect to other techniques such as intrauterine insemination (86, 78), zygote intrafallopian transfer (ZIFT) (87), or GIFT (70, 80) in the treatment of infertility. The latter two have the same indications as intrauterine insemination, but patient recruitment differs considerably, depending on the teams and the criteria for inclusion. Intrauterine insemination has variable success, from a 0% pregnancy rate per cycle (88) to 8.3% (79). GIFT has yielded good results for certain authors (89, 90), although, statistically speaking, GIFT administered to a randomized patient group has not led to good results (18%) in comparison to treatment by in vitro fertilization (91, 92). The three techniques (GIFT, DIPI, and intrauterine insemination) have several common denominators: indications, preliminary examinations, eligibility, and prerequisites such as absence of tubal pathology and ovulation induction. Sperm preparation differs slightly due to the methodology of insemination. The volume and quality of the fluid placed in PF, the uterus, or the fallopian tubes is quite different. In our opinion, intrauterine insemination and DIPI are to be favored over GIFT, which requires a relatively major operation. It is quite probable that, thanks to PFMT, a hostile peritoneal environment will be recognized. This will permit orientation of patients to the most suitable treatment. Apart from further strict statistical data, the decision to choose a particular technique will also depend greatly on the working habits and the preferences of each team.

Table 9.3.
Results of Direct Intraperitoneal Insemination (DIPI)

Author	Duration of Infertility[a]	Type of Infertility						Cycles of Treatment	Pregnancy Rate (%)	
		UI	OATS	CF	M	TD	E		Per Patient	Per Cycle
Buzzoni	2–12, 5.1	16	8	4	8	0	0	58	22.2	13.8
Curson	5	10	0	0	0	0	0	10	10	10
Guastella	6–14	1	4	1	0	0	0	6	33.3	33.3
Schimberni	5–11	26	15	0	0	7	0		12.5	12.5
Studd	5	9	0	1	0	0	1	17	35	18

[a]duration of infertility: range of values and/or mean.
[b]UI, unexplained infertility; OATS, oligoasthenoteratozoospermia; CF, cervical factors; M, multifactorial: cervical factor + oligoasthenoteratozoospermia; TD, tubal disease; E, endometriosis.

Acknowledgment

The invaluable contributions of Mrs. Rachel Price Kreitz for the translation of this text and Mrs. Helga Mury for preparation of the manuscript are gratefully acknowledged.

References

1. Ahlgren M: Migration of spermatozoa to the fallopian tubes and the abdominal cavity in women including some immunological aspects. Thesis University of Lund, Sweden, 1969
2. Ahlgren M: Sperm transport to and survival in the human fallopian tube. Gynecol Invest 6:206, 1975
3. Templeton AA, Mortimer D: Laparoscopic sperm recovery in infertile women. Br J Obstet Gynecol 87:1128, 1980
4. Templeton AA, Mortimer D: The development of a clinical test of sperm migration to the site of fertilization. Fertil Steril 37:410, 1982
5. Menard A: Liquide péritoneal et fertilité—insémination intrapéritonéale par culdocentèse Paris: Thèse, 1986
6. Forrler (Menard) A, Dellenbach P, Nisand I, Moreau L, Cranz C, Clavert A, Rumpler Y: Direct intraperitoneal insemination in unexplained and cervical infertility. Lancet i: 916, 1986
7. Forrler (Menard) A, Badoc E, Moreau L, Nisand I: Direct intraperitoneal insemination: first results confirmed. Lancet i:1468, 1986
8. Conill Serra V: La fonction tubaire et ses troubles Paris: Masson, 1955, p 188
9. Pauerstein CJ, Hodgson BJ, Young RJ, Chatkoff ML, Carlton AE: Use of radioactive microspheres for studies of tubal ovum transport. Am J Obstet Gynecol 122:655, 1975
10. Novak J: Uber ursache und bedeutung des physiologishe ascites beim weibe. Zentralbl Gynäkol 46:854, 1922
11. Bissel D: Observation on the cyclical pelvic fluid in the female. Am J Obstet Gynecol 24:271, 1932
12. Rizzuti A, Olivelli F: Variazioni quantitative del liquido peritoneale e affezioni ginecologiche. Minerva Ginecologica 25:335–337, 1950
13. Decker A: Culdoscopic observations on the tuboovarian mechanism of ovum reception. Fertil Steril 2:253, 1951
14. Doyle JB: Tuboovarian mechanism: observation at laparotomy. Obstet Gynecol 8:686, 1956
15. Doyle JB: Exploration culdotomy for observation of tuboovarian physiology at ovulation time. Fertil Steril 2:475, 1957
16. Rubenstein BB, Strauss H, Lazarus ML, Hankin H: Sperm survival in women. Fertil Steril 2:15, 1951
17. Horne HH, Thibault JP: Sperm migration through the human female reproductive tract. Fertil Steril 13:135, 1962

18. Settlage DS, Motoshima M, Tredway DR: Sperm transport from the external cervical os to the fallopian tubes in women: a time and quantitative study. Fertil Steril 24:655, 1973
19. Maathuis JB, Houx PCW, Bastiaans LA, Mastboom JL: Some properties of peritoneal fluid obtained by laparoscopy from fertile and infertile women. J Reprod Fertil 35:630, 1973
20. Maathuis JB, Van Look PFA, Michie EA: Changes in volume total protein and ovarian steroid concentrations of peritoneal fluid throughout the human menstrual cycle. J Endocrinol 76:123, 1978
21. Koninckx PR, Heyns W, Verhoeven G, Van Baelen H, Lissens WD, De Moor P, Brosens IA: Biochemical characterization of peritoneal fluid in women during the menstrual cycle. J Clin Endocrinol Metab 51:1239, 1980
22. Badawy SZA, Marshall L, Gabal AA, Nusbaum ML: The concentration of 13,14-dihydro-15-keto prostaglandin $F2\alpha$ and prostaglandin E2 in peritoneal fluid of infertile patients with and without endometriosis. Fertil Steril 38:166, 1982
23. Dhont M, Serreyn R, Duvivier P, Vanluchen E, De Boever J, Vandekerckhove D: Ovulation stigma and concentration of progesterone and oestradiol in peritoneal fluid: relation with fertility and endometriosis. Fertil Steril 41:872, 1984
24. Drake TS, Metz SA, Grunert GM, O'Brien W: Peritoneal fluid volume in endometriosis. Fertil Steril 34:280, 1980
25. Drake TS, O'Brien WF, Ramwell PW, Metz SA: Peritoneal fluid thromboxane B2 and 6-keto-prostaglandin $F1\alpha$ in endometriosis. Am J Obstet Gynecol 140:401, 1981
26. Halme J, Hammond MG, Hulka JF, Raj SG, Talbert LM: Retrograde menstruation in healthy women and in patients with endometriosis. Obstet Gynecol 64:151, 1984
27. Haney A F, Handwerger S, Weinberg JB: Peritoneal fluid prolactin in infertile women with endometriosis: lack of evidence of secretory activity by endometrial implants. Fertil Steril 42:935, 1984
28. Joshi SG, Zamah NM, Raikar RS, Buttram VC, Henriques ES, Gordon M: Serum and peritoneal fluid proteins in women with and without endometriosis. Fertil Steril 46:1077, 1986
29. Suginami H, Yano K, Watanabe K, Matsuura S: A factor inhibiting ovum capture by the oviductal fimbriae present in endometriosis peritoneal fluid. Fertil Steril 46:1140, 1986
30. Ylikorkala O, Koskimies A, Laatkainen T, Tenhunen A, Viinikka L: Peritoneal fluid prostaglandins in endometriosis, tubal disorders and unexplained infertility. Obstet Gynecol 63:616, 1984
31. Donnez J, Langerock S, Thomas K: Peritoneal fluid volume and 17 β-estradiol and progesterone concentrations in ovulatory, anovulatory and postmenopausal women. Obstet Gynecol 59:687, 1982
32. Koninckx PR, Ranaer M, Brosens IA: Origin of peritoneal fluid in women: an ovarian exudation product. Br J Obstet Gynaecol 87:177, 1980
33. Koninckx PR, De Moor P, Brosens IA: The importance of peritoneal fluid for reproductive physiology and for the management of infertility in women. Ann Endocrinol 41:143, 1980
34. Lesorgen PR, Wu CH, Green PJ, Gocial B, Lerner LJ: Peritoneal fluid and serum steroids in infertility patients. Fertil Steril 42:237, 1984
35. Syrop CH, Halme I: Peritoneal fluid environment and infertility. Fertil Steril 48:1, 1987
36. Mudge TJ, James MJ, Jones WR, Walsh JA: Peritoneal fluid 6-keratoprostaglandin F1 α levels in women with endometriosis. Am J Obstet Gynecol 152:901, 1985
37. Rock JA, Dubin NH, Ghodgaonkar RB, Bergquist CA, Erozan YS, Kimball AW: Cul-de-sac fluid in women with endometriosis: fluid volume and prostanoid concentration during the proliferative phase of the cycle—days 8 to 12. Fertil Steril 37:747, 1982
38. Olive DL, Weinberg JB, Haney AF: Peritoneal macrophages and infertility: the association between cell number and pelvic pathology. Fertil Steril 44:772, 1985
39. Drake TS, O'Brien WF, Ramwell PW: Elevated peritoneal fluid prostanoïds in unexplained infertility: a possible biochemical marker for microscopic endometriosis. Fertil Steril 37:302, 1982
40. Menezo Y: Uterus et fécondité Paris: Masson, 1981, p 3
41. Lippes J, Krasner J, Alfonso LA, Dacalos E, Lucero R: Human oviductal fluid proteins. Fertil Steril 36:623, 1981
42. Abeille JP, Tomikowski J, Legros R, Tallobre P, Borgard JP, Doussin A: Dosages péritonéaux percoelioscopiques et sériques de l'orosomucoïde et d'autres marqueurs de l'inflammation dans l'étude des processus inflammatoires pelviens. Gynécologie 34:519, 1983
43. Miyamoto H, Chang MC: The importance of serum albumin and metabolic intermediates for capacitation of spermatozoa and fertilization of mouse eggs in vitro. J Reprod Fertil 32:193, 1973
44. Bouckaert PXJM, Evers JLH, Doesburg WH, Schellekens LA, Rolland R: Patterns of changes in glycoproteins, polypeptides and steroids in the peritoneal fluid of women during the periovulatory phase of the menstrual cycle. J Clin Endocrinol Metab 62:293, 1986

45. Kruitwagen RFPM, Janssen Caspers HAB, Wladimiroff JW, Schats R, De Jong FH, Drogendijk AC: Oestradiol 17 β and progesterone level changes in peritoneal fluid around the time of ovulation. Br J Obstet Gynaecol 94:548, 1987
46. Crain JL, Luciano AA: Peritoneal fluid evaluation in infertility. Obstet Gynecol 61:159, 1983
47. Devroey P, Naaktgeboren N, Traey E, Wisanto A, Van Steirteghem AC: Follicular rupture changes the endocrine profile of peritoneal fluid. Acta Eur Fertil 16:237, 1985
48. Donnez J, Langerock S, Thomas K: Peritoneal fluid volume and 17 β estradiol and progesterone concentrations in women with endometriosis and/or luteinized unruptured follicle syndrome. Gynecol Obstet Invest 16:210, 1983
49. Loumaye E, Donnez J, Thomas K: Ovulation instanteously modifies women's peritoneal fluid characteristics: a demonstration from an in vitro fertilization program. Fertil Steril 44:827, 1985
50. Edwards RG: Follicular fluid. J Reprod Fertil 37:189, 1974
51. Dawood MY, Khan Dawood FS, Wilson L: Peritoneal fluid prostaglandins and prostanoids in women with endometriosis, chronic pelvic inflammatory disease and pelvic pain. Am J Obstet Gynecol 148:391, 1984
52. Sgarlata CS, Hertelendy F, Mikhail G: The prostanoid content in peritoneal fluid and plasma of women with endometriosis. Am J Obstet Gynecol 147:563, 1983
53. Halme J, Becker S, Wing R: Accentuated cyclic activation of peritoneal macrophages in patients with endometriosis. Am J Obstet Gynecol 148:85, 1984
54. MacGowan L, Bunnag B: A morphologic classification of peritoneal fluid cytology in women. Int J Gynaecol Obst 11:173, 1973
55. Haney AF, Muscato JJ, Weinberg JB: Peritoneal fluid cell populations in infertility patients. Fertil Steril 35:696, 1981
56. Halme J, Becker S, Haskill S: Altered maturation and function of peritoneal macrophages: possible role in pathogenesis of endometriosis. Am J Obstet Gynecol 156:783, 1987
57. Muscato JJ, Haney AF, Weinberg JB: Sperm phagocytosis by human peritoneal macrophages: a possible cause of infertility in endometriosis. Am J Obstet Gynecol 144:503, 1982
58. Chacho KJ, Stronkowski Chacho M, Anderson PJ, Scommegna A: Peritoneal fluid in patients with and without endometriosis: prostanoids and macrophages and their effect on the spermatozoa penetration assay. Am J Obstet Gynecol 154:1290, 1986
59. Halme J, Hammond MG, Syrop CH, Talbert LM: Peritoneal macrophages modulate human granulosa luteal cell progesterone production. J Clin Endocrinol Metab 61:912, 1985
60. Halme J, Hall JL: Effect of pelvic fluid from endometriosis patients on human sperm penetration of zona free hamster ova. Fertil Steril 37:573, 1982
61. London SN, Haney AF, Weinberg JB: Macrophages and infertility: enhancement of human macrophage mediated sperm killing by antisperm antibodies. Fertil Steril 43:274, 1985
62. Bartosik D, Jacobs SL, Kelly LJ: Endometrial tissue in peritoneal fluid. Fertil Steril 46:796, 1986
63. Portuondo JA, Herran C, Echanojauregui AD, Riego AG: Peritoneal flushing and biopsy in laparoscopically diagnosed endometriosis. Fertil Steril 38:538, 1982
64. Halme J, Becker S, Hammond MG, Raj S: Pelvic macrophages in normal and infertile women: the role of patent tubes. Am J Obstet Gynecol 142:890, 1982
65. Oak MK, Chantler EN, Williams CAV, Elstein M: Sperm survival studies in peritoneal fluid from infertile women with endometriosis and unexplained infertility. Clin Reprod Fertil 3:297, 1985
66. Koninckx PR, Ranaer M, Brosens IA: Origin of peritoneal fluid in women: an ovarian exudation product. Br J Obstet Gynaecol 87:177, 1980
67. Morcos RN, Gibbons WE, Findley WE: Effect of peritoneal fluid on in vitro cleavage of 2-cell mouse embryos: possible role in infertility associated with endometriosis. Fertil Steril 44:678, 1985.
68. Wiegerinck MA, De Laat WN, Moret E: A new culdocentesis system. Fertil Steril 45:434, 1986
69. Menard-Forrler A, Dellenbach P, Moreau L, Rouard M, Cranz L, Clavert A: Apport du test de migration peritoneal à l'exploration de la stérilité du couple: triathlon du spermatozoïde ou comparaison des résultats de 130 spermogrammes, test de migration peritoneal. Presented at the XXXIII Assises de Société Française de Gynécologie, Poitiers, May 29–30, 1987
70. Asch RH, Ellsworth LR, Balmaceda JP, Wong PC: Pregnancy following translaparoscopic gamete intrafallopian transfert. Lancet ii:1034, 1984
71. Garcia J, Acosta A, Andrews ML, Jones HR, Mantzavinos T, Mayer J, McDowell J, Sandow B, Veeck L, Whilbley T, Wilkes C, Wright G: In vitro fertilization in Norfolk, Virginia, 1980–1982. J In Vitro Fertil Embryo Trans 1:24, 1984
72. Dellenbach P, Nisand I, Moreau L, Feger B, Plumere C, Gerlinger P: Transvaginal sonographically controlled follicle puncture for oocyte retrieval. Fertil Steril 44:656, 1985

73. Manhes H, Hermabessiere J: Fécondation intrapéritoneale: première grossesse obtenue sur indication masculine. Communication au 3e Forum International d'Andrologie, Paris, 18–19 juin 1985
74. Pampiglione JS, Davies MC, Steer C, Kingsland C, Mason BA, Campbell S: Factors affecting direct intraperitoneal insemination. Lancet i:1336, June 11, 1988
75. De Almeida M, Herry M, Testart J, Belaisch Allart J, Frydman R, Jouannet P: In vitro fertilization results from thirteen women with antisperm antibodies. Hum Reprod 2:599, 1987
76. Steptoe PC, Edwards RG: Birth after the reimplantation of a human embryo. Lancet ii:336, 1978
77. Hewitt J, Cohen J, Krishnaswamy V, Fehilly CB, Steptoe PC, Walters DE: Treatment of idiopathic infertility, cervical mucus hostility, and male infertility, artificial insemination with husband's semen or in vitro fertilization, Fertil Steril 44:350, 1985
78. Kerin JFP, Peek J, Warnes GM, Kirby C, Jeffrey R, Matthews CD, Cox LW: Improved conception rate after intrauterine insemination of washed spermatozoa from men with poor quality semen. Lancet i:533, 1984
79. Sunde A, Kahn J, Molne K: Intrauterine insemination. Human Reproduction 3:97, 1988
80. Asch RH, Ellsworth LR, Balmaceda JP, Wong PC: Birth following gamete intrafallopian transfer. Lancet ii:163, 1985
81. Buzzoni P, Noci I, Saltarelli O, Criscuoli L, Pellegrini S, Coccia E, Dubini V, Cozzi C: Intraperitoneal insemination as a treatment for infertility. Communication, 6th Forum of International Andrology May 3–4, 1988
82. Curson R, Parson J: Disappointing results with direct intraperitoneal insemination. Lancet i:112, 1987
83. Guastella G, Cimino C: Intraperitoneal insemination (I.P.I.) in couples with infertility unrelated to female organic pelvic disease. Acta Eur Fertil 17:377, 1986
84. Schimberni M, Giallonardo A, Figliolini M, Cerza S, Arcuri GV, Palma E, Aragona C: Direct intraperitoneal insemination in infertility treatment. First Congress of the International Society of Gynecological Endocrinology, Crane, Montana, March 6–12, 1988
85. Studd J, Lim Howe D, Dooley M, Savvas M: Direct intraperitoneal insemination. Lancet i:326, 1987
86. Allen NC, Herbert CM, Maxson WS, Rogers BJ, Diamond MP, Wentz AC: Intrauterine insemination: a critical review. Fertil Steril 44:569, 1985
87. Devroey P, Braeckmans P, Smitz J, Van Waesberghe L, Wisanto A, Van Steiregheme A, Heytens L, Camu F: Pregnancy after translaparoscopic zygote intrafallopian transfer in a patient with sperm antibodies. Lancet i:1329, 1986
88. Thomas EJ, McTighe L, King H, Lenton EA, Harper R, Cooke ID: Failure of high intrauterine insemination of husband's semen. Lancet i:693, 1986
89. Molloy D, Speirs AL, du Plessis Y, McBain J, Johnston I: A laparoscopic approach to a program of gamete intrafallopian transfer. Fertil Steril 47:289, 1987
90. Yovich JL, Matson PL, Turner SR, Richardson PA, Yovich JM: Limitation of gamete intrafallopian transfer in the treatment of male infertility. Med J Aust 14:444, 1980
91. Leeton J, Rogers P, Caro C, Healy D, Yates C: A controlled study between the use of gamete intrafallopian transfer (GIFT) and in vitro fertilization and embryo transfer in the management of idiopathic and male infertility. Fertil Steril 48:605, 1987
92. Dodson WC, Whitesides DB, Hughes CL, Easley HA, Haney AF: Superovulation with intrauterine insemination in the treatment of infertility: a possible alternative to gamete intrafallopian transfer and in vitro fertilization. Fertil Steril 48:441, 1987

CHAPTER 10

Role of Spermatozoa Cryopreservation in Assisted Reproduction

MARY CONDON MAHONY, M.S., MAHMOOD MORSHEDI, PH.D., RICHARD T. SCOTT, M.D., AMANDA DE VILLIERS, M.C.T., AND EVELYN ERASMUS, M.S.

As early as 1776, Lazzaro Spallanzani reported the effects of cryopreservation on human semen. Ninety years later, Paolo Mantegazza suggested the establishment of a sperm bank for veterinary use and, in addition, for human use to produce legitimate children after a husband's death on the battlefield (1). Human spermatozoa were among the first living cells to be studied for the effects of freezing-thawing (2). The recent history of cryopreserved human semen began in 1953 with the demonstration that thawed semen was capable of fertilization and the induction of normal embryonic development (3, 4).

In the cryobiology laboratories at the Jones Institute for Reproductive Medicine in Norfolk and at the Tygerberg Infertility Clinic in South Africa, semen is cryopreserved for several purposes. The procedure is invaluable for men who are about to undergo surgery of the reproductive system, as well as cancer treatment, including radiation and chemotherapy, all of which can potentially render them infertile (5). Also, the sperm of the male partner in an IVF couple is cryopreserved when (*a*) the patient is concerned about the stress of having to collect semen on demand; (*b*) a history of poor specimens collected for IVF has been established; or (*c*) the husband will be out of town for the IVF procedure. Since Norfolk has a large military population, husbands often face extended deployment. Wives can be artificially inseminated with their husbands' cryopreserved semen during their absence. In Parow, South Africa, oligozoospermic samples are accumulated for homologous insemination.

Our donor sperm banks offer semen for artificial insemination by donor (AID) when it is indicated (6). Freezing and storage of semen provides a way to retest donors after sufficient quarantine for acquired immune deficiency syndrome (AIDS), hepatitis B, and other sexually transmitted diseases. This should prove invaluable in dealing with the concern about AIDS and its transmission in AID specimens (7, 8) and for complying with the revised guidelines of the American Fertility Society (9). This chapter examines the factors affecting successful cryopreservation of human sperm.

Mechanism of Cryopreservation

As a liquid is being frozen, the temperature falls steadily to slightly below 0°C, at which time ice appears and the temperature concurrently returns to and remains at 0°C until all liquid is frozen. Once total solidity is attained, the temperature resumes a steady decline. This supercooling (a process wherein the temperature of a liquid falls below the freezing point without solidifying the liquid) is due to the release of the heat of fusion necessary to form the molecular lattice structure of solid water (10).

Solutions freeze at lower temperatures than a pure solvent. The freezing point for water is depressed 1.86°C for each mole of solute contained in 1 kg of solvent.

The successful cryopreservation of cells is affected by the rates of freezing, both above and below the freezing point, and the composition of the solution in which the cells are frozen (11). Cold shock—injury to cells by a fluctuation of temperature above the freezing point—is cell-specific and species-specific (12). Human spermatozoa are resistant to cold shock (13) with respect to motility and oxygen consumption (14, 15). However, concern for cold shock has resulted in protocols which freeze at slow rates (1° to 2°C per minute) from room temperature to the freezing point (12).

As the cells approach the freezing temperature, the water outside the cell freezes first, removing liquid solvent from the extracellular broth and resulting in increased extracellular osmolarity. Water then leaves the cells to follow the osmotic gradient, concentrating the intracellular components sufficiently to eliminate supercooling. Supercooling results when cells are cooled too rapidly, in which case the cells do not lose water fast enough to avoid intracellular freezing and are thereby damaged (16). At appropriate rates of cooling, extracellular ice formation is favored over intracellular formation; thus the concentration of extracellular solutes increases. Because of this osmotic differential, more water leaves the cells, resulting in cell shrinkage (17). If the rate of freezing is too slow, cells may also be damaged because ice forms so slowly outside the cell that unfrozen extracellular channels are produced. As the temperature continues to decrease, these channels decrease in size and may damage cell membranes (18, 19). The damage may result from the exposure of cells to elevated concentrations of extracellular solutes during the freezing process (20). The most significant injuries to spermatozoa appear to be plasma membrane swelling and acrosomal leakage and breakdown (21). To prevent injury to sperm, even at controlled rates of freezing, cryoprotectants and extenders are added to the freezing medium.

Cryoprotectants

When human spermatozoa are subjected to freezing-thawing without the addition of a cryoprotectant, cell survival is <15% (22). Sperm remain viable after freezing if glycerol is included (23–25), and this is now the most common cryoprotectant added to whole semen or semen diluted with an extender (26). Weidel examined various cryoprotectant buffers and saw the most significant decrease in post-thaw progressive motility when glycerol was absent (27). When 5% to 10% glycerol was added, adequate protection was provided (28). (One group suggested that 7.5% offers maximal survival of spermatozoa (29)). Neither the method of adding the glycerol (drop by drop or the total amount at once) nor the temperature at which it is added (room temperature or 5°C) has an effect on human sperm survival (29). Spermatozoa from other species (e.g., the bull and boar) are affected by such changes (30).

The protective action of glycerol may be due to its ability to depress the freezing point and to reduce the electrolyte concentration to which the cells are exposed during freezing procedures (31). It moderates the effect of slow-cooling injury (32). Glycerol is also beneficial in maintaining the pH and in changing the temperature at which the liquid-to-solid phase change is reached (33). Cryoprotectants in general may also bind to sensitive sites on the cell membrane (34), increasing membrane stability (35).

In contrast, Jeyendran (26) indicated that spermatozoa may become dependent on glycerol so that once it is removed—by in vitro washing or in vivo passage through the cervix—motility rapidly decreases. Furthermore, glycerol may increase osmotic shock to spermatozoa by permeating the cell membrane during the freezing process (36). Both theoretical considerations indicate the need for a buffering system that will outperform glycerol.

Dimethyl sulfoxide (DMSO), another cryoprotectant, has been compared to glycerol (21, 37, 38) with success for some cell types (39), including mouse and human embryos (40, 41). The sperm penetration assay (SPA) and electron microscopy have been used to evaluate specimens frozen-thawed with either DMSO or glyercol as the cryoprotectant (21). Addition of 10% glycerol resulted in significantly higher SPA results and a higher percentage of intact sperm heads as viewed by ultrastructure, when compared with DMSO.

In Norfolk the semen specimens are allowed to liquefy for approximately 30 minutes, after which a basic semen analysis is completed with the CellSoft Automated Semen Analyzer (Cryo Resources, Ltd., New York, N.Y.). In Parow a small portion (0.5 ml) of the liquefied specimen is removed for non-automated analysis. Glycerol is the cryoprotectant in both laboratories. It is added to the medium which is used as an extender of the semen.

Extenders

Although glycerol is the most widely used cryoprotectant for freezing human spermatozoa, several more complex media containing a variety of compounds have been reported to result in higher cryosurvival than glycerol alone (27). While many of these formulas preserve sperm function, the means of their doing so are often not well understood. These various media, termed extenders, assist glycerol during cryopreservation by (a) optimizing the osmotic pressure and pH; (b) providing an energy source to prevent the sperm's undesirable use of its own intracellular phospholipid; (c) preventing bacterial contamination when an antibiotic is included; and (d) allowing for dilution of the semen while offsetting the deleterious effect on survival produced by high dilution (42).

The choice of an extender for human spermatozoa should be based on its ability to maintain cellular integrity and function during cryopreservation. Zwitterion (dipolar) buffers containing TRIS [(hydroxymethyl) aminomethane], TES [N-TRIS (hydroxymethyl) methylaminoethane sulfonic acid], or a combination of these has been suggested for preservation (26, 27, 43–45). These substances may improve motile sperm recovery by their ability to bind heavy metals such as copper, zinc, or gold, which can decrease the motility of human sperm (46). The mechanism involved may be the capacity of the divalent ion to bind free hydrogen and hydroxyl ions in the surrounding medium to aid the dehydration process. Sodium citrate, another substance added to extending buffers, may have a similar effect (33).

Besides zwitterion buffers, other substances have been suggested as extenders. A modified Tyrode's medium with sucrose and human serum albumin has also been used (29), as well as a chemically defined medium containing human serum albumin, glycerol, and kallikrein (47). The discovery that egg yolk in semen extenders has a beneficial effect on fertility led to its widespread use in bull semen extenders (48). Early researchers reported that egg yolk aided the sperm cell in resisting cold shock (49, 50), and others have suggested that this more complex medium is more effective in cryopreservation than glycerol alone (24, 25, 51). Subsequent studies have shown that the lipoprotein fraction of egg yolk may be responsible for protecting sperm against cold shock by minimizing the loss of lipids from sperm during freezing (52). More specifically, egg yolk may alter the physical properties of sperm membranes by forming loose interactions with membrane lipids or proteins or through alteration of sperm membrane properties by modification of its lipid composition (42). Cholesterol transfer from egg yolk to the sperm membrane could be the stabilizing mechanism (53). However, Holt (54) indicated that cholesterol stabilization did not provide more effective cryopreservation.

A combination of zwitterions, TES, and TRIS with sodium citrate and egg yolk has been suggested by two groups (26, 27) as the optimal extender. However, they disagree on the beneficial effects of adding glycerol.

In Norfolk we make our own zwitterion-citrate-egg yolk extender (Table 10.1). It contains TES and TRIS, both of which have an osmolarity of 325 mOsm and a pH of 7.2. Sodium citrate at 12.5% and fresh egg yolk at 20% are added to the zwitterion solution. It is stored in liquid nitrogen or at $-20°C$ for up to 6 months. Just before use, the extender is brought to room temperature, mixed with glycerol (12%), and added to the semen sample. With equally good results we also use an extender obtained from Irvine Scientific (Santa Ana, Calif.; Cat. no. 9971), to which 12% glycerol has already been added. In both types, the extender:semen ratio is usually 1:1, which gives a final glycerol concentration of 6% in this mixture. However, the ratio is determined by the original semen parameters and the final motile concentration of thawed sperm desired (25 $\times$ 10^6 motile sperm per thawed vial).

In Parow an equal volume of human semen preservation medium containing glycerol and sucrose with a pH of 6.5 is slowly added to and mixed with the semen.

Freezing and Thawing Rates

Cryopreservation is cell-specific, since cells may differ both in the amount of intracellular water and the permeability of the cell membrane (55). The optimal freezing rates of mammalian spermatozoa—with their small volume, large surface, and small amount of intracellular water—are usually in the range of 10° to 100°C per minute (56). However, there is desagreement concerning the methods used to freeze specimens within this range. The standard technique of vapor freezing was introduced by Sherman (4). The specimens are suspended 15 cm from the liquid nitrogen meniscus for 50 minutes. A programmable freezer to control the rate of freezing can also be used (57–61). In Norfolk

Table 10.1.
Preparation of 100 ml of TESTCY (TES-TRIS-Citrate-Yolk) Buffered Egg Yolk Medium (26)

Chemicals
1. TES: N-TRIS (hydroxymethyl) methylaminoethanesulfonic acid (Sigma T6022);
2. TRIS: (hydroxymethyl) aminomethane (Ultra Pure AMRESCO, Solon, Ohio);
3. Sodium citrate (crystals) $Na_3C_6H_5O_7 \cdot 2H_2O$ (Fisher Scientific, Springfield, N.J.);
4. Penicillin (10,000 units)/streptomycin (10 mg) solution (Sigma P0781; Sigma, St. Louis, Mo.);
5. Three fresh eggs;
6. Ultrapure water for making medium and rinsing glassware.

Procedure
1. Rinse two 150-ml beakers with ultrapure water.
2. In one beaker dissolve 4.83 g of TES and 1.16 g of TRIS in 100 ml of ultrapure water.
3. In the other beaker dissolve 1.78 g of sodium citrate in 50 ml of ultrapure water.
4. Filter each solution separately into sterile containers. Refrigerate overnight, if necessary.
5. Clean three eggs with 70% ethyl alcohol (EtOH). Be sure that the eggs are dry before you begin. Put on sterile non-powdered gloves. Separate the egg yolks from the whites by cracking each egg with a sterile rod or pipette and manipulating the yolks into a sterile container.
6. Mix the yolks thoroughly with a sterile rod.
7. Combine 70 ml of the TES-TRIS solution, 12.5 ml of the sodium citrate solution, and 17.5 ml of the egg yolks, mixing thoroughly.
8. Transfer the solution into two 50-ml centrifuge tubes.
9. Centrifuge the solution at 10,000 × g (8.5 K) for 60 minutes.
10. Pour off and save the supernatant. Discard the pellets. Do not filter the supernatant.
11. Add 1 ml of the penicillin-streptomycin solution.
12. Store the solution in desired aliquots at −20°C or below until needed. The medium can be maintained at −20°C for up to 6 months.
13. The medium is quality controlled on blood agar and eosin methylene blue (EMB) and MacConkey media.

we have noted comparable results between standard vapor freezing and computer-controlled freezing. In Parow a programmable freezer is the method of choice. Specimens are routinely stored in glass ampules, cryovials, or plastic straws. Use of a plastic tuberculin syringe, 10 cm in length, for freezing and storage has also been suggested.

Methods of thawing vary. Both our laboratories and others have noted better survival rates when specimens are slow-thawed in 20° to 35°C air on a laboratory bench than in 5° or 75°C water baths (58).

In Norfolk we usually use a Linde BF-5 liquid nitrogen freezer or a Handi-freeze Tray (Taylor-Wharton Cryogenic Equipment, Theodore, Ala.) to permit more controlled vapor cooling without the expense of the computerized, programmable freezer (used primarily for research projects in our laboratory) with its use of large amounts of liquid nitrogen (62). The Linde BF-5 and the Handi-freeze Tray both fit into the neck of most storage tanks. The level of the specimens relative to the meniscus of the liquid nitrogen is adjustable, and this distance controls the rate of freezing (Table 10.2).

After the addition of an extender with glycerol, the specimens are aliquotted into 2-ml freezer tubes and placed in the freezer following a 60-minute equilibration in a

Table 10.2.
Norfolk Freezing Protocol

1. Semen is collected by masturbation following 2 to 3 days of abstinence.
2. The sample is allowed to liquefy at room temperature for 30 minutes.
3. One vial of cryoprotectant plus extender is thawed and brought to room temperature or to 37°C.
4. The liquefied sample is transferred to a sterile 15-ml conical centrifuge tube. The volume is determined, and the medium is added drop by drop until a 1:1 sample:medium ratio is achieved.[a]
5. Aliquot the sample-medium mixture into labeled 2-ml cryotubes. Do not add more than 0.8 ml per tube.[b]
6. The sample-medium mixture is refrigerated at 2° to 4°C to allow a slow cooling (0.5°C per minute). After 60 minutes the sample is ready to freeze.
7. Freeze with a programmable freezer or manually on a freezing tray (Handi-freeze, Union Carbide). For the programmable freezer, the cooling rate is −0.5°C/min from room temperature to −4°C and −10°C/min from −4°C to −90°C. For manual freezing, vials can be placed 20 cm above liquid nitrogen (approximately −2°C) for 25 minutes, 13.5 cm above liquid nitrogen (approximately −40°C) for 10 minutes, and 12 cm above liquid nitrogen (approximately −90°C) for 10 minutes. The sample is then taken to −196°C by plunging it directly into the liquid nitrogen.

[a]Samples displaying high viscosity may require the additional step of repeated pipetting or passage through an 18-gauge needle to ensure thorough mixing.
[b]Volumes between 0.5 ml and 0.8 ml seem to freeze and thaw with higher motility retention.

refrigerator at 2° to 4°C. Samples are manually frozen following the procedure outlined in Table 10.2.

In Parow, extending medium containing glycerol is added to the semen, and a 20-minute equilibration is allowed. The interval between ejaculation and the beginning of freezing is never more than 4 hours and is preferably 1 hour. The mixture of semen and cryoprotectant is then drawn into 0.25-ml plastic straws for freezing. These straws are sealed with a moisture-sensitive powder plug and labeled for identification. The sealed straws are then placed horizontally in the chamber of the electronically controlled biological freezer. The cooling rate between room temperature and +4°C is −0.5°C per minute. From +4° to −90°C, the straws are cooled at −10°C per minute. When this final temperature is reached, the straws are plunged directly into liquid nitrogen for storage at −196°C (Table 10.2). Levels of liquid nitrogen in the storage tanks are measured each week to maintain an adequate amount for tube immersion.

The Parow group thaws specimens on a dry countertop for 15 to 30 minutes at room temperature just prior to use. The Norfolk group, however, prefers a 45-minute thawing time at room temperature.

Conclusion

Freezing, storage, and the concentration of a husband's semen are now possible (4). Not only are human spermatozoa resistant to freezing-thawing; they also survive various methods of freezing-thawing and storage (63). However, more research on sperm cryopreservation is needed. For example, there is insufficient knowledge of the possible deleterious effects of cyropreservation on sperm morphology.

Use of a donor sperm bank in the treatment of infertility is another important clinical application of semen cryopreservation. With concern over the transmission of AIDS, fresh semen is no longer an alternative for AID or in vitro fertilization. Further investigation to optimize the cryopreservation process is necessary for a balance to be reached between improved sperm survival, effort expended, and clinical application.

References

1. Triana V: Artificial insemination and semen banks in Italy. In David G, Price W (eds): Human Artificial Insemination and Semen Preservation. NY: Plenum, 1980, p 51
2. Sherman JK: Cryopreservation of human semen. In Hafez ESE (ed): Techniques of Human Andrology. Amsterdam: Elsevier, 1977, p 399
3. Bunge RG, Sherman JK: Fertilizing capacity of frozen human spermatozoa. Nature 172:767, 1953
4. Bunge RG, Keettal WC, Sherman JK: Clinical use of frozen semen. Fertil Steril 5:520, 1954
5. Rothman C: Clinical aspects of sperm bank. J Urol 119:511, 1978
6. Alexander NJ, Ackerman S: Therapeutic insemination. Obstet Gynecol Clin North Am 14:905, 1987
7. Sherman JK: Frozen semen: efficiency in artificial insemination and advantage in testing for acquired immune deficiency syndrome. Fertil Steril 47:19, 1987
8. Peterson EP, Alexander NJ, Moghissi KS: AID and AIDS—too close for comfort. Fertil Steril 49:209, 1988
9. American Fertility Society: New guidelines for the use of semen donor insemination. Fertil Steril 46:95s, 1986
10. Lee GL, VanOrden HO: General Chemistry: Inorganic and Organic, 2nd ed. Philadelphia: WB Saunders, 1965, p 130
11. Farrant J: General principles of cell preservation. In Richardson DW, Joyce D, Symond EM (eds): Frozen Human Semen. Boston: Martinus Nijhoff, 1980, p 6
12. Mayer JF, Lanzendorf SE: Cryopreservation of gametes and pre-embryos. In Jones HW Jr, Jones GS, Hodgen GD, Rosenwaks Z (eds): In Vitro Fertilization—Norfolk. Baltimore: Williams & Wilkins, 1986, p 260
13. Sherman JK: Temperature shock in human spermatozoa. Proc Soc Exp Biol Med 88:6, 1955
14. Sawada Y, Ackerman D, Behrman SJ: Motility and respiration of human spermatozoa after cooling to various low temperatures. Fertil Steril 10:775, 1967
15. Sherman JK: Improved methods of preservation of human spermatozoa by freezing and freeze-drying. Fertil Steril 14:49, 1963
16. Mazur P: The role of intracellular freezing in the death of cells cooled at supraoptimal rates. Cryobiology 14:251, 1977
17. Mazur P: Freezing of living cells: mechanism and implications. Am J Physiol 247:C125, 1964
18. Rapatz GL, Merz LJ, Luyet BJ: Anatomy of the freezing process in biological materials. In Meryman HT (ed): Cryobiology. NY: Academic Press, 1966, p 139
19. HyClone Laboratories: Freezing and thawing serum and cells: optimal procedures minimize damage and maximize shelf life. Art to Sci 5:1, 1986
20. Lovelock JE: The mechanism of the protective action of glycerol against hemolysis by freezing and thawing. Biochem Biophys Acta 11:28, 1953
21. Serafini PC, Hauser D, Moyer D, Marrs RP: Cryopreservation of human spermatozoa: correlations of ultrastructural sperm head configuration with sperm motility and ability to penetrate zona-free hamster ova. Fertil Steril 46:691, 1986
22. Lucena E, Obando H: Comparative analysis of different glycerol levels when used as cryoprotective agents on human spermatozoa. In Paulson JD (ed): Andrology: Male Fertility and Sterility. NY: Academic Press, 1986, p 553
23. Polge C, Smith AU, Parkes AS: Revival of spermatozoa after vitrification and dehydration at low temperatures. Nature 166:666, 1949
24. Behrman SJ, Ackerman DR: Freeze preservation of human sperm. Am J Obstet Gynecol 103:654, 1969
25. Matheson GW, Calborg L, Gemze C: Frozen human semen for artificial insemination. Am J Obstet Gynecol 104:495, 1969
26. Jeyendran RS, van der Ven HH, Kennedy W, Perez-Pelaez M, Zaneveld LJD: Comparison of glycerol and a zwitterion buffer system as cryoprotective media for human spermatozoa. J Androl 5:1, 1984

27. Weidel L, Prins GS: Cryosurvival of human spermatozoa frozen in eight different buffer systems. J Androl 8:41, 1987

28. Sherman JK: Synopsis of the use of frozen semen since 1964: state of the art of human semen banking. Fertil Steril 24:397, 1973

29. Mahadevan M, Trounson AO: Effect of cryoprotective media and dilution methods on the preservation of human spermatozoa. Andrologia 15:355, 1983

30. Graham EF, Grabo BG: Some methods of freezing and evaluating human spermatozoa. In Integrity of Froizen Spermatozoa: Proceedings of a Round-Table Conference, Washington, DC, 1976. Washington, DC: National Academy of Sciences, 1978, p 274

31. Lovelock JE, Polge C: The immobilization of spermatozoa by freezing and thawing and the protective action of glycerol. Biochem J 58:618, 1954

32. Mazur P: Slow-freezing injury in mammalian cells. Ciba Found Symp 52:19, 1977

33. Graham EF: Fundamentals of the preservation of spermatozoa. In Integrity of Frozen Spermatozoa: Proceedings of a Round-Table Conference, Washington DC, 1976. Washington, DC: National Academy of Sciences, 1978, p 4

34. Greiff D, Seifert P: Cryotolerance of selected sites on the surfaces of membrances of cells. Cryobiology 4:295, 1968

35. Meryman HT: Review of biologic freezing. In Meryman HT (ed): Cryobiology. NY: Academic Press, 1966, p 1

36. Zavos PM: Opisthosmotic shock of frozen-thawed human spermatozoa. Infertility 5:247, 1982

37. Zimmerman SJ, Maude MB, Moldawer M: Freezing and storage of human semen in 50 healthy medical students: a comparative study of glycerol and dimethyl sulfoxide as a preservative. Fertil Steril 15:505, 1964

38. Sherman JK: Dimethyl sulfoxide as a protective agent during freezing and thawing of human spermatozoa. Proc Soc Exp Biol Med 117:261, 1964

39. Lovelock JE, Bisdhop MWH: Prevention of freezing damage to living cells by dimethyl sulphoxide. Nature 183:1394, 1959

40. Leibo SP: Cryobiology: preservation of mammalian embryos. In Evans JW, Hollaender A (eds): Genetic Engineering of Animals: An Agricultural Perspective. NY: Plenum, 1985, p 251

41. Trounson AO, Mohr L: Human pregnancy following cryopreservation, thawing, and transfer of an eight-cell embryo. Nature 305:707, 1983

42. Foote RH: Physiological aspects of artificial insemination. In Cole HH, Cupps PT (eds): Reproduction in Domestic Animals. NY: Academic Press, 1969, p 313

43. Graham EF, Grabo BF, Brown KI: Effect of some zwitterion buffers on the freezing and storage of spermatozoa. I. Bull. J Dairy Sci 55:372, 1972

44. Davis IS, Bratton RW, Foote RH: Livability of bovine spermatozoa at 5, -25, and $-85°C$ in TRIS buffered and citrate buffered yolk glycerol extenders. J Dairy Sci 46:333, 1963

45. Yassen AM, Foote RH: Freezability of bovine spermatozoa in TRIS buffered yolk extenders containing different levels of TRIS, Na^+, K^+, and Ca^{++}. J Dairy Sci 50:867, 1967

46. Kerreru EE, Leon F: Effect of different solid metals and metallic pairs of human sperm motility. J Fertil 19:81, 1974

47. Kaden R, Klippel FF, Datzorke T, Propping D, Schone D: A new instant cryoprotectant for human sperm. Arch Androl 14:133, 1985

48. Phillips PH: The preservation of bull semen. J Biol Chem 130:415, 1939

49. Bogart R, Mayer DT: The effects of egg yolk on the various physical and chemical factors detrimental to spermatozoan viability. J Anim Sci 9:143, 1950

50. Lasley JF, Mayer DT: Available physiological factors necessary for the survival of bull spermatozoa. J Anim Sci 3:129, 1944

51. Beck WW, Silverstein I: Variable motility recovery of spermatozoa following freeze preservation. Fertil Steril 26:863, 1975

52. Holt WV, North RD: Thermotropic phase transitions in the plasma membrane of ram spermatozoa. J Reprod Fertil 78:447, 1986

53. Karnovsky MJ, Kleinfeld AM, Hoover RL, Dawidowicz EA, McIntyre DG, Salzman EA, Klausner RD: Lipid domains in membranes. Ann NY Acad Sci 401:61, 1982

54. Holt WV, North RD: The role of membrane-active lipids in the protection of ram spermatozoa during cooling and storage. Gamete Res 19:77, 1988

55. Mazur P: Cryobiology: freezing of biological systems. Science 168:939, 1970

56. Polge C: Principles and practice of freezing animal semen. In Richardson DW, Joyce D, Symond EM (eds): Frozen Human Semen. Boston: Martinus Nijhoff, 1980, p 18

57. Serafini P, Marrs RP: Computerized stage-freezing technique improves sperm survival and preserves penetration of zona-free hamster ova. Fertil Steril 45:854, 1986

58. Mahadevan M, Trounson AO: Effect of cooling, freezing, and thawing rates and storage conditions on preservation of human spermatozoa. Andrologica 16:52, 1984

59. Matheson CW, Carlburg L, Gemzell C: Frozen human semen for artificial insemination. Am J Obstet Gynecol 104:495, 1969

60. Taylor PJ, Wilson J, Laycock R, Weger J: A comparison of freezing and thawing methods for the cryopreservation of human semen. Fertil Steril 37:100, 1982

61. Cohen J, Felten P, Zeilmaker GH: In vitro fertilizing capacity of fresh and cryopreserved human spermatozoa: a comparative study of freezing and thawing procedures. Fertil Steril 36:356, 1981

62. Hammond MG, Jordan S, Sloan CS: Factors affecting pregnancy rates in a donor insemination program using frozen semen. Am J Obstet Gynecol 155:480, 1986

63. Ackerman DR: Damage to human spermatozoa during storage at warming temperatures. Int J Fertil 13:220, 1968

CHAPTER 11

Predictive Value of Spermatozoa Morphology in Natural Fertilization

JOHANNES A. VAN ZYL, M.D., THEUNS J. VAN W.
KOTZE, PH.D., AND ROELOF MENKVELD, PH.D.

The role of sperm morphology as a predictor of fertilization and pregnancy is controversial. Amann (1) and Afzelius (2) were confronted by this problem, as we were at the Tygerberg Unit. In 1976 minimum values were established for semen parameters below which the occurrence of natural fertilization would be extremely unlikely (Table 11.1) (3). This chapter directs attention to the significance of sperm morphology in fertile and subfertile semen.

Differentiation between Normal and Abnormal Spermatozoa

In a survey from 1976 to 1987, 1004 couples were treated at the Infertility Clinic at Tygerberg Hospital; 323 conceptions occurred. Semen specimens were examined according to the authors' criteria (4). Sperm morphology was singled out for special attention, slides were carefully evaluated, and patients were then classified into groups based on the strict normal sperm morphology outlined in Chapter 5. The patients were divided according to the percentage of normal morphology: 0% to 9%, 10% to 19%, 20% to 29%, 30% to 39%, 40% to 49%, 50% to 59%, 60% to 69%, and 70% to 79%.

In this study only data from the strict normal morphology groups were used. At least two, preferably three, semen specimens were examined before treatment or spontaneous conception. If conception occurred before two semen specimens could be examined, the couple was excluded from the survey.

Based on these preliminary semen examinations, a spermiogram that showed the average value of each semen parameter was compiled and was regarded as a guideline for treatment and prognosis. Follow-up semen examinations after treatment and/or conception were carried out to see whether any significant changes occurred in the various parameters (Fig. 11.1).

319

Table 11.1.
A Prognostic Criterion for Minimum Values of Semen Parameters Below Which Natural Fertilization Became Uncertain: 1880 Cases and 304 Conceptions

Semen Parameter	Minimum Value[a]	Borderline Value[b]	International Value
Count/ml (millions)	2.0	10.0	>20.0
Motility percentage	10	30	>40
Forward progression (FP)	1.0	2.0	>3.0
Normal cell morphology (%)	10	20	>40
Volume (ml)	—	—	2–6

[a]Unpublished data.
[b]Data taken from van Zyl JA, Menkveld R, Kotze JvW, Van Niekerk WA: The importance of spermiograms that meet the requirements of international standards and the most important factors that influence semen parameters. In: Proceedings of the 17th Congress of the International Society of Urology. Paris: Diffusion Doin 1976, p 263.

The average, maximum, and minimum values of five main semen parameters (volume, count per milliliter, motility percentage, speed of forward progression, and percentage of normal sperm morphology) were noted. These values, represented on spermiograms, were compiled at about the time of fertilization. Only data obtained about 3 months before and/or after conception were used for statistical purposes in this study. These data most closely resembled the ejaculate by which natural conception occurred (Fig. 11.1).

Results and Discussion

The spermiogram results of the 1004 patients showed that 254 patients (25.3%) had a normal morphology of <20%, 194 (19.3%) had a normal sperm morphology of 20% to 29%, 188 (17.9%) had 30% to 39%, 16.7% had 40% to 49%, 12.5% had between 50% and 59%, 8.1% had 60% to 69%, and 0.2% had 70% to 79%. In this study, 628 of the patients (62.5%) showed a normal sperm morphology of <40% (Fig. 11.2).

Pregnancy Rate

Since research into sperm morphology started—and even now in the era of in vitro fertilization (IVF)—controversy has existed. According to Jeulin (5) and Kruger (6), sperm morphology has a definite influence on IVF, whereas Alper (7) and Tarlatzis (8) have expressed the opposite opinion. In the English-language literature of the past 10 years, no reference to sperm morphology in relation to natural (in vivo) fertilization could be found.

When minimum values were established in 1976 for semen parameters which could be expected to produce natural fertilization (Table 11.1), it was obvious that the conception rate declined markedly when the value was less than the established minimum. It was also significant that if the speed of forward progression became <2.0, the conception rate declined to 3% (unpublished data). This finding confirmed the importance of this semen parameter in natural fertilization.

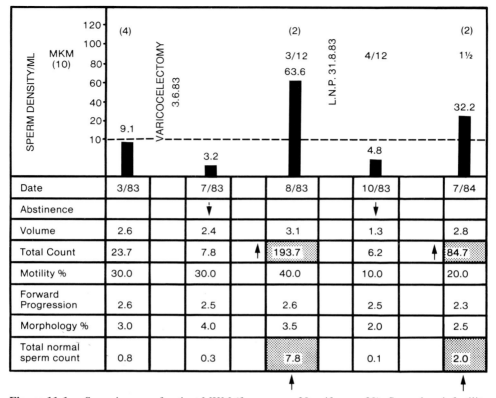

Date	3/83		7/83		8/83		10/83		7/84
Abstinence			▼				▼		
Volume	2.6		2.4		3.1		1.3		2.8
Total Count	23.7		7.8	↑	193.7		6.2	↑	84.7
Motility %	30.0		30.0		40.0		10.0		20.0
Forward Progression	2.6		2.5		2.6		2.5		2.3
Morphology %	3.0		4.0		3.5		2.0		2.5
Total normal sperm count	0.8		0.3		7.8		0.1		2.0

Figure 11.1. Spermiogram of patient MKM (farmer, age 30; wife, age 29). Secondary infertility for 2 years. Previous diagnosis elsewhere: left varicocele, of which correction could have no benefit to fertility, and sperm count too low to ever result in fertilizaton. Varicocele corrected: fertilization 5 months later (last normal period, August 31, 1983). Follow-up spermiograms (July 1983, August 1983, October 1983, July 1984) differed remarkably from spermiogram based on average values for semen parameters of initial semen examinations (March 1983). A favorable outburst of certain semen parameters occurred at fertilization (see August 1983). The compensating factor? Following treatment, the count per milliliter, total count, and total number of normal spermatozoa per ejaculate increased (*arrows* and *dotted areas*) and compensated for the unchanged low percentage of normal sperm morphology. Numbers between brackets indicate number of semen examinations. Time lapses between semen examinations following varicocelectomy indicated by *3/12* (3 months), *4/12* (4 months), and 1½ (1½ years).

We found a linear increase in natural fertilization corresponding with a rise in the percentage of normal sperm morphology. This is illustrated by the distribution of the 323 natural fertilizations that occurred in the study group. In patients with <10% normal sperm morphology, a decline in the natural fertilization rate occurred in 13 of 93 patients (14%) (Fig. 11.3).

Since the study on the 1004 patients was completed, more data became available on the group of patients with a normal sperm morphology <10%. In Table 11.2 we discuss the pregnancy results of a combination of patients. The 93 patients in the study group were combined with 163 patients with a normal sperm morphology <10% who were studied between 1984 and 1987. A total of 256 patients with a normal morphology <10% were evaluated, 49 of whom achieved a pregnancy (19.14%). We divided the

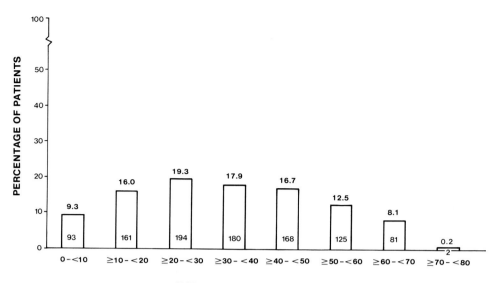

Figure 11.2. Distribution, according to morphology, of 1004 males complaining of infertility.

patients into groups according to the P and G patterns (6): those with a normal sperm morphology ≤4% (P pattern) and those with 5% to 14% normal forms (G pattern). The pregnancy rate in the P-pattern group was 11.47% (seven of 61); in the G-pattern group it was 21.53% (42 of 195).

When we look at the data (Fig. 11.1 and Table 11.2), a line of demarcation or a threshold is established below which the chance of fertilization is less. The threshold is

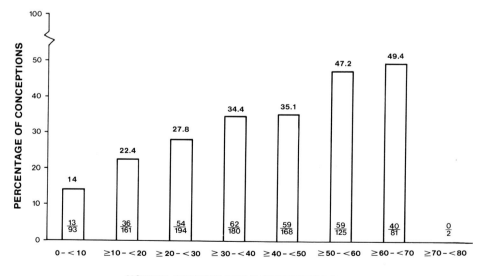

Figure 11.3. Conception rate in relation to morphology (323 fertilizations) in a group of 1004 male patients complaining of infertililty.

Table 11.2.
Conceptions in Relation to Percentage of Normal Spermatozoa in a Group of Patients with Less than 10% Normal Spermatozoa (Combined Data)[a]

| Classification | Percentage of Normal Spermatozoa[b] | | | | | Total |
	0–2	2–4	4–6	6–8	8–10	
Not pregnant	18	36	38	63	52	207
Pregnant	1	6	16	11	15	49
TOTAL	19	42	54	74	67	256

[a]Conception rate at <4%: 11.47% (7/61); conception rate at >4%: 21.53% (42/195); total conception rate at <10%: 19.14% (49/256).
[b]Upper boundary not included in interval.

the percentage of normal morphology below which the rate of natural fertilization decreases faster than the linear relationship established over the interval of 10% to 70% normal morphology. According to Table 11.2, this cutoff score can be established at <4% normal forms, since with <4% normal morphology, a faster-than-linear decline in fertilization rate occurred.

In spite of this dramatic decline, 11.5% natural fertilization occurred in the P-pattern group (Table 11.2). Starting at 4% normal sperm morphology, a linear rise in fertilization rate is obvious. In a series of IVF cases (6) it was also found that the critical dividing score is 4% normal sperm morphology. In that study the fertilization rate was 7.6% in the P-pattern group and 63.9% in the G-pattern group. In this series the lowest percentage of normal sperm morphology resulting in a pregnancy was 3%. When the concentration or total count near the last normal period was considered, the total number of normal spermatozoa per ejaculate was approximately 800,000 (Fig. 11.1). The first author feels that this study strongly suggests that an interaction between semen volume, total sperm count, and motility percentage takes place to compensate for the low percentage of normal sperm morphology. This was obvious in the group with <10% normal sperm morphology (Figs. 11.1 and 11.3).

An important semen parameter in this compensating interaction is sperm motility, especially if forward progression is exceptionally good or at least within normal limits. The importance of sperm motility was pointed out by Mahadevan (9). In the current study it was shown that, in 98% of natural fertilizations, the motility exceeded 30%, and the speed of forward progression was 2 or more on a scale of 1 to 4.

In terms of prognosis in in vivo fertilization, speed of forward progression and percentage of motility can be regarded as cornerstones. If these are good or within normal limits, any other semen parameter also found to be within normal limits is an asset. Not only does a critical level of normal spermatozoa have a good potential for natural fertilization, but also slightly amorphous (borderline) spermatozoa assist in establishing the prognosis and in predicting the fertilization rate (6).

Another important aspect of a fertility workup is thorough evaluation of the female, who should have a full examination and treatment, if required, to increase the chances of success in couples where a male factor is the initial cause of infertility.

It is also important to point out that in cases with <10% normal sperm morphology, the total sperm count is very important. The higher the total count, the more spermatozoa with normal morphology will be available for fertilization.

Conclusion

In our series of infertility patients, 25% showed <20% normal sperm morphology, 62.5% showed <40%, and 9.3% showed <10%. A normal morphology of 20% to 30% was seen in 19.3% of the patients, while only 8.3% showed >60% normal morphology.

A linear increase in natural fertilization occurred in correspondence with an increased percentage of normal morphology. It was statistically determined that the critical threshold of normal sperm morphology for success in natural fertilization was 4%. Although total sperm count and the percentage of motility and forward progression are combined compensating factors among semen parameters to achieve fertilization, normal sperm morphology can be singled out for its fundamental contribution.

Under no circumstances is it justified to use a single spermiogram variable as the decisive prognostic factor in male infertility. No matter how meticulously tests are done and calculations are validated by statistical analysis, in most cases the degree of male fertility is constantly changing. The male's ability to procreate is greatly influenced by his female partner. Prognosis can very seldom be a cut-and-dried decision.

References

1. Amann RP: A critical review of methods for evaluation of spermatogenesis from seminal characteristics. J Androl 2:39, 1981
2. Afzelius BA: Abnormal human spermatozoa including comparative data from apes. Am J Primatol 1:175, 1981
3. van Zyl JA, Menkveld R, Kotze TJvW, Van Niekerk WA: The importance of spermiograms that meet the requirements of international standards and the most important factors that influence semen parameters. In: Proceedings of the 17th Congress of the International Society of Urology. Paris: Diffusion Doin, 1976, p 263
4. van Zyl JA: The infertile comple. Part II. Examination and evaluation of semen. S Afr Med J 57:485, 1980
5. Jeulin C, Feneux D, Serres C, Jouannet P, Guillet-Rosso F, Belaisch-Allart J, Freedman R, Testart J: Sperm factors related to failure of human in vitro fertilization. J Reprod Fertil 76:735, 1986
6. Kruger TF, Acosta AA, Simmons KF, Swanson RJ, Matta JF, Oehninger S: Predictive value of abnormal sperm morphology in in vitro fertilization. Fertil Steril 49:112, 1988
7. Alper MM, Lee GS, Seibel MM, Smith D, Oskowaity SP, Rausil BJ, Taymor ML: The relationship of semen parameters to fertilization in patients participating in a program of in vitro fertilization. J In Vitro Fertil Embryo Trans 2:217, 1985
8. Tarlatzis BC, De Cherney AH, Amster S, Laufer N, Graebe RA, Boyers S, Huszar G, Naftolin F: Semen characteristics and in-vitro fertilization of human oocytes (Abstract). 3rd International Congress of Andrology. Boston, MA, April 27–May 2, 1985. J Androl 6 (Suppl): N55, 1985
9. Mahadevan MM, Trounson AO: The influence of seminal characteristics on the success rate of human in vitro fertilization. Fertil Steril 42:400, 1984

CHAPTER 12

Oocyte Donation

DAVID KREINER, M.D., AND ZEV ROSENWAKS, M.D.

The 1980s have brought technological advances in reproductive medicine that provide novel therapies for infertility and make the achievement of pregnancy possible in patients who in the past were considered to be irreversibly sterile.

Female sterility due to absent or irreparable fallopian tubes has been overcome through in vitro fertilization (IVF). Success with IVF has allowed extension of this technique to any etiological infertility factor that has failed conventional therapy, as long as the couple involved have normal gametes and the wife has a normal uterus. Recently the successful transfer of donated embryos (1–3) and of donated oocytes fertilized in vitro has extended the use of IVF technology to conditions where no oocytes are present or where oocytes are inaccessible to harvest (4–10), or where previous failure with IVF occurs secondary to oocyte abnormalities.

Although oocyte donation is medically analogous to sperm donation, the relative inaccessibilty of oocytes and the relative difficulty of synchronizing the ovulatory process in the donor with endometrial maturation in the recipient make the procedures quite different technically.

Historical Aspects and Animal Experimentation

Embryo transfer technology has been investigated since the first successful embryo transfer was performed in rabbits in 1891 (11). Over the past 100 years, embryo transfers have resulted in pregnancies in many species, including the mouse, rabbit, sheep, and cow. Indeed, advancement in embryo transfer technology has made this a useful tool for the cattle industry (12). The protocol includes superovulation of donors with gonadotropins, insemination in vivo, uterine flushing to recover the embryos, followed by embryo transfer to the uterus of a recipient (Fig. 12.1). Alternatively, embryos may be cryopreserved for subsequent transfer into a suitable recipient.

Experience in the bovine has demonstrated that success is greatest—with a nearly 70% pregnancy rate per embryo transfer—when the asynchrony between the donor and recipient estrus cycles is less than 2 days in the luteal phase (13, 14). In mice, synchrony between donor and recipient must be within 0.25 day for implantation to occur (15). The

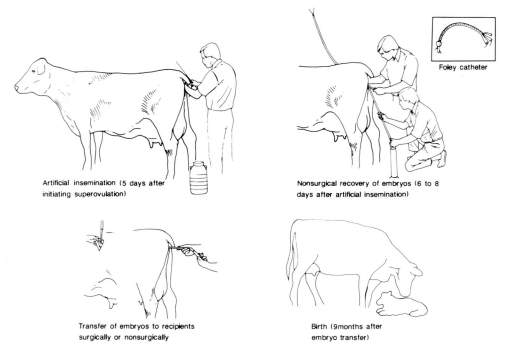

Foley catheter

Artificial insemination (5 days after initiating superovulation)

Nonsurgical recovery of embryos (6 to 8 days after artificial insemination)

Transfer of embryos to recipients surgically or nonsurgically

Birth (9months after embryo transfer)

Figure 12.1. Schema for bovine in vivo fertilization.

importance of luteal synchronization between donor and recipient is also seen in sheep, where the pregnancy rate is 75% per embryo transfer when there is exact synchronization. However, implantation efficiency drops to 8% when the asynchrony is 3 or more days (16). In the monkey a 36% pregnancy rate was demonstrated when the degree of asynchrony was 3 days or less in oophorectomized recipient monkeys treated with subcutaneous estradiol (E_2) and progesterone (P) capsules (17).

Indications

Candidates for oocyte donation fall into two major categories: those with and those without functioning ovaries. Oocyte donation may be considered in the presence of ovarian function in the following conditions: (*a*) anatomically inaccessible ovaries (with the newly developed techniques of oocyte retrieval, this has become a very infrequent situation); (*b*) IVF failure due to oocyte abnormalities; (*c*) hereditary disorders, including genetic abnormalities and autosomal-dominant or sex-linked disorders and autosomal recessive traits where the couple is reluctant to use donor insemination; (*d*) a medical contraindication to surgical ovum harvest; and (*e*) a history of recurrent or persistent ovarian cysts precluding use of ovarian stimulation. The following causes of ovarian failure have been seen in patients desiring oocyte donation in the Norfolk program: (*a*) gonadal dysgenesis (13.9%, of whom 58.8% have an abnormal karyotype); (*b*) insensitive ovary syndrome (2.3%); (*c*) autoimmune ovarian failure (15.1%); (*d*) premature ovarian failure of any etiology, including surgical extirpation (61.6%), exposure to chemotherapy (3.5%), and radiation (1.16%) (18).

Workup of Donors and Recipients

In Norfolk oocyte donors are screened in accordance with the American Fertility Society (AFS) guidelines (19), which include (*a*) minimal genetic screening for gamete donors based on the donor's family medical history; (*b*) historical screening for sexually transmitted diseases; and (*c*) testing for hepatitis-B surface antigen and antibody and human immunodeficiency virus (HIV). In addition, potential donors are screened by a psychiatrist for any underlying emotional disorders or ambivalence which may affect the donor in making a rational decision or may be predictive of future regret. Donors may be IVF patients who agree to donate excess oocytes. With the availability of cryopreservation as an option, most patients choose to freeze any excess concepti. Consequently, the donor program must depend upon the availability of specific donors. In some instances a sister has provided oocytes; at other times a patient requesting tubal ligation will agree to undergo superovulation and oocyte retrieval prior to the procedure. The program has a policy of discouraging payment to donors (as recommended by the AFS Ethics Committee). All designated donors have been stimulated with a combination of follicle-stimulating hormone (FSH) (Metrodin, Serono Laboratories, Randolph, Mass.) and human menopausal gonadotropin (hMG; Pergonal, Serono) (20, 21). Gonadotropin stimulation is begun on days 3 and 4 of the menstrual cycle with the administration of two ampules of FSH in the morning, followed by two ampules of hMG in the afternoon. Beginning on day 5, two ampules of hMG are administered daily until critical follicular development is achieved, as judged by daily serum E_2, ultrasonograms, and cervical mucus changes (20, 21). Typically, human chorionic gonadotropin (hCG) is administered in the evening of day 9, and oocyte harvest is scheduled approximately 34 to 36 hours later (22). After harvest, the oocytes are inseminated with the sperm of the infertile woman's husband, as described for our basic IVF insemination procedures (23). Typically, transfer of concepti occurs 44 to 74 hours after insemination, depending upon the recipient's luteal day and the previously defined endometrial histology for the day of transfer, thus allowing for maximum synchronization of endometrium and conceptus.

Potential recipients undergo a more rigorous workup that includes determining the indication and the suitability of the patient for the procedure, as well as the correct hormone replacement protocol to adequately support the endometrium in patients with ovarian failure. A hysterosalpingogram is performed to determine the adequacy of the uterine cavity in all recipients.

Oocyte donation may be performed in three clinical situations. If a patient has ovarian failure, the cause of her gonadal dysfunction is determined, and she is placed on hormone replacement and monitored to determine the adequacy of therapy. Serum E_2 and P are monitored on an almost daily basis to ensure adequate absorption. An endometrial biopsy is performed on days 21 and 26 to determine the adequacy of the endometrium for implantation and for sustaining a pregnancy. If E_2 and P levels and endometrial biopsies are adequate, embryo transfer is performed during an ensuing similarly replaced cycle. Although several steroid replacement protocols have been proposed, they all endeavor to mimic the steroidal milieu of the natural cycle. If a patient is to receive oocyte donation during a natural, monitored cycle, then serum E_2 and luteinizing hormone (LH) assays are performed during the early follicular phase and daily in the periovulatory phase of the menstrual cycle. It is recommended that a basal body temperature (BBT) chart, as well as daily P determinations in the early luteal phase, be used to confirm the timing of the LH surge and ovulation. Recent information suggests that synchronization of donor and recipient should be aimed at furnishing a 4- to 16-cell embryo for transfer on days 16 to 19 of the recipient's cycle, where day 14 is arbitrarily defined as the day of LH surge, and day 15 is designated as the day of ovulation.

The third clinical situation in which oocyte donation may occur is during a failed IVF cycle. In women in whom IVF attempts have failed repeatedly, one can be prepared to use donor oocytes during an anticipated failed cycle. Repeated IVF failures may be due to abnormalities of the ovaries and/or gametes. In such patients, previous attempts are characterized by deficient E_2 responses to ovarian stimulation in successive cycles, by recurrently poor oocyte harvests, and—more infrequently—by the collection of abnormal oocytes. Oocyte abnormalities include failure of final maturation and repetitive failure of fertilization by seemingly normal sperm. A cytoplasmic refractile body has been associated with lack of fertilization in some women (24). To maintain the anonymity of potential recipients, it is preferable to use predesignated donors rather than excess oocytes from women who are co-participants in the IVF program. Gonadotropin stimulation of donor recipients must coincide to allow optimal synchrony of oocyte retrievals and embryo transfers. If no oocytes are obtained from the potential recipient, one can inseminate the donor oocytes with the sperm of the recipient's husband, aiming at a transfer day which is within 1 to 2 days of the previously anticipated transfer day.

Hormone Replacement Protocols

The first pregnancy using oocyte donation in an ovarian failure patient was achieved with oral E_2 valerate (Progynova, Schering, Sydney, Australia) and vaginal P suppositories for hormone replacement (4). Following embryo transfer, intramuscular P injections were used. Navot (10) modified this protocol by using intramuscular P for luteal phase replacement. Briefly, 1 mg/day of E_2 valerate was administered orally on days 1 to 5. This was increased to 2 mg/day for days 6 to 9 and to 6 mg/day on days 10 to 13. The dosage was reduced to 2 mg/day on days 14 to 17, then increased to 4 mg/day on days 18 to 26 (10). Reduction of E_2 valerate on days 14 to 17 was used to mimic the drop in E_2 that is observed in the natural cycle after the LH surge. Intramuscular P, 25 mg, was administered on days 15 and 16, and 50 mg on days 17 to 26. This protocol (10) appears to result in satisfactory serum levels of E_2 and P, as well as adequate endometrial maturation, as judged by luteal biopsy.

A number of replacement protocols have been evaluated in Norfolk. E_2 has been delivered by the vaginal route using polysiloxane-impregnated E_2 rings provided by Paul Stumpf (25, 26) (Jersey Shore Medical Center, Neptune, N.J.), or by the oral route using micronized E_2 (Estrace, Mead Johnson, Evansville, Ind.), following a modification of the Lutjen protocol (4), or most recently by the transdermal route (Estraderm, Ciba-Geigy, Summit, N.J.) (27). P has been administered most frequently by vaginal suppository or by IM injection. Although early studies suggested that 2000-mg intravaginal polysiloxane cylinders, also provided by Stumpf, were adequate for achieving appropriate P blood levels, their use was soon abandoned because of vaginal discomfort and/or infection. The surface area necessary for delivery of nanogram levels of P made the cylinder too cumbersome and impractical.

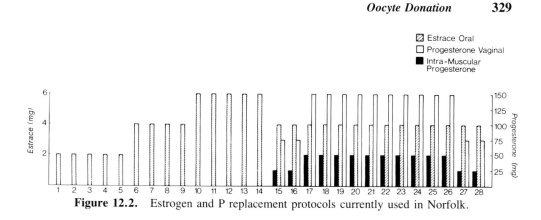

Figure 12.2. Estrogen and P replacement protocols currently used in Norfolk.

E₂ REPLACEMENT

Two milligrams of micronized E_2 are administered orally on cycle days 1 to 5. Dosage is increased to 4 mg/day (given at 12-hour intervals) on days 6 to 9, and to 6 mg/day (given at 8-hour intervals) on days 10 to 13. The dosage is then decreased to 4 mg/day on days 15 to 28 (Fig. 12.2). Serum E_2 and estrone (E_1) levels are measured to ensure adequate absorption and to permit dose modification as necessary. The alternative method of E_2 replacement uses E_2-impregnated vaginal rings, which provide a steady release of E_2 into the bloodstream. The replacement schedule is highly individualized to ensure optimal stimulation of the menstrual cycle hormonal milieu. It may be necessary to monitor patients for two or three cycles before adequate hormonal replacement is achieved. A typical replacement protocol is represented in Figure 12.3. Note that a new ring is placed on days 1, 9, 11, and 13. Absorption data reveal that, with each insertion of a new ring, one observes a burst of E_2 before a steady state of absorption is maintained. One can use this phenomenon to achieve super-high E_2 levels at the simulated mid-cycle by introducing a new ring every other day. It soon became evident, however, that vaginal P suppositories inhibit the absorption of E_2, probably by coating the ring surface. Therefore, it was necessary to add oral E_2 to achieve adequate E_2 levels in the luteal phase. The transdermal E_2 protocol was established in an attempt to maintain steady E_2 levels throughout the day rather than experience the peaks and troughs seen with both the oral and vaginal routes of administration. Additionally, oral E_2 is exposed to the intestinal wall, where a proportion of E_2 is metabolized to E_1 (28). E_2 and E_1 are carried to the liver via the portal circulation, where additional metabolism converts the E_2 and E_1 to estriol (E_3) (29), or they are conjugated to glucuronide and sulfated forms, thereby becoming unavailable for target organ stimulation. Approximately 30% of orally administered E_2 is metabolized prior to reaching the systemic circulation (30), thereby effectively reducing the estrogen effect. The potential adverse effect of orally administered E_2 by virtue of the effect on the liver is an additional reason to use a transdermal route of administration, especially since these patients often require several months of therapy prior to achieving a transfer. The protocol we have developed (27) is the following, as seen in Figure 12.4: 50 μg applied to the lower abdomen on days 1 to 6, with a patch changed every 3 days. On days 7 to 9, 100-μg patches were applied, with an increase to 200 μg on days 10 to 11. On days 12 to 14, the dosage was increased to 400 μg, then reduced to 100 μg on days 15 to 17. On days 18 to 28, the dosage was once

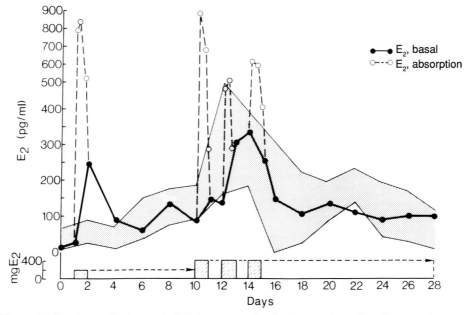

Figure 12.3. Protocol with vaginal E_2-impregnated polysiloxane rings. Baseline morning serum levels. *Open circles,* Absorption levels at 1, 2, and 6 hours after ring insertion. *Shaded area* represents E_2 ranges in normally cycling women.

more increased to 200 μg. A significantly higher E_2 value was found on days 12 to 14 in patients on transdermal E_2 than in those on orally administered E_2 ($P<0.01$). Additionally, the $E_2:E_1$ ratio of 1.59 ± 0.16 was significantly greater for transdermal E_2 patients compared to 0.13 ± 0.4 for orally administered E_2 patients ($P<0.05$). No significant difference was noted with respect to endometrial histology.

To date, nine transfers have been performed between days 17 and 19 with the transdermal protocol, with viable intrauterine pregnancies confirmed in five.

PROGESTERONE REPLACEMENT

Adequate P levels can be achieved by vaginal suppository or by intramuscular administration. We have used 75 mg of vaginally administered P (given every 8 hours in divided doses) on days 15 and 16. Dosage was then increased to 150 mg (given every 8 hours in divided doses) on days 17 to 26, and decreased to 25 mg three times a day on days 27 and 28. Absorption studies confirmed the adequacy of replacement compared to normal control luteal phase levels, as illustrated in Figure 12.5. P replacement can also be accomplished by intramuscular injection, as demonstrated by Navot (Fig. 12.6) (10). Alternatively, P suppositories can be used during the monitored, simulated preparatory cycles (to assess the adequacy of endometrial maturation), later to be supplemented or changed to the intramuscular route during the cycle of transfer.

Final judgment on the suitability of a given replacement protocol depends on the histological assessment of the endometrium. Secretory changes which compare favorably with the expected natural cycle-day histology would be the desirable end point.

We have observed that early biopsies performed on days 20 to 22 display day 17 to 18 glandular architecture, along with a characteristic day 21 to 23 stroma. A typical early biopsy performed on day 21 is depicted in Figure 12.7. Note the subnuclear vacuoliza-

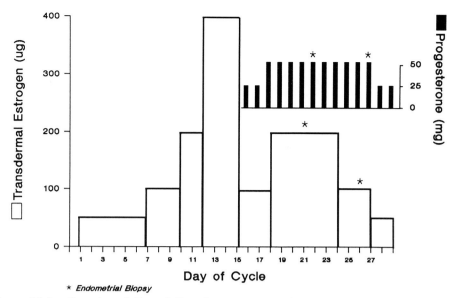

Figure 12.4. Transdermal E_2 and P replacement protocol used in Norfolk. (Adapted from Droesch K, Navot D, Scott R, Kreiner D, Liu H-C, Rosenwaks Z: Transdermal estrogen replacement in ovarian failure for ovum donation. Fertil Steril 50:931, 1988.)

tion and linear arrangement of nuclei characteristic of day 18 architecture, juxtaposed with edematous stroma suggestive of day 21 to 22 endometrium. This asynchrony occurs despite seemingly adequate P absorption. In contrast, biopsies performed on day 26 reveal the characteristic pseudo-decidual changes in the stroma of a day 25 to 26 endometrium. Thus, early gland development seems to lag behind the stroma, although the endometrium appears to catch up in the late luteal phase. It should be emphasized that the early luteal phase biopsy findings were confirmed on repeated biopsies, suggesting that the lag in glandular maturation was not due to first-cycle exposure to steroids; rather, this lag may indicate that the glands may require a longer—albeit lower-threshold—exposure to P in order to achieve prompt and timely secretory changes. It is possible that during the natural cycle the early rise of P on day 14 allows the gradual development of the glandular endometrial compartment, whereas during replacement therapy the endometrium is exposed to P 1 to 2 days later, thus explaining the disparity between glands and stroma in the day 20 and 21 biopsies. Conversely, the stroma may mature more rapidly when exposed to a threshold level of P. This apparent lag in development of the glands does not appear to interfere with implantation, as pregnancies have occurred after transfer of concepti on days 17 to 19 of the replaced cycle, suggesting that the retarded glandular development may not be as critical for implantation as the stromal development stage. It should be noted that Navot (10) found a greater conformity between the day of biopsy and the expected histological architecture in women receiving intramuscular P for luteal phase replacement. Similarly, Lutjen (7) reported that endometrial biopsies obtained on luteal day 21 or 22 in patients treated with P vaginal suppositories (50 mg on days 15 and 16, followed by 100 mg on days 17 to 26) were histologically dated as day 20 ± 2.1 endometrium (mean ± SD; range, 17 to 23) in nine women with ovarian failure (31). The disparity in endometrial dating between the Norfolk and Melbourne findings, despite Norfolk's high P dosage, may represent a different interpretation of similar histological

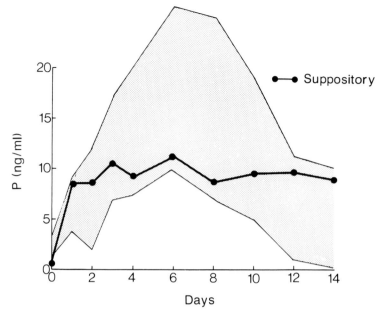

Figure 12.5. Representative daily P concentrations after treatment with P vaginal suppositories in the simulated luteal phase. Shaded area depicts the luteal range of P levels in normally cycling women. Dosage is 75 mg of P on days 15 and 16 in three divided doses, 150 mg on days 17 to 25 in divided doses, then 75 mg on days 27 and 28.

findings. Conversely, the delayed glandular development observed in the Norfolk series may be secondary to the somewhat lower serum E_2 concentrations seen in some women who had hormonal replacement with oral E_2. It may be that inadequate or suboptimal E_2 replacement could result in diminished glandular proliferation, decreased induction of P receptors in the glands, and consequently delayed endometrial maturation.

Temporal Window of Transfer

By transferring concepti into histologically defined environments, we can determine the width of the window of transfer at implantation in the human. Navot (10) transferred concepti into eight women on days 16 to 21 of the E_2 and P replacement cycles, with pregnancies occurring from a day 18 and a day 19 transfer. The Monash group (7) typically performed embryo transfers on day 17 ± 1 of the replacement cycle. In Norfolk 21 transfers were performed with multiple concepti, and seven patients became pregnant. All seven (7/14) underwent transfer on days 17 to 19, while none of the remaining seven patients who underwent transfer on day 20 or later became pregnant. These observations, taken together with the reported world experience, suggest that in a hormone replacement cycle, the transfer of 4- to 8-cell embryos into an endometrium histologically developed to day 17 to 19 is likely to produce the best results. Limited data regarding embryo transfer during hormonally replaced cycles on day 16 preclude any conclusion regarding transfer on this day. However, data from our cryopreservation program, in which we transfer concepti (usually 4-cell) after 30 to 38 hours of incubation post-insemination, approximately 28 to 48 hours after documented ovulation, suggest

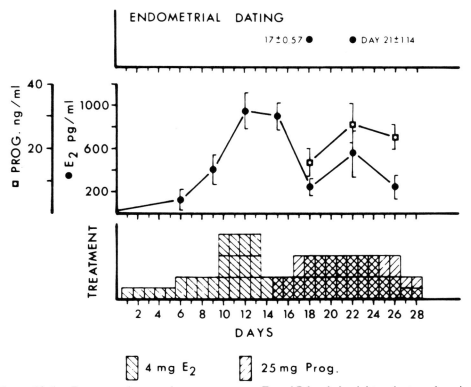

Figure 12.6. Exogenous hormonal treatment, serum E_2 and P levels in eight patients undergoing E_2 and P replacement. (Adapted from Navot D, Laufer N, Koplovic J, Rabinowitz R, Birkenfeld A, Lewin A, Granat M, Margalioth E, Schenker JG: Artificially induced endometrial cycles and establishment of pregnancies in the absence of ovaries. N Engl J Med 314:806, 1986.)

that an earlier transfer in a natural cycle is at least equally successful, as we have had six of 30 embryos successfully implanted in this program.

Synchronization of Donors and Recipients

As discussed above, success with oocyte donation may be optimized by close synchronization between donor and recipient so that a conceptus may be transferred into a recipient uterus that has been appropriately timed within the window of transfer. In the natural cycle, patients are monitored for their LH surge with periovulatory serum E_2, LH, and P so that embryo transfer may be timed at 3 to 5 days after the LH surge. Monitoring in a natural cycle restricts the recipient to oocytes available on those 3 days of her menstrual cycle, approximately 48 to 72 hours prior to the window of transfer. Recipients undergoing hormone replacement are similarly restricted to available oocytes, according to their protocol on those same 3 days. Unfortunately, the availability of donor oocytes may be unpredictable; therefore, perfect synchronization may be impossible to achieve. One program to solve the problem of synchronization has evolved into a simplified protocol of continuous E_2 valerate (6 to 8 mg/day) whether or not a patient has ovarian failure, with administration of intramuscular P, 100 mg, 1 day before oocytes are

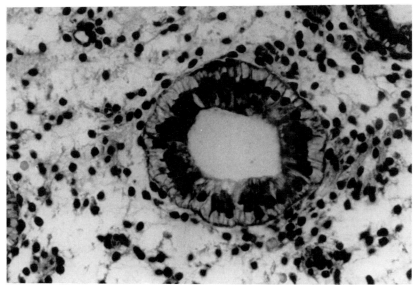

Figure 12.7. Histology of day 21 endometrial biopsy after E_2 and P replacement in an ovarian failure patient. Note the subnuclear vacuolization and linear arrangement of nuclei characteristic of day 18 glands, juxtaposed with edematous stroma characteristic of day 21 to 22 endometrium.

made available (32). These investigators have reported 14 patients undergoing transfer, with six pregnancies. In the Norfolk program, we have investigated the effects of shortening and lengthening follicular phases, as well as accelerated luteal differentiation (33). Based on our study, prolonged, unopposed E_2 stimulation has no apparent adverse effect on endometrial morphology. The glandular delay in secretory transformation was similar to that of the basic protocol, while the stroma seemed to be in phase with the chronological age of the endometrium. The known mitogenic and proliferative effects of E_2 were not apparent on histologic examination. Similarly, a relatively short (6-day) exposure to moderate E_2 levels appeared to be adequate for the induction of endometrial P receptors and allowed for normal luteal differentiation. Very high P levels obtained by 75-mg P intramuscular injections seemed to abolish the glandular-stromal disparity observed in the early biopsies. In fact, by cycle day 24, stromal changes characteristic of day 25 to 26 were obtained.

Furthermore, surface negativity proved similar in galactose residues and glycocalyx intensity—histochemical markers for endometrial normalcy—and was greatest during the implantation interval, comparing favorably with similar histochemical analyses of endometrial biopsies obtained from normally cycling women of proven fertility (34, 35). It seems reasonable, therefore, to assume that endometrial changes induced by these protocols are compatible with successful implantation. These protocols have been used in the following fashion. The shortened follicular phase is commenced in the recipient 3 days after the establishment of menstrual flow in the donor. The lengthened follicular phase allows for continuous E_2 stimulation until the onset of menstruation in the donor. Similarly, if unexpected donor oocytes become available, P may be administered at regular or high dose to the recipient at the time of oocyte harvest to allow the endometrium to mature to day 16 or 17 by the time of embryo transfer. Alternatively, one can delay the donor's menstrual cycle by a variety of agents, including gonadotropin-releasing hormone agonist (GnRH-a), P, and oral contraceptives. A study in which norethindrone was used to time retrievals by timing the onset of menses did demonstrate some success (36) in that 82% had their retrieval on the expected day. Experience with GnRH-a and oral conceptives has been somewhat more disappointing. Stimulation with GnRH-a is not very predictable in cycle length, with a 20% coefficient of variation in 26 cases in our program. Pretreatment with oral contraceptives, as with norethindrone, may affect the ability and quality of ovarian stimulation. It has been our preference, therefore, to manipulate the recipient's cycle if necessary, rather than the donor's. Most recently, success with cryopreservation has allowed ideal synchronization without manipulation of the donor or the recipient. In view of our pre-zygote survival rate of 73% and a pregnancy rate of 20% per embryo transferred, we believe that this may be a reasonable solution to the synchronization problem.

Maintenance of Pregnancy in the Ovarian Failure Patient

Detailed experience in the requirements for pregnancy maintenance has been reported by several investigators. A positive β-hCG titer can be expected on approximately days 26 to 28, or 10 to 12 days after embryo transfer. If the pregnancy test is negative, one tapers the E_2 and P dosage to allow endometrial shedding and menstruation to occur. If the test is positive, most investigators have immediately and substantially increased the E_2 dosage. Lutjen (7) maintained patients on 2 mg of E_2 valerate per day in the luteal phase of the transfer cycle, increasing the dosage to 8 or 9 mg/day as soon as the β-hCG titer became positive. At the same time, he placed the patient on intramuscular P at 50 to 100 mg/day. He suggested that this regimen maintains the plasma steroid levels at concentrations that are within the normal range for pregnancy. The goal was to maintain E_2 concentrations at 100 to 500 pmol/liter and P within the 100 to 200 nmol/liter range. Lutjen (7) discontinued E_2 treatment at 12 weeks of pregnancy, whereas P injections were maintained through week 16. Withdrawal of medication was predicated on observing a rise in endogenous steroids from the placenta. From the observations of Csapo (37) in luteectomized women, one would expect adequate placental steroid production after day 50 to 60 of pregnancy. Navot (10) maintained steroid concentrations at supraphysiological levels. At the time of transfer, he increased the intramuscular P dosage from 50 to 100 mg/day. He then increased the P dosage by 25 mg/week to a maximum of 200 mg/day by week 8. The E_2 valerate dosage was increased by 4 to 6 mg/week until week 7, when the dosage reached 24 mg/day. In contrast to the described Australian (4) and Israeli (10) protocols, the Norfolk pregnancy maintenance protocol is highly individualized. Dosage adjustment is liberal and highly dependent on the measured serum steroidal concentration. The intramuscular P dose is maintained at 50 mg/day, rarely exceeding 75 mg/day. The E_2 (Estrace) dose has ranged from 3 to 10 mg/day. We have attempted to minimize the dosage of replaced E_2 in view of the observations in the rhesus monkey by Meyer (38) and Hodgen (39) which suggested that E_2 replacement might not be necessary in the primate. In our first ovarian failure pregnancy, however, we attempted to maintain the pregnancy with P injections alone; the E_2 levels remained between 10 and 30 pg/ml during the luteal phase. No attempt was made to appreciably increase the E_2 levels. Although the β-hCG titers were increasing properly for 7 days after pregnancy diagnosis, they soon began to drop in the ensuing week, finally decreasing to zero by week 6.

During a second established pregnancy in the same patient, E_2 rings were used for follicular phase E_2 replacement. Micronized E_2 was administered in a dosage of 3 mg/day during the luteal phase, increasing to 5 mg/day by week 7, then decreasing until week 12 of pregnancy to 1 mg/day, with discontinuation of Estrace by week 13. E_2 levels were maintained at 100 to 300 pg/ml, and endogenous placental E_2 began to rise during week 8 of gestation. Maintenance of a fixed steroid dosage allowed the assessment of the onset of endogenous E_2 production by the placenta. Extrapolation of the data from five of our donor oocyte pregnancies reveals that placental secretion of E_2 can be recognized by 7 weeks and that of P by 8 weeks of gestation (40). Navot (10) observed an E_2 surge during week 11 and began stepwise withdrawal of E_2 at that time. P appeared to rise during week 12 of pregnancy. Lutjen (7) reported earlier increases in steroid production, with withdrawal of steroids started on days 65 to 38 of pregnancy in two recent patients, respectively. Cessation of replacement was completed on day 80. In comparison, earlier patients required varied dosages for replacement, and steroids were withdrawn in the second trimester (4). It appears that, in the human, E_2 concentration requirements for implantation and early pregnancy maintenance may be less than previously used. Further investigations are needed to determine specifically the ideal E_2:P ratio necessary for implanation and pregnancy maintenance in the human.

Summary

There have been few published reports (6, 7, 10) of pregnancies after donation of in vitro fertilized oocytes. The Monash group has widely reported on their experience with ovarian failure patients who were treated with oral E_2 valerate and P vaginal suppositories. Lutjen reported six ongoing pregnancies after 28 embryo transfers (unpublished data). Approximately 60% of transfers were with fresh embryos, with the remainder constituting cryopreserved-thawed embryos. Navot (10) reported on two successful pregnancies in eight ovarian failure patients who were treated with oral E_2 and intramuscular P. Asch (41) reported on six clinical pregnancies in eight ovarian failure patients treated with orally administered E_2 and intramuscular P and treated by gamete intrafallopian transfer (GIFT). All cases of GIFT were performed on days 12 to 15. In Norfolk 18 pregnancies have resulted from 47 transfers of embryos to E_2- and P-replaced women (a 38.3% rate). Two pregnancies occurred from transfers with replacement by E_2 vaginal rings, whereas eight occurred after 15 transfers with oral E_2 (a 32.0% rate), and five occurred after nine transfers with transdermal E_2 (a 55.5% rate). Three other pregnancies have resulted from 10 transfers of in vitro fertilized donated oocytes during the natural cycle (a 30.0% rate), and two have resulted from transfer of cryopreserved-thawed concepti in four of these hormonally replaced cycles. The reported world IVF experience with donated oocytes is depicted in Table 12.1. An alternative to oocyte donation through IVF is the use of non-surgical recovery and transfer of concepti (Fig. 12.8). This procedure, which involves lavage of the donor uterus performed transcervically on days 5 to 7 after the donor's LH peak, was first described by Seed and Seed in 1980 (42). Success of the non-surgical recovery and transfer of in vivo fertilized ova must depend on the efficiency of concepti recovery and the consistency of synchronization in donor and recipient. Since Buster (1) used the natural cycle with its limitation of single embryo recovery, his efficiency was not optimal.

Table 12.1.
In Vitro Fertilization of Donated Oocytes: The World Experience[a]

Author	No. of Embryo Transfers	Days of Transfer (%)[b]	No. of Pregnancies (%)	No. of Viable Pregnancies
Rosenwaks (9)	21	17–19	8(38)	6(28.6)
Rosenwaks (9)	11	20–24	0(0)	0(0)
Lutjen (4)	31	16–18	6(19)	4(13)
Navot (10)	8	16–21	2(25)	2(25)
Levran[c]	27	17	10(37)	4(15)
Feichtinger (43)	4	17	1(25)	1(25)
Devroey (44)	31	—	3(9.7)	2(6.5)
Asch (41)	8	—	6(75)	

[a]Fresh oocytes only.
[b]First day of P administration is day 15. Day of spontaneous LH surge is normalized to day 14.
[c]Unpublished data.

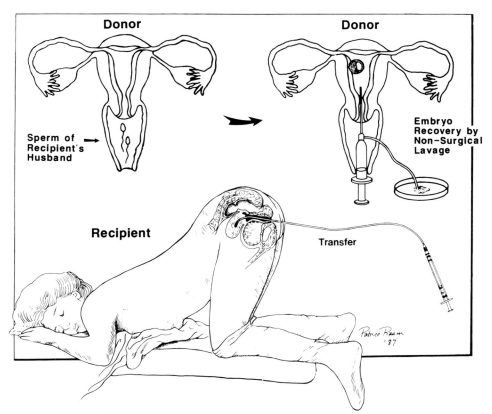

Figure 12.8. Schema for human in vivo fertilization. Lavaged embryos are transferred to synchronized donors.

Conclusions

Oocyte donation has extended our ability to treat women previously thought to be irreversibly sterile. The transfer of embryos into a defined endometrial environment continues to provide critical scientific information on the window of receptivity of the human endometrium. Although the quality of transferred embryos remains an enigma and confounds the interpretation of the data, our results strongly suggest that the window of transfer in the human for the 4- to 16-cell embryo extends from day 16 to day 19 of the idealized 28-day cycle. If one assumes that the 4- to 16-cell conceptus becomes a blastula within 2 to 3 days in vivo, it can be surmised that the window of implantation in the human does not extend beyond day 22 or 23 of the menstrual cycle.

E_2 and P replacement in ovarian failure patients allows assessment of the relative roles of these steroids in endometrial proliferation and differentiation. The transfer of defined, staged concepti into specific endometria has enabled the assessment of the window of implantation in the human. Clearly, precise manipulation of endometrial proliferation and differentiation by varying E_2 and P regimens in ovarian failure patients will allow the separation of endometrial from ovarian factors. The ability to manipulate the E_2 and P dosages during pregnancy in ovarian failure patients will precisely define the roles of these steroids in the establishment and maintenance of pregnancy.

A donor oocyte program, while being an exciting and gratifying treatment modality for infertility, has provided a unique human model for the study of conceptus, endometrial, and steroidal interaction. It may elucidate previously unapproachable questions of human reproduction and infertility.

References

1. Buster JE, Bustillo M, Thorneycroft IH, Simon JA, Boyers SP, Marshall JR, Louw JA, Seed RW, Seed RG: Nonsurgical transfer of in vivo fertilized donated ova to five infertile women: report of two pregnancies. Lancet 2:223, 1983
2. Bustillo M, Buster JE, Cohen SW, Thorneycroft IH, Simon JA, Boyers SP, Marshall JR, Seed RW, Louw JA, Seed RG: Nonsurgical ovum transfer as a treatment in infertile women: preliminary experience. JAMA 25:1171, 1984
3. Bustillo M, Buster JE, Cohen SW, Hamilton F, Thorneycroft IH, Simon JA, Rodi IA, Boyers SP, Marshall JR, Louw JA: Delivery of a healthy infant following nonsurgical ovum transfer. JAMA 251:889, 1984
4. Lutjen P, Trounson A, Leeton J, Findlay J, Wood C, Renov P: The establishment and maintenance of pregnancy using in vitro fertilization and embryo donation in a patient with primary ovarian failure. Nature 307:174, 1984
5. Trounson A, Leeton J, Besanka M, Wood C, Conti A: Pregnancy established in an infertile patient after transfer of a donated embryo fertilized in vitro. Br Med J 286:835, 1983
6. Rosenwaks Z, Veeck LL, Liu H-C: Pregnancy following transfer of in vitro fertilized donated oocytes. Fertil Steril 45:417, 1986
7. Lutjen PJ, Leeton JF, Findlay JK: Oocyte and embryo donation in IVF programs. Clin Obstet Gynaecol 12:799, 1985
8. Leeton J, Trounson A, Wood C: The use of donor eggs and embryos in the management of human infertility. Aust NZ Obstet Gynaecol 24:265, 1984
9. Rosenwaks Z: Donor eggs: their application in modern reproductive technologies. Fertil Steril 47:895, 1987
10. Navot D, Laufer N, Kopolovic J, Rabinowitz R, Birkenfeld A, Lewin A, Granat M, Margalioth E, Schenker JG: Artificially induced endometrial cycles and establishment of pregnancies in the absence of ovaries. N Eng J Med 314:806, 1986

11. Heape W: Preliminary note on the transplantation and growth of mammalian ova within a uterine foster mother. Proc R Soc Lond 48:457, 1890

12. Seidel GEJ Jr: Superovulation and embryo transfer in cattle. Science 211:351, 1981

13. Newcomb R, Rowson LW: Conception rate after uterine transfer of cow eggs in relation to synchronization of oestrus and age of eggs. J Reprod Fertil 43:539, 1975

14. Rowson LEA, Lawson RAS, Moor RM, Baker AA: Egg transfer in the cow: synchronization requirements. J Reprod Fertil 28:427, 1982

15. Beatty RA: Transplantation of mouse eggs. Nature 168:2995, 1951

16. Rowson LEA, Moore RM: Embryo transfer in the sheep: the significance of synchronizing oestrus in the donor and recipient animal. J Reprod Fertil 11:210, 1966

17. Hodgen GD: Surrogate embryo transfer combined with estrogen-progesterone therapy in monkeys: implantation, gestation and delivery without ovaries. JAMA 250:2167, 1983

18. Kreiner D, Droesch K, Navot D, Scott R, Rosenwaks Z: Spontaneous and pharmacologically induced remissions in patients with premature ovarian failure. Obstet Gynecol 72:926, 1988

19. Ethics Committee, American Fertility Society: Ethical considerations of the new reproductive technologies. Fertil Steril (Suppl 1):1s, 1986

20. Muasher SJ, Garcia JE, Rosenwaks Z: The combination of follicle-stimulating hormone and human menopausal gonadotropin for the induction of multiple follicular maturation for in vitro fertilization. Fertil Steril 44:62, 1985

21. Rosenwaks Z, Muasher SJ, Acosta AA: Use of hMG and/or FSH for multiple follicle development. Clin Obstet Gynecol 29:148, 1986

22. Rosenwaks Z, Muasher SJ: Recruitment of fertilizable eggs. In Jones HW Jr, Jones GS, Hodgen GD, Rosenwaks Z (eds): In Vitro Fertilization—Norfolk. Baltimore: Williams & Wilkins, 1986, p 30

23. Veeck LL, Maloney M: Insemination and fertilization. In Jones HW Jr, Jones GS, Hodgen GD, Rosenwaks Z (eds): In Vitro Fertilization—Norfolk. Baltimore: Williams & Wilkins, 1986, p 168

24. Veeck LL: Atlas of the Human Oocyte and Early Conceptus. Baltimore: Williams & Wilkins, 1986, p 314

25. Stumpf PG, Maruca J, Santen RJ, Demers LM: Development of a vaginal ring for achieving physiologic levels of 17 β-estradiol in hypoestrogenic women. J Clin Endocrinol Metab 54:208, 1982

26. Stumpf PG: Selecting constant serum estradiol levels achieved by vaginal rings. Obstet Gynecol 67:91, 1986

27. Droesch K, Navot D, Scott R, Kreiner D, Liu H-C, Rosenwaks Z: Transdermal estrogen replacement in ovarian failure for ovum donation. Fertil Steril 50:931, 1988

28. Ryan KJ, Engel LL: The interconversion of estrone and estradiol by human tissue slices. Endocrinology 52:287, 1953

29. Murad F, Haynes RC Jr: Estrogens and progestins. In Goodman AG (ed): Goodman and Gilman's Pharmacological Basis of Therapeutics, 7th ed. NY: Macmillan, 1985, p 1412

30. Campbell S, Whitehead MI: Potency and hepato-cellular effects of estrogen after different routes of administration. In van Keep PA, Utian W, Vermeulan A (eds): The Controversial Climacteric. Lancaster, England: MTP, 1982, p 103

31. Lutjen PJ, Findlay JR, Trouson AO, Leeton FJ, Chan LK: Effects on plasma gonadotropins of cyclic steroid replacement in women with premature ovarian failure. J Clin Endocrinol Metab 62:419, 1985

32. Craft I, Brinsden P, Serhal P: Ovum donation: a simplified and flexible approach using IVF or tube-sperm egg transfer (T-SET/GIFT). Presented at the Vth World Congress on In Vitro Fertilization and Embryo Transfer; Norfolk, VA 1987

33. Navot D, Anderson TL, Droesch K, Scott RT, Kreiner D, Rosenwaks Z: Hormonal manipulation of endometrial maturation: J Clin Endocrinal Metab 68:801, 1989

34. Anderson T, Coddington C, Shen M, Hodgen G: Defining the window of uterine receptivity: biochemical evaluation of the endometrium. Presented at the Fifth World Congress on In Vitro Fertilization and Embryo Transfer, Norfolk, VA, 1987

35. Jansen RPS, Turner M, Johannisson E, Landgren B-M, Dicfalusy E: Cyclic changes in human endometrial surface glycoproteins: a quantitative histochemical study. Fertil Steril 44:85, 1985

36. Wardle PG, Foster PA, Mitchell JD, McLaughlin EA, Williams JAC, Corrigan E, Ray BD, McDermott A, Hull MGR: Norethisterone treatment to control timing of the IVF cycle. Hum Reprod 1:455, 1986

37. Csapo AI, Pulkinnen KO, Wiest WG: Effects of luteectomy and progesterone replacement therapy in early pregnant patients. Am J Obstet Gynecol 115:759, 1973

38. Meyer RK, Wolf RC, Arsland M: Implantation and maintenance of pregnancy in progesterone-treated ovariectomized monkeys (*Macaca mulatta*). Presented at the Second International Congress of Primatology, Atlanta, GA, 1968

39. Hodgen GD: Managing ovarian response to gonadotropins: GnRH agonists versus antagonists. Presented at the IVth World Congress on In Vitro Fertilization and Embryo Transfer, Melbourne, Australia, 1985

40. Scott R, Navot D, Droesch K, Kreiner D, Liu H-C, Rosenwaks Z: A unique human in vivo model for studying early placental steroidogenesis and pregnancy maintenance. Presented at the 35th Annual Meeting, Society for Gynecologic Investigation, Baltimore, 1988

41. Asch RH, Balmaceda JP, Ord T, Barrero C, Cefalu E, Gastaldi C, Rojas F: Oocyte donation and gamete intrafallopian transfer in premature ovarian failure. Fertil Steril 49:263, 1988

42. Seed RG, Seed RW: Artificial embryonation—human embryo transplant. Arch Androl 5:90, 1980

43. Feichtinger W, Kemeter P: Pregnancy after total ovariectomy achieved by ovum donation. Lancet 2:722, 1985

44. Devroey P, Braeckmans P, Camus M, Khan I, Smitz J, Staessens C, Van Der Abbeel E, Van Waesberghe L, Wisanto A, Van Steirteghen AC: Pregnancies after replacement of fresh and frozen-thawed embryos in a donation program. In Feichtinger W, Kemeter P (eds): Future Aspects of Human In Vitro Fertilization. Berlin: Springer-Verlag, 1987, p 133

CHAPTER 13

Research on Spermatozoa in Assisted Reproduction

Part One—Spermatozoa Microinjection

SUSAN E. LANZENDORF, PH.D., AND GARY D. HODGEN, PH.D.

Medical indications for in vitro fertilization (IVF) have been extended to include the treatment of couples where male factor infertility is present. "Male factor" refers to the impaired fertilizing capacity of a male with one or more semen abnormalities. As discussed in Chapters 4 and 5, such abnormalities can include abnormalities of semen volume, liquefaction, sperm motility, sperm morphology and concentration, and the ability of sperm to penetrate eggs; the presence of antisperm antibodies in the semen; infection in the reproductive tract; and abnormal concentrations of biochemicals in the semen.

Because fertilization can occur in the presence of diminished numbers of motile sperm cells (1–4), IVF benefitted men selected for very low sperm concentrations. However, studies show that patients with less than 1.5×10^6 total sperm with rapidly progressive motility recovered by separation techniques do not achieve fertilization in vitro (5). Therefore, some male factor infertility patients may still have a basic semen quality level too low to achieve fertilization by the IVF procedure.

Other means of assisting these male factor infertility patients have been suggested. These include mechnical techniques such as the removal of cumulus cells from around the egg or the addition of enzymes that weaken the zona pellucida in an attempt to enhance egg penetration. Direct placement of a spermatozoon into the perivitelline space, bypassing the egg investments (zona pellucida and surrounding cumulus cells), has been attempted (6–9). The microinjection of a spermatozoon directly into the ooplasm has also been examined as a means of achieving fertilization and pregnancy (10–13).

Mammalian fertilization, whether it takes place within the female reproductive tract or within a laboratory dish, involves a specific sequence of processes, including: (a) binding of spermatozoa to the zona pellucida; (b) penetration of egg investments by the spermatozoon; (c) incorporation of the spermatozoon into the ooplasm; (d) activation of the egg to complete the second meiotic division; (e) transformation of the egg chromosomes and sperm nucleus to create the male and female pronuclei; and (f) syngamy, the pairing of the male and female chromosomes (14–17). It follows that an abnormality in one or more of these processes will result in a failure of fertilization to occur.

Extensive studies have been performed to examine the various semen abnormalities and to learn how they relate to failures in fertilization. Insufficient concentrations of motile spermatozoa may result in the failure of dispersion of cumulus cells, preventing contact between spermatozoa and the zona pellucida. Morphologically abnormal sperm are thought to be impeded in their passage through the cumulus oophorus (18). Sperm head anomalies, such as the absence of the acrosome (19) or postacrosomal sheath anomalies (20), are known to prevent both binding (21) and passage of spermatozoa through the zona pellucida and fusion with the egg plasma membrane. Therefore, impediments at the level of gamete interaction may prevent the successful penetration and subsequent fertilization of an egg by a spermatozoon.

This chapter will discuss both past and current research in the area of assisted IVF. Two major techniques are currently under investigation: (*a*) the microinjection of spermatozoa into the perivitelline space, and (*b*) the microinjection of spermatozoa into the egg cytoplasm. Both techniques are designed to bypass potential barriers to the fertilizing potential of some sperm types.

Microinjection of Spermatozoa: A Review of the Literature

MICROINJECTION OF SPERMATOZOA INTO THE PERIVITELLINE SPACE

To penetrate the zona pellucida, bound spermatozoa must first complete the acrosome reaction. The acrosome reaction is believed to be induced by sperm receptors located on the surface of the zona pellucida. During the acrosome reaction, fusion and vesiculation occur between the outer acrosomal membrane and the plasma membrane of the spermatozoon, resulting in the release of acrosomal enzymes. These enzymes, in combination with sperm motility, soften or dissolve the material of the zona pellucida, thereby aiding the spermatozoon in its passage. The spermatozoon passes through the zona pellucida and enters the perivitelline space. The two cells make contact; fusion of the spermatozoon and the egg plasma membrane takes place. Following this, the sperm head is incorporated into the egg cytoplasm (14).

Sperm-egg binding and fusion are thought to occur between the plasma membrane of the egg and the inner acrosomal and/or post-acrosomal region of the sperm (14). Therefore, during sperm penetration, the egg is interacting with a spermatozoon which has previously undergone the acrosome reaction, which exposes the sperm surface required for fusion.

The microinjection of spermatozoa into the perivitelline space has been studied as a means of increasing the fertilizing potential of spermatozoa of infertile males. In this technique a spermatozoon is injected beneath the zona pellucida into the perivitelline space in an attempt to enhance its proximity to the egg plasma membrane to allow normal fusion events. Should this procedure prove successful, it would eliminate the need for large numbers of motile sperm cells during fertilization in vivo or in vitro. In addition, this technique may result in fewer injuries to the egg when compared to the direct microinjection of a spermatozoon into the egg cytoplasm.

In 1985 Lassalle (6) microinjected motile spermatozoa into the perivitelline space of hamster eggs. In this study the penetration rate of the injected eggs was found to be low when fewer than five spermatozoa were injected beneath the zona pellucida of each egg. An elevated penetration rate was achieved when the number of spermatozoa injected was increased to between five and 12. The authors propose that the failure of some sperm to penetrate the injected eggs was due to the inhibition of the acrosome reaction. Increasing the number of sperm injected into the perivitelline space improved the probability of introducing a sperm capable of fertilization.

Using the same technique, Barg (8) microsurgically injected mouse spermatozoa beneath the zona pellucida of mouse eggs to study the relationship of sperm motility to gamete fusion and to evaluate the technique for future use in assisting fertilization in animals of impaired fertility. Samples of spermatozoa used were shown to be acrosome-reacted and were rendered immotile prior to their use. The results of the study suggest that immotile spermatozoa were incapable of fertilizing eggs following their insertion beneath the zona pellucida, even though they had undergone the acrosome reaction.

Metka (7) attempted this procedure in the human for treatment of male infertility. In this study human spermatozoa were microinjected into the perivitelline space of human eggs. The methods of sperm preparation were not discussed in this report. Of the nine eggs injected, one pronucleus formed in one egg, while development to the four-cell stage was achieved in another. No pregnancy resulted from this work.

More recently, Laws-King (9) reported the injection of a single human spermatozoon into the perivitelline space of human eggs, followed by confirmation of fertilization in 8 of the 19 eggs injected. Prior to injection, spermatozoa were induced to undergo capacitation by exposure to calcium-depleted medium containing strontium chloride, as previously reported by Mortimer (22). The treatment of spermatozoa in this manner is believed to increase the population of capacitated, and possibly acrosome-reacted, spermatozoa in the sample, thereby enhancing the chance of selecting a spermatozoon for microinjection which is capable of fusing with the egg. In addition, this study reports the injection of both normal, motile spermatozoa and non-motile but live spermatozoa. Successful fertilization of human eggs using spermatozoa without forward motility may suggest that motility is not a prerequisite to fusion between the egg and sperm, as previously reported (8).

These studies provide important information on the use of this technique for the treatment of infertility. The microinjection of a spermatozoon into the perivitelline space to achieve fertilization may assist those individuals with reduced motility or low sperm concentrations to fertilize eggs in vitro. These studies also demonstrate that merely injecting a spermatozoon beneath the zona pellucida does not insure fusion of sperm and egg, and subsequent penetration. It is now understood that use of this procedure requires the preselection of spermatozoa in terms of capacitation status and possibly even the acrosome reaction. Though this procedure bypasses such events as sperm passage through the cumulus mass, zona binding, acrosome reaction, and penetration through the zona pellucida, the remaining fertilization events, namely sperm-egg fusion and penetration of the egg, have to occur as during normal fertilization.

MICROINJECTION OF SPERMATOZOA INTO THE EGG CYTOPLASM

In the early 1900s, G. L. Kite first microinjected spermatozoa into the eggs of starfish. Although it is known that cleavage in the injected eggs did not occur, the complete results of the experiment were never published (23). Many years later,

Hiramoto (24) reported microinjecting live spermatozoa into the unfertilized eggs of sea urchins in an attempt to determine if spermatozoa can participate in fertilization without interaction between the sperm and egg membranes. Hiramoto worked under the assumption that the trigger of fertilization is transferred from the fertilizing sperm to the egg following its reaction with the egg surface. Using a self-designed microinjection device, he penetrated the surface membranes of the eggs with a micropipette and succeeded in injecting sperm directly into the egg cytoplasm. Successful penetration was measured by the direct contact of a spermatozoon with the cytoplasm of the egg. The spermatozoa injected into unfertilized sea urchin eggs exhibited no change; sperm head membranes remained intact and egg activation did not occur. Based on this information, the investigator concluded that the ''substance in the spermatozoon'' responsible for egg activation must directly react with the egg surface from outside the egg (24).

In addition, this study attempted the insemination of eggs before and after the injection of a spermatozoon into the egg cytoplasm. These results revealed a high percentage of polyspermic division in both groups. The author concluded that injected spermatozoa can participate in fertilization regardless of when the injection occurs, as long as the cytoplasm of the egg is in the activated state and the interaction of the spermatozoon itself with the egg surface is not necessary for it to participate in fertilization. Penetration of the inseminated egg by more than one spermatozoon was ruled out because the rate of polyspermy in control eggs injected with sea water was low following insemination. Although pronuclear formation by an injected spermatozoon was not demonstrated by this procedure, injected eggs were later found capable of undergoing normal fertilization and cleavage.

These results show that it is possible to penetrate the membranes of an egg without destroying its functional capacity. This observation in mammals was supported by the work of Lin (25), who showed that fertilized mouse eggs are capable of developing into living fetuses following membrane puncture and the injection of known amounts of bovine γ-globulin into the ooplasm. In this study the eggs were injected using an injection pipette with an outside diameter no greater than the head of a mouse spermatozoon. Control eggs underwent either no pipette puncture or puncture with no injection of fluid. Following treatment, all eggs were transferred to the oviducts of pregnant recipient females. The investigator reported that fetuses developing from injected eggs were frequently found to be smaller than their untreated littermates (in six of 32 cases compared to one of 19 control fetuses). No gross external abnormalities were observed in the fetuses undergoing the study treatment. A higher rate of degeneration following implantation was also observed in eggs following injection, even in eggs which had undergone puncture but not injection. It was concluded that mouse eggs at the pronuclear stage can survive membrane puncture and the injection of foreign material, although it appears that some decrease in viability may occur in these eggs.

In a study designed to investigate whether mammalian sperm cells or sperm nuclei can form male pronuclei following their injection, Uehara (26) microinjected hamster sperm nuclei, isolated by tissue homogenization, into unfertilized hamster eggs. Fresh, frozen-thawed, and freeze-dried human spermatozoa were also injected into hamster eggs to determine whether sperm nuclei can develop into pronuclei within the cytoplasm of an egg of another species and to determine the stability of sperm nuclei following various forms of storage. It was found that even without the egg and sperm interactions required for normal fertilization, eggs injected with both hamster and human sperm nuclei, regardless of prior storage conditions, were capable of undergoing resumption of meiosis with the successful formation of both male and female pronuclei. Exocytosis of the cortical granules in these eggs was also reported. These investigators concluded from this study that (*a*) the nuclei of mammalian spermatozoa are very stable, demonstrated by their ability to develop into male pronuclei following freeze-thawing or freeze-drying and mechanical disruption; (*b*) transformation of a sperm nucleus into a male pronucleus is not species-specific; and (*c*) surgical fertilization results in the activation of the eggs, as demonstrated by the exocytosis of the cortical granules, the extrusion of the second polar body, and the formation of the female pronucleus. It was also postulated that it was the mechanical stimulation of the injection pipette on the plasma membrane or egg cytoplasm which induced egg activation. This was later demonstrated when mature hamster eggs were "pricked" with a glass needle in an effort to induce activation (27). The results showed that activation occurred in approximately 80% of eggs thus mechanically stimulated, provided calcium ions were present in the medium and the size of the needle was large enough to provide adequate stimulation to the egg.

Still another study by these researchers (28) demonstrated that hamster sperm nuclei isolated from different regions of the male reproductive tract behaved differently following microinjection into hamster eggs. Hamster sperm nuclei were isolated from the testis caput and cauda epididymis, and injected into unfertilized eggs. Following an incubation time of 7 to 9 hours, it was observed that the sperm from all three groups decondensed within the eggs, regardless of whether the eggs were activated or not. The nuclei of testicular and cauda epididymal sperm were capable of forming pronuclei in activated eggs, while the nuclei of caput epididymal spermatozoa were incapable of pronuclear formation in activated eggs. The authors postulated that the failure of caput epididymal sperm nuclei to form pronuclei could be due to the presence of an inhibiting factor. This factor is absent from spermatozoa of testicular origin and is either inhibited or removed from spermatozoa in the cauda epididymis. It was noted that not all injected eggs were activated, and it was believed that activation was associated with adequate stimulation by the micropipette during the procedure. If the microinjection process failed to fully activate the egg, the formation of the male pronucleus from the decondensed sperm did not occur.

It is known that sperm pronuclei form only in mature eggs. To determine whether the sperm penetration seen during normal fertilization is required for sperm to respond to an egg undergoing maturation, Thadani (29) injected mouse sperm heads into rat eggs at the germinal vesicle stage (prophase I). These injected sperm heads remained in the condensed state until the germinal vesicle of the eggs had broken down, at which time they decondensed. Injected sperm nuclei did not form pronuclei in eggs undergoing maturation, a finding which replicated those reported for IVF of immature eggs. Because sperm nuclei fail to undergo decondensation until egg maturation occurs, it was concluded that substances released during germinal vesicle breakdown may be required for sperm decondensation and subsequent male pronucleus formation.

In a later study, Thadani (30) reported that the injection of the mouse spermatozoa into the cytoplasm of the rat egg results in activation of the egg, with the formation of both the male and female pronuclei, supporting the earlier work of Uehara (26). In addition a small percentage of the eggs fertilized by this procedure developed to the two-cell stage. The study also reported that capacitated and uncapacitated spermatozoa reacted alike following injection.

A study by Markert (31) reported no correlation between the phenotype (physical morphology) of injected mouse spermatozoa and their fertilizing capacity. Immotile and morphologically defective spermatozoa were found capable of decondensation and pronuclear formation within the egg. In addition, the ability of acrosome-reacted motile spermatozoa to decondense and form pronuclei was similar to that achieved when sonicated sperm heads (flagella and membranes removed) were used.

The injection of a sperm nucleus directly into the cytoplasm of the egg has also been used as a tool to study the biochemical aspects of fertilization. For example, to determine whether the proteinase (associated with sperm nuclei) is necessary for sperm decondensation, Perreault and Zirkin (32) treated sperm nuclei with proteinase inhibitors prior to their injection into hamster oocytes. The results demonstrated that these sperm nuclei were capable of decondensation and pronuclear formation, leading the investigators to conclude that if proteinase(s) is required for sperm decondensation, it must be supplied by the egg.

The sperm injection procedure has also been used to investigate whether sperm decondensation and pronuclear formation depend on the ability of the egg to reduce the disulfide bonds of the sperm nucleus (33). In this study mature hamster eggs were treated with iodoacetamide or diamide to inhibit or deplete glutathione. In these eggs no sperm decondensation was observed following injection. When sperm nuclei were treated in vitro to reduce the disulfide bonds and then microinjected into eggs treated with iodoacetamide or diamide, sperm nuclear decondensation did occur. In addition, germinal vesicle-intact and parthenogenetically activated pronuclear eggs were injected with untreated sperm nuclei and nuclei treated with dithiothreitol to reduce disulfide bonds. Untreated sperm nuclei were unable to decondense in these two groups of eggs, while the disulfide-poor sperm nuclei were capable of decondensation. These results support the belief that, following sperm penetration, the egg reduces the disulfide bonds of the sperm nucleus to achieve decondensation and that germinal vesicle-intact (prophase I) eggs and pronuclear eggs both lack the ability to effect sperm decondensation.

A variation of the sperm injection procedure has also been used to study biochemical reactions during egg activation (34). In this study an immunological analog to the human pregnancy-associated plasma protein-A (PAPP-A) was isolated and an antiserum produced. Guinea pigs injected with this antiserum to the PAPP-A analog did not conceive, indicating some type of contraceptive action. In an attempt to identify the site of action, the antiserum was applied in indirect immunofluorescent studies on the gametes and embryos of the golden hamster. Fluorescence staining was not demonstrated with intact gametes (eggs or sperm) or control samples. However, fertilized eggs from the pronuclear stage to the blastocyst were strongly fluorescent, suggesting that after fertilization, eggs may secrete stored antigen(s). To determine whether the ability of the egg to produce this antigen is a function of sperm penetration, hamster eggs were injected with a minute amount of culture medium, followed by gentle disruption of the cytoplasm to induce parthenogenic activation. After this treatment it was found that eggs exhibiting two polar bodies and a single pronucleus also demonstrated fluorescence, suggesting that release of the antigen is solely dependent on the mechanisms of egg activation.

The microinjection of human spermatozoa into hamster eggs has been performed to determine the ability of spermatozoa obtained from infertile individuals to react to an egg and participate in the early events of fertilization (10, 11). The spermatozoa studied had previously been incapable of penetrating zona-free hamster eggs in the sperm penetration assay or of fertilizing human eggs in vitro. The studies revealed that these spermatozoa are capable of decondensation and pronuclear formation following their direct injection into the cytoplasm of the hamster eggs. Therefore, the defect(s) in the spermatozoa of these individuals is restricted to fertilization events preceding successful incorporation of the spermatozoon into the ooplasm. These observations indicate that such defective sperm, once mechanically introduced into the egg, are able to participate in the subsequent events of fertilization.

The technique of sperm microinjection into the ooplasm may also be useful in circumventing various sperm abnormalities. An example of such a sperm population is the acrosomeless spermatozoon typically found in infertile men with ''round head syndrome,'' first described by Schirren in 1971 (35). The most evident malformation of these spermatozoa is the complete absence of both an acrosome and a post-acrosomal sheath. This sperm head abnormality is believed to be caused by the loss of the acrosome as it is forming during spermiogenesis (36). The most apparent reason then for the infertility of these individuals would be the inability of the spermatozoon to pass through the zona pellucida due to the absence of acrosomal enzymes. Studies have also shown that spermatozoa lacking both an acrosome and a post-acrosomal sheath are incapable of binding to and penetrating zona-free hamster eggs (37, 38). Because the acrosome reaction is thought to be a necessary prerequisite to sperm-egg fusion, the absence thereof may prevent normal fertilization, even of eggs stripped of their zonae pellucidae. It is also thought that sperm-egg fusion during normal fertilization is initiated between the egg plasma membrane and the inner acrosomal membrane and/or post-acrosomal region of the spermatozoon, regions which are absent from these spermatozoa (14, 16). Courtot (20) demonstrated that spermatozoa with postacrosomal sheath anomalies have a significantly decreased ability to bind and penetrate zona-free hamster eggs.

Using the technique of sperm injection into hamster eggs, it has been demonstrated that spermatozoa obtained from individuals with ''round head syndrome'' are capable of sperm decondensation and pronuclear formation following their direct microinjection into the egg cytoplasm (12). The diagnosis of round-head syndrome allows the clinician to determine the underlying cause of the infertility, but in this instance there is no known treatment or means of assisting the couple to achieve a pregnancy. The technique of sperm injection allows the investigator to bypass egg surface barriers and permits the study of the interaction of certain abnormal spermatozoa with an egg. These events have previously been difficult, if not impossible, to study. The findings of such experiments provide insight into future use of the surgical fertilization technique as a means of overcoming various forms of male infertility.

An initial evaluation of the clinical usefulness of this procedure in the human was attempted by the injection of human spermatozoa into human eggs (13). Following injection, eggs were cultured in vitro for a total of 13 hours and assessed for egg activation and pronuclear formation, followed by a more detailed evaluation with light and electron microscopy. The results demonstrated that human eggs are capable of surviving the mechanical insertion of a spermatozoon directly into the ooplasm. Eggs reacted to the microinjection as demonstrated by the resumption of the second meiotic division and formation of the male and female pronuclei.

Microinjection of Spermatozoa: Equipment and Methodology

Investigators in the IVF program at the Jones Instutitute for Reproductive Medicine have performed extensive preclinical evaluations of the sperm before the microinjection technique is used in the treatment of male factor infertility. The procedures discussed here are as previously reported (12, 13) and were adapted from the techniques described by Thadani (29) and Perreault (32).

EQUIPMENT

The microsurgical fertilization procedure requires an inverted microscope equipped with a micromanipulation system by which the very fine movements of the micropipettes can be controlled when handling the gametes. The experimental procedures performed in Norfolk use equipment obtained from Narishige USA, Inc. (Greenvale, N.Y.). Injection procedures are performed on a Nikon Diaphot inverted microscope with phase contrast optics (Image Systems, Inc., Columbia, Md.) (Fig. 13.1).

Micropipettes used in the injection of spermatozoa or sperm nuclei are prepared from thin-walled glass capillary tubes (Drummond Scientific, Broomall, Pa.; outer and inner diameters of 0.9 and 0.6 mm, length 150 mm) using a Narishige PB-7 micropipette puller and Narishige MF-9 microforge. The injection micropipette tips are opened by dipping them into 25% hydrofluoric acid, followed by washes in distilled water and acetone. The inside diameter of the microinjection pipette tip is 5 to 8 μm. Egg-holding micropipettes are prepared in a similar manner but with an inner diameter of approximately 20 μm. To achieve a smooth, blunt surface, the tips of the egg-holding pipettes are fire-polished using the microforge.

Control of suction and pressure in the injection and egg-holding micropipettes is achieved by air-tight Hamilton syringes fitted with polyethylene tubing connected to the micropipettes. Syringes and tubing are filled with heavy mineral oil.

Coarse positioning of the micropipettes is provided by two Narishige MN-2 three-dimensional manipulators mounted directly on the microscope. The very fine, controlled movements necessary for the microinjection procedure are performed with two Narishige MO-202 joystick hydraulic micromanipulators.

PREPARATION OF SPERMATOZOA AND SPERM NUCLEI FOR MICROINJECTION

Spermatozoa used for microinjection are often prepared by sonication to remove the sperm flagella before injection. Flagellar removal facilitates the handling of sperm during the procedure and permits the use of a smaller injecting pipette. Sonication also removes the outer membranes surrounding the sperm head, membranes which (with their associated enzymes) are required during normal fertilization for the penetration of the sperm through the zona pellucida. It is suggested that because sonication typically removes sperm membranes and because the injection procedure makes the penetration of the zona pellucida unnecessary, sonicated spermatozoa qualify as "functionally equivalent" to sperm which normally fertilize an egg (30). Previous studies support the fact that sonicated sperm, referred to as sperm nuclei, are capable of normal functioning in early development following injection (26, 31).

To obtain hamster spermatozoa, mature animals are sacrificed by cervical dislocation; the cauda of the epididymis is removed and rinsed in phosphate-buffered saline (PBS) to remove blood and debris. Holding the cauda epididymis under approximately 2.0 ml of PBS, each tube is minced, and sperm cells are dispersed into the medium. The sperm solutions are then sonicated by three 1-minute bursts at 30-W power output using a Kontes cell disrupter (Vineland, N.J.). Nuclei are isolated from the suspensions by a two-step filtration through columns of glass wool. The resulting solution containing the nuclei is divided into 0.1-ml aliquots and stored at $-70.0°C$ until just before use.

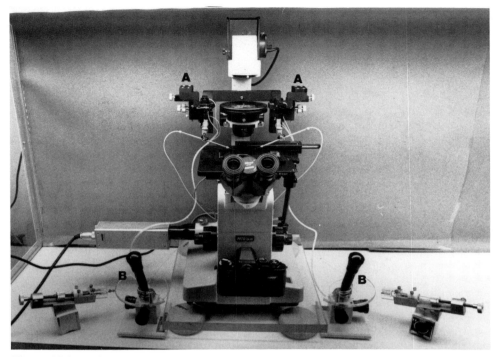

Figure 13.1. Microinjection is performed using a Nikon Diaphot inverted microscope equipped with two Narishige MN-2 three-dimensional manipulators (*A*) and two Narishige MO-202 joystick hydraulic micromanipulators (*B*).

Human semen samples, collected by masturbation, are allowed to liquefy at room temperature and then washed twice by centrifugation with PBS at 270 × g for 10 minutes to remove seminal plasma. The washed semen pellets are resuspended in 1.0 ml of PBS. Sperm cells then can be sonicated (two 1-minute bursts at 30-W power output) or used whole with tails and membranes intact. Nuclei are isolated from the sonicated suspensions, as previously discussed. Sperm suspensions, sonicated or whole, are divided into 0.1-ml aliquots and stored at −70.0°C until just before use.

Before microinjection, spermatozoa or sperm nuclei are diluted 1:5 volume/volume (v/v) with 10% polyvinylpyrrolidone (PVP; molecular weight, 90,000) in phosphate-buffered saline. The addition of PVP to the sperm preparation aids in the handling of the sperm during microinjection and coats the injection micropipette, preventing sperm from sticking to its inner surface during the procedure.

COLLECTION AND PREPARATION OF EGGS FOR MICROINJECTION

Most experiments at the Jones Institute have been performed using ovulated hamster eggs or excess donated human eggs. To obtain mature hamster eggs for surgical fertilization, female golden hamsters are superovulated by intraperitoneal injections of 25 IU of pregnant mare serum gonadotropin (PMSG) between 8:00 and 10:00 AM on day 1 of the animal's estrous cycle. Fifty-six hours following PMSG administration, the animals are given an intraperitoneal injection of 25 IU of human chorionic gonadotropin (hCG) to induce ovulation. Animals are sacrificed by cervical dislocation 15 to 17 hours post-hCG and the eggs harvested from the excised oviducts into TALP-HEPES medium (39). Cumulus cells are removed from the eggs by treatment with 0.1% hyaluronidase in TALP-HEPES medium under heavy mineral oil and incubated (37°C, 5% CO_2) prior to microinjection. Removal of the cumulus cells increases visibility for observation of the egg during the microinjection procedure.

Human eggs used in the microinjection procedure were typically obtained at the germinal vesicle-bearing stage. Eggs were cultured (37°C, 5% CO_2) in a modified (40) Ham's F-10 medium supplemented with 7.5% human fetal cord serum (HFCS) (Ham's F-10 + 7.5% HFCS) in vitro until extrusion of the first polar body, when the egg was said to be at the metaphase II stage of development (41). If necessary, cumulus cells were removed from eggs with 0.1% hyaluronidase in Ham's F-10 + 7.5% HFCS supplemented with HEPES buffer to give a final concentration of 10 mM.

MICROINJECTION OF SPERMATOZOA OR SPERM NUCLEI INTO EGGS

Microinjection is performed in a 50-μl drop of medium, buffered with HEPES to prevent rapid pH changes during the procedure. Drops of the prepared sperm suspensions in PVP are also placed inside the dish, and the dish is filled with heavy mineral oil to prevent evaporation (Fig. 13.2).

Mercury and a small amount of air are placed in the microinjection pipette to act as a pressure transducer and to increase the accuracy of control. Both the microinjection and egg-holding pipettes are attached to the tubing, and oil is introduced into the body of each micropipette by the controlled action of the syringes.

Just before the injection of an egg, the tip of the injection micropipette is snapped off inside the egg-holding pipette to create the sharp, bevelled point required for penetration of the zona pellucida and egg membrane. The injection micropipette is moved to the drop containing the sperm, and a single sperm is drawn into the tip of the micropipette. Both pipettes are then moved to the drop of medium containing the eggs. An egg is picked up and held securely by suction. The injection of the sperm is achieved by firmly pushing the injection micropipette through the zona pellucida and deep into the egg cytoplasm (Fig. 13.3). A small amount of cytoplasm is drawn into the micropipette and then released back into the egg along with the spermatozoon or sperm nucleus. The injection micropipette is withdrawn, and the egg is released from the egg-holder, washed, and cultured in the appropriate medium for the egg species being injected.

In the examination of microinjected eggs, an egg is said to be activated if the second polar body is extruded into the perivitelline space, an event occurring approximately 2 hours post-injection in the hamster. An egg is considered to be fertilized if two pronuclei form. Male and female pronuclei are typically visible. In the hamster, formation of male and female pronuclei is easily observed 4 hours after microinjection of the sperm nucleus (Fig. 13.4). Following a 6-hour incubation, successfully microinjected human eggs contain a second polar body. Formation of both male and female pronuclei can be observed in human eggs approximately 13 hours post-microinjection. To facilitate viewing, eggs can be slightly compressed beneath a coverslip supported at the corners with small amounts of a paraffin-vaseline mixture. Observation of all planes of the egg can be acomplished by gently pushing the edge of the coverslip, allowing the egg to be "rolled." If further evaluation of an egg is required, it can be fixed and stained. This is achieved by drawing the fixative, 2.5% glutaraldehyde in 0.1-M cacodylate buffer, beneath the coverslip, followed by the stain 1% aceto-lacmoid.

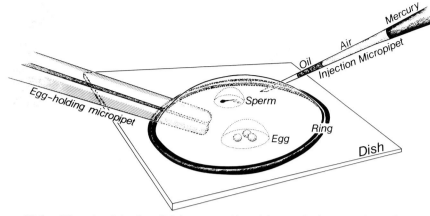

Figure 13.2. The microinjection dish is prepared by gluing an O-ring to a glass slide. A drop of medium is placed within the depression to contain the eggs during the procedure. A drop of the prepared sperm suspension is also placed within the well, which is then filled with heavy mineral oil.

Conclusion

Initial studies in assisted reproduction have advanced the feasibility of incorporating microinjection techniques into standard IVF use. The potential value of these procedures is obvious in the treatment of male factor fertility disorders.

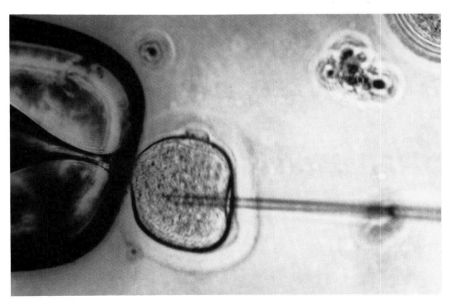

Figure 13.3. Phase-contrast micrograph of the microsurgical injection of sperm into the cytoplasm of a hamster egg ($\times 400$). (From Lanzendorf S, Maloney M, Ackerman S, Acosta A, Hodgen G: Fertilizing potential of acrosome-defective sperm following microsurgical injection into eggs. Gamete Res 19:329, 1988.)

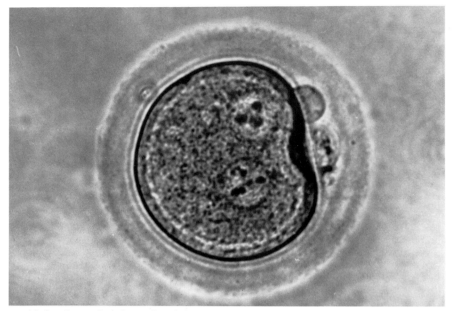

Figure 13.4. Pronuclear formation following microinjection of a hamster sperm nucleus into a hamster egg incubated for 4 hours. Male and female pronuclei and two polar bodies are visible (× 400).

Further studies may yield additional data on the relationships of sperm-oolemma contact, egg activation, sperm decondensation, and pronuclear formation, as well as the timing and completion of these events in the human. Results of studies such as these may be valuable in determining the future treatment and categorization of infertility. Knowledge thus obtained may serve the double purpose of developing a viable microinjection technique for clinical use and charting the early events of human fertilization at the intracellular level.

Scarcely 10 years ago, the ability to perform IVF in the human became a reality. Hundreds of infertile couples now have children because of a medical technology which assists in the process of fertilization. Although the techniques of assisted fertilization presented here are still in the early stages of research, the knowledge gained may one day assist both basic scientists in their understanding of fertilization and clinicians in their ability to assist the infertile.

References

1. Jones HW Jr, Acosta AA, Andrews MC, Garcia JE, Jones GS, Mayer J, McDowell JS, Rosenwaks Z, Sandow BA, Veeck LL, Wilkes CA: Three years of in vitro fertilization at Norfolk. Fertil Steril 42:826, 1984
2. Cohen J, Edwards R, Fehilly C, Fishel S., Hewitt J, Purdy J, Rowland G, Steptoe P, Webster J: In vitro fertilization: a treatment for male infertility. Fertil Steril 43:422, 1985
3. Battin D, Vargyas JM, Sato F, Brown J, Marrs RP: The correlation between in vitro fertilization of human oocytes and semen profile. Fertil Steril 44:835, 1985
4. Hirsch I, Gibbons WE, Lipshultz LI, Rossavik KK, Young RL, Poindexter AN, Dodson MG, Findley WE: In vitro fertilization in couples with male factor infertility. Fertil Steril 45:659, 1986

5. Van Uem JFHM, Acosta AA, Swanson RJ, Mayer J, Ackerman S, Burkman LJ, Veeck L, McDowell JS, Bernardus RE, Jones HW: Male factor evaluation in in vitro fertilization: Norfolk experience. Fertil Steril 44:375, 1985

6. Lassalle B, Courtot AM, Testart J: Fertilization of hamster oocyte by injection of human sperm in the perivitelline space. In Testart J, Frydman R (eds): Human In Vitro Fertilization, Actual Problems and Prospects. New York: Elsevier, 1985, p 209

7. Metka M, Harmony T, Huber J: Milkromamipulatorishe spermainjektion ein neur weg in der behandlung infertiler manner? Wien Med Wochenschr 3:55, 1985

8. Barg PE, Wahrman MZ, Talansky BE, Gordon JW: Capacitated, acrosome reacted but immotile sperm, when microinjected under the mouse zona pellucida, will not fertilize the oocyte. J Exp Zool 237:365, 1986

9. Laws-King A, Trounson A, Sathananthan, H, Kola I: Fertilization of human oocytes by microinjection of a single spermatozoon under the zona pellucida. Fertil Steril 48:637, 1987

10. Lanzendorf SE, Mayer JF, Swanson J, Acosta AA, Hamilton M, Hodgen GD: The fertilizing potential of human spermatozoa following microinjection into hamster oocytes. Abstract presented at the Vth World Congress on In Vitro Fertilization and Embryo Transfer, Norfolk, VA, April 1987

11. Lanzendorf SE, Maloney M, Rosenwaks Z, Hodgen GD: The fertilizing potential of human spermatozoa microinjected into hamster ova: a study of semen samples utilized for human in vitro fertilization (Abstract). Presented at American Fertility Society, 43rd Annual Meeting, September, 1987

12. Lanzendorf S, Maloney M, Ackerman S, Acosta A, Hodgen G: Fertilizing potential of acrosome-defective sperm following microsurgical injection into eggs Gamete Res 19:329, 1988

13. Lanzendorf SE, Maloney MK, Veeck LL, Slusser J, Hodgen GD, Rosenwaks Z: A preclinical evaluation of pronuclear formation by microinjection of human spermatozoa into human oocytes. Fertil Steril 49:835, 1988

14. Yanagimachi R: Mechanisms of fertilization in mammals. In Mastroianni L, Biggers JD (eds): Fertilization and Embryonic Development In Vitro. New York: Plenum, 1981, p 81

15. Austin CR: The egg. In Austin CR, Short RV (eds): Reproduction in Mammals: Germ Cells and Fertilization. New York: Cambridge University Press, 1982, p 48

16. Bedford JM: Fertilization. In Austin CR, Short RV (eds): Reproduction in Mammals: Germ Cells and Fertilization. New York: Cambridge University Press, 1982, p 128

17. Wassarman PM: The biology and chemistry of fertilization. Science 235:553, 1987

18. Krzanowska H: The passage of abnormal spermatozoa through the uterotubal junction of the mouse. J Reprod Fertil 38:81, 1974

19. Weissenberg R, Eshkol A, Rudak E, Lunenfeld B: Inability of round acrosomeless human spermatozoa to penetrate zona-free hamster ova. Arch Androl 11:167, 1982

20. Courtot AM, Escalier D, Jouannet P, David G: Impaired ability of human spermatozoa to penetrate zona-free hamster oocytes: is a postacrosomal sheath anomaly involved? Gamete Res 17:145, 1987

21. Kot MC, Handel MA: Binding of morphologically abnormal sperm to mouse zonae pellucidae in vitro. Gamete Res 18:57, 1987

22. Mortimer D, Curtis EF, Dravland JE: The use of strontium-substituted media for capacitating human spermatozoa: an improved sperm penetration method for the zona-free hamster egg penetration test. Fertil Steril 46:97, 1986

23. Lillie FR: Studies of fertilization. VI. The mechanisms of fertilization in arbacia. J Exp Zool 16:523, 1914

24. Hiramoto Y: Microinjection of the live spermatozoa into sea urchin eggs. Exp Cell Res 27:416, 1962

25. Lin TP: Microinjection of mouse eggs. Science 151:333, 1966

26. Uehara T, Yanagimachi R: Microsurgical injection of spermatozoa into hamster eggs with subsequent transformation of sperm nuclei into male pronuclei. Biol Reprod 15:467, 1976

27. Uehara T, Yanagimachi R: Activation of hamster eggs by pricking. J Exp Zool 199:269, 1977

28. Uehara T, Yanagimachi R: Behavior of nuclei of testicular, caput and cauda epididymal spermatozoa injected into hamster eggs. Biol Reprod 16:315, 1977

29. Thadani VM: Injection of sperm heads into immature rat oocytes. J Exp Zool 210:161, 1979

30. Thadani VM: A study of hetero-specific sperm-egg interactions on the rat, mouse, and deer mouse using in vitro fertilization and sperm injection. J Exp Zool 212:435, 1980

31. Market CL: Fertilization of mammalian eggs by sperm injection. J Exp Zool 228:195, 1983

32. Perreault SD, Zirkin BR: Sperm nuclear decondensation in mammals: role of sperm-associated proteinase in vivo. J Exp Zool 224:253, 1982

33. Perreault SD, Wolf RA, Zirkin BR: The role of disulfide bond reduction during mammalian sperm nuclear decondensation in vivo. Dev Biol 101:160, 1984

34. Sinosich MJ, Lanzendorf S, Bonifacia MD, Saunders DM, Hodgen GD: Immunofluorescent studies of pregnancy-associated elastase inhibitor (PAEI) expression by activated gametes and preimplantation hamster embryos (Abstract). In: 1988 Annual Program of the Society for Gynecologic Investigation

35. Schirren CG, Holstein AF, Schirren C: Uber die morphogenese rundkopfiger spermatozoen des menschen. Andrologie 3:117, 1971

36. Holstein AF, Schirren C, Schirren CG: Human spermatids and spermatozoa lacking acrosomes. J Reprod Fertil 35:659, 1973

37. Weissenberg R, Eshkol A, Rudak E, Lunenfeld B: Inability of round acrosomeless human spermatozoa to penetrate zona-free hamster ova. Arch Androl 11:167, 1982

38. Syms AJ, Johnson AR, Lipshultz LI, Smith RG: Studies on human spermatozoa with round head syndrome. Fertil Steril 42:431, 1984

39. Bavister BD, Leibfried ML, Lieberman G: Development of preimplantation embryos of the golden hamster in a defined culture medium. Biol Reprod 28:235, 1983

40. Veeck LL, Maloney M: Insemination and fertilization. In Jones HW Jr, Jones GS, Hodgen GD, Rosenwaks Z (eds): In Vitro Fertilization—Norfolk. Baltimore: Williams & Wilkins, 1986, p 168

41. Veeck LL: Morphological estimation of mature oocytes and their preparation for insemination. In Jones HW Jr, Jones GS, Hodgen GD, Rosenwaks Z (eds): In Vitro Fertilization—Norfolk. Baltimore: Williams & Wilkins, 1986, p 81

Part Two—Human Hemizona Attachment Assay

Assay

DANIEL R. FRANKEN, PH.D., LANI J. BURKMAN, PH.D., CHARLES C. CODDINGTON, M.D., SERGIO OEHNINGER, M.D., AND GARY D. HODGEN, PH.D.

The current high incidence of male factor infertility has promoted an intense search for reliable means to predict human sperm fertilizing potential in vivo and in vitro. For ethical reasons scientists and physicians have frequently hesitated to perform direct diagnostic functional assessments; that is, binding of human spermatozoa to intact viable human oocytes has usually been regarded as an inappropriate test (1). However, reliable and discriminating prognostic assays are needed to determine which infertile men are likely to achieve fertilization in vitro or in vivo.

Tight binding of human spermatozoa to the human zona pellucida is an early critical event in gamete interaction leading to fertilization. This binding step may provide unique information predictive of ultimate sperm fertilizing potential. Due to species specificity, human spermatozoa will bind firmly to no other zonae pellucida except the human (2). The feasibility of tight human sperm binding to the zonae pellucidae of non-living human oocytes was first examined by Overstreet and Hembree (1). Sperm binding and zona penetration were tested using oocytes recovered from postmortem ovarian tissue and later from ovaries removed for surgical indications (3). These studies, however, did not investigate the kinetics of zona binding or the specific relationship between the binding event and male fertility. Yanagimachi (4) showed that highly concentrated salt solutions provided effective storage of hamster and human oocytes which could then be used in sperm penetration assays.

We have developed a new sperm function assay based on the relative binding of patient versus control spermatozoa to the matching halves of a bisected human oocyte (5–8). This hemizona assay (HZA) assessed tight binding of sperm to the outer surface of the zona hemisphere. The HZA has three clear advantages: (*a*) the two halves (hemizonae) are functionally (qualitatively) equal zona surfaces, allowing a controlled comparison of binding; (*b*) the very limited number of recovered human oocytes is amplified, since an internally controlled test can be carried out on a single oocyte; and (*c*) ethical objections to possible inadvertent fertilization of a viable oocyte are eliminated by first cutting the egg into halves.

During the developmental stages, we first addressed the feasibility of cutting the zonae and then obtaining normal sperm binding. It was then imperative to examine the time-dependent pattern of sperm binding to the hemizonae and establishing an optimal assay protocol. The most recent work has methodically tested HZA results against known in vitro fertilization (IVF) outcomes for the same patients.

Sources, Storage, and Cutting of Oocytes for the HZA

All oocytes used in these studies were non-living, with no developmental potential. Oocytes were obtained from three sources: (*a*) ovarian tissue that was collected post-mortem; (*b*) ovarian tissue that was surgically removed; and (*c*) donated immature oocytes from the IVF treatment program. In the first two instances, the ovarian tissue was excised within 24 hours of death or surgery and stored at +4°C in phosphate-buffered saline (PBS; Gibco, Grand Island, N.Y.). Between 2 and 48 hours later, manual dissection was carried out following the protocol of Overstreet (3). Zona-intact oocytes denuded of granulosa cells were recovered and placed into capillary tubes containing a 2-M solution of dimethyl sulfoxide (DMSO) in PBS. The tube ends were sealed with Critoseal (Fisher Scientific, Springfield, N.J.) and immediately frozen at −70°C. DMSO-treated oocytes were stored for 1 to 6 months before use.

A smaller number of immature or non-fertilizable oocytes were donated by in vitro fertilization (IVF) patients (informed consent was obtained). Such oocytes had been collected by follicular aspiration following ovarian stimulation using exogenous gonadotropin for IVF therapy (9). Approximately 50% of these eggs were frozen in the DMSO solution on the same day they became available (24 to 48 hours after aspiration). The remaining eggs were stored briefly under oil (at +4°C) until they were cut by micromanipulation. These minor differences in handling had no discernible effect on hemizona performance in tight sperm binding. In later studies oocytes were placed in salt solution (4) within small plastic vials, each containing 0.5 ml of 1.5-M magnesium chloride (Mallinckrodt Chemical Works, St. Louis, Mo.) with 0.1% polyvinylpyrrolidone (PVP, MW 36000, Sigma Chemical Co., St. Louis, Mo.). All salt-treated oocytes were stored at room temperature. Salt storage is now our preferred method, as modified by Yoshimatsu (10) to include 40-mM HEPES in the salt solution for necessary buffering.

CUTTING THE OOCYTE INTO HEMIZONAE BY MICROMANIPULATION

The eggs were prepared for micromanipulation after retrieving them from the salt solution or thawing those eggs which were stored in DMSO. Both types of stored oocytes were rinsed in PBS and cut by micromanipulation into nearly equal halves—the matched hemizonae. The cutting was performed on the day before HZA testing. A complete micromanipulation system (Narishige, Tokyo, Japan) was used for bisecting the eggs. An inverted phase contrast microscope (Nikon Diaphot, Garden City, N.Y.) was equipped with a pair of Narishige micromanipulators (model MO 102). In most of the work, a number 11 microscalpel blade was glued to the side of a metal bar (12 cm long, 3 mm in diameter). The bar was bent to give a sigmoidal shape; the tip of the bar had a flat, vertical face for attachment of the blade. More recently a one-piece ophthalmological blade assembly was used (Beaver, no. 1767; Katena Products, Denville, N.J.).

A 100-ml plastic petri dish (Falcon No. 25362) served as the cutting chamber and was partially filled with any of several media supplemented with serum or albumin (Ham's F-10, PBS, etc.). The cutting blade was positioned at the center and bottom of the dish. The egg was then transferred to the working area of the dish using a finely drawn glass pipette. The oocyte was held at the tip of a special egg-holding pipette by gentle suction while the blade was centered over the egg. Alternatively, use of the egg-holding pipette could be avoided by first etching a shallow groove into the bottom of the dish and then positioning the egg over the groove by nudging it with the flat side of the cutting blade.

Using a total magnification of 200×, the blade was lowered slowly, until it rested on top of the egg. The egg was rolled slightly until the blade appeared to be centered over it. The blade was then lowered smoothly, first flattening the egg, and finally initiating a midline cut through the zona. A further lowering of the blade, along with one to two side-to-side excursions, produced two cleanly cut hemizonae (Fig. 13.5). The ooplasm inside was then dislodged by pipetting the hemizona through a small-bore tip. Each hemizona pair was placed in a separate 50-µl droplet of medium in a petri dish, covered with mineral oil (Fisher Scientific, Springfield, N.J.), and stored overnight at +4°C.

Sperm Handling in Preparation for the HZA

For all semen samples examined by the HZA, a basic semen analysis was performed using a computerized analysis system (CellSoft Semen Analysis System, Labsoft Division of Cryo Resources, Ltd., New York, N.Y.). Cytological assessment of sperm morphology was carried out, as detailed in Chapters 4 and 5.

In cases with extremely low sperm counts or decreased motility, the sperm concentration was calculated using a hemocytometer. Percentage of motility was assessed by scoring 100 spermatozoa per microscopic slide. The following parameters were evaluated: sperm concentration, percentage of normal motility, and percentage of normal morphology. Semen was classified as normal when (*a*) sperm concentration was >20 ×10^6 cells per milliliter; (*b*) sperm motility exceeded 40%, and (*c*) normal sperm morphology exceeded 14% according to the new strict criteria of evaluation described in Chapters 4 and 5.

An aliquot of semen (0.5 ml) was mixed with 1 ml of Ham's F-10 culture medium, supplemented with 7.5% heat-inactivated human fetal cord serum, then centrifuged (5 minutes, 300 × g). After a second wash the final sperm pellet was overlaid with 0.5 ml of Ham's F-10 medium and incubated (37°C, 5% CO_2 in air) to effect a "swim-up" separation of vigorously motile spermatozoa (11). After 1 hour the sperm supernatant was recovered and used for the HZA evaluations.

For the preliminary experiments described below, sperm droplets were prepared using a motile concentration of 0.1 × 10^6 to 0.25 × 10^6/ml. For all other HZA work we used 0.5 × 10^6 motile sperm per milliliter.

Preliminary Studies on HZA Feasibility

PRECISION OF ZONA CUTTING

Accuracy in producing matched hemizonae of nearly equal size was assessed for 12 cut oocytes (5). Bisecting of the zona by surgical micromanipulation showed small deviations from an exact 50:50 cut. When the sizes of matching hemizona halves were compared using a reticle, the mean difference in the depth of the concave hemizona shells was 10% ± 2.0% (mean ± SEM; median difference, 8.1%).

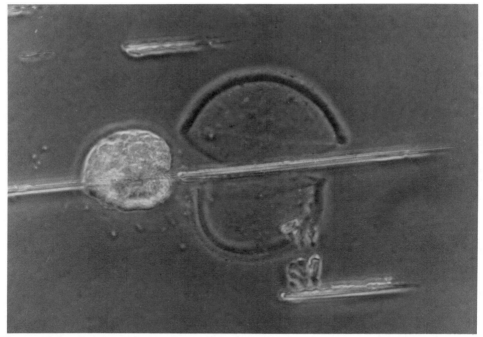

Figure 13.5.   Two matching hemizonae from a newly cut non-viable oocyte. The degenerated ooplasm has been pulled away from the hemizonae ($\times 200$).

USE OF THAWED POSTMORTEM OOCYTES VERSUS IVF ZONAE

The use of oocytes from postmortem tissue versus immature eggs from IVF did not significantly influence sperm binding potential of the zona pellucida (Fig. 13.6). After vigorous pipetting, the number (mean $\pm$ SEM) of firmly bound spermatozoa was not statistically different for the intact postmortem zonae (5.0 ± 1.9, $n = 6$) than for the intact IVF zonae (5.4 ± 2.1, $n = 7$).

SPERM BINDING TO INTACT VERSUS BISECTED ZONAE

During the developing stages of the HZA, we wished to test whether potential release of ooplasmic contents during cutting would alter sperm binding (5). In five experiments a 50-μl droplet of swim-up sperm (250,000 motile sperm per milliliter) was placed under oil. For each experiment one to two intact zonae and two to three hemizonae were placed in the sperm droplet. After 2 to 3 hours of coincubation, the total number of spermatozoa associated with the outer zona surface was first counted in the insemination droplet, *before* disturbing the intact eggs or hemizonae. Thus, sperm with loose association as well as those bound tightly were included. This approach seemed preferable, since it was not known whether the spherical intact egg versus the hemizona shell could be pipetted with the same shear force to remove loose sperm. For each experiment, therefore, a single pipette was used to vigorously rinse the intact eggs and hemizonae five times. For statistical comparisons between intact zona and hemizona, the number of hemizona attachments was doubled in each experiment. The number of sperm bound to the inner surface of the hemizona was also counted after rinsing.

Figure 13.6. Comparison of the intact zona of a *postmortem* egg versus the intact zona of an *IVF* egg with respect to the number of tightly bound (attached) sperm ($\bar{x} \pm$ SEM; number of zonae shown in parentheses).

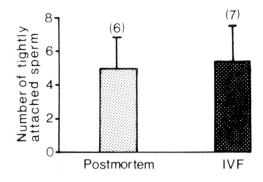

When assessed before pipetting, total sperm association (loose and tight binding) with the outer surface of cut hemizonae was not different from that observed for the intact zonae. When the total number of associated spermatozoa was doubled for all hemizonae, the means were not statistically different: hemizonae (57 ± 16, $n = 12$) versus the intact egg (64 ± 21, $n = 8$).

Some tight sperm binding occurred on the inner zona surface of the hemizona. Following rinsing, the mean number attached to the outer surface was 10.4 ± 5.1 ($\bar{x} \pm$ SEM) compared to 1.6 ± 0.8 on the inner surface ($n = 8$). We do not know the significance of this inner attachment (12).

SPERM BINDING TO MATCHING HEMIZONAE

During preliminary experiments we tested eight matched hemizona pairs using the sperm of five different men (5). The two matching hemizonae were exposed to equivalent sperm droplets from the same male. After 2 to 3 hours of coincubation, tight binding was assessed. Matching hemizonae showed no detectable difference in their capacity for tight sperm binding to the outer zona surface (3.5 ± 0.6 for one set of hemizonae versus 2.6 ± 0.4 for the matching halves).

Kinetics of Sperm Binding to Hemizonae: Establishing Optimal Assay Conditions

The literature contains no concrete information on the kinetics of human sperm binding to the zona pellucida. Therefore, we first clarified the time-dependent nature of tight binding to the zona in our in vitro HZA system.

The sperm of four known fertile men were coincubated with hemizonae for periods up to 8.5 hours (5). Two hemizonae were analyzed per time interval (duplicate testing). The hemizonae were assigned so that matching halves were used at different times, permitting comparison of sperm attachment over time for the same egg. All hemizonae began coincubation at the same time. After periods of 1, 2.5, 4, 5.5, and 8.5 hours, the hemizonae were removed to assess sperm binding. They were pipetted five times to dislodge loosely associated sperm, and the number of tightly bound sperm on the outer surface was counted. Care was taken to identify matching hemizonae for later statistical evaluation.

The spermatozoa of all men showed similar trends for binding to the hemizonae over the 8.5-hour period. The kinetic curves for two representative experiments are depicted in Figure 13.7, illustrating a high and a low binding pattern. As shown there, the differences in binding capacity between fertile men may reflect variability in the efficiency of sperm binding to the zona. Uniformly, tightly bound sperm were present on the hemizona surface within 1 hour of coincubation. The number ($\bar{x} \pm$ SEM) of bound sperm was 39.1 $\pm$ 12 (four men, nine hemizona pairs). In this study maximal binding occurred at approximately 3.5 hours for one man, at 4.0 hours for two others, and at 5.5 hours for the fourth donor. Interestingly, there was a consistent decline in the number of sperm tightly bound to the hemizonae at the first observation time beyond the binding peak. Thereafter, the number for tightly bound sperm remained almost constant through 8.5 hours.

The change in sperm binding over time between matching hemizonae was also assessed in this initial kinetics study. Paired data were analyzed for three coincubation intervals (1 vs. 4 hours, 2.5 vs. 5.5 hours, and 4 vs. 8.5 hours, with 4 to 6 hemizona pairs per interval). The paired data are illustrated in Figure 13.8. During the 1 vs. 4 hour interval, all binding slopes rose dramatically. The overall binding increase was 17.5 $\pm$ 4.4 sperm per hour ($\bar{x} \pm$ SEM).

CHARACTERIZATION OF THE SPERM BINDING PATTERN DURING THE FIRST 4 HOURS OF COINCUBATION

Data above on the kinetics of sperm binding indicated the need for more detailed information on the early coincubation period, specifically the 1- to 4-hour interval. For each experiment (five different fertile males studied), one sperm droplet was prepared under oil and two matching hemizonae were added (5). Coincubation was briefly interrupted at the end of 1, 2, 3, 4, and 5.5 hours, with a final reading of tightly bound sperm numbers at 8.5 hours. At these times the two hemizonae were quickly recovered and placed in a warm droplet of rinsing medium (Ham's F-10) under oil. The sperm dish was immediately returned to the incubator, and the hemizonae were rinsed five times to dislodge loosely associated spermatozoa before counting. During the counting, the microscopic stage area was warmed (35°C to 37°C) using a stream of air (Arenberg Sage Air Curtain Incubator, model 279, Forma Scientific, Jamaica Plain, Mass.). After determining the number of sperm bound to the outer surface, the matched pair was then transferred back to the original sperm drop for further coincubation. The counting procedure was carried out during the final 10 minutes of each assessment interval. All rinsing and counting steps were performed by a single investigator.

Representative sperm binding curves from three of six experiments are shown in Figure 13.9. In all six experiments, the means for the matched pairs of hemizonae revealed a consistent peak in sperm binding after about 4 hours of coincubation. Longer incubation showed a slight decline through 8.5 hours. Importantly, by the use of frequent counts, our observations typically revealed a nearly linear increase in tight sperm binding between 1 and 4 hours.

Reproducibility of binding for matched hemizonae was high. In five of the six cases, differences between paired hemizonae ranged from 8% to 20% for the number of sperm bound at 4 hours. The paired curves showed very similar slopes for the rising phase of sperm binding.

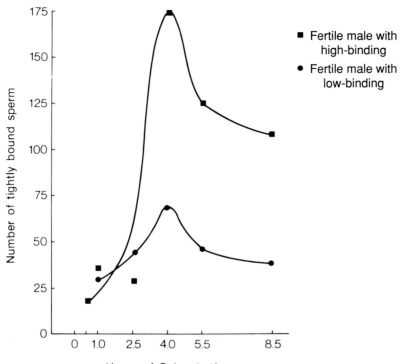

Figure 13.7. The kinetics for tight binding of sperm from fertile men to the hemizonae of different eggs during coincubation of 1 through 8.5 hours; representative curves for a high-binding male (*closed boxes*) versus a low-binding male (*closed circles*) ($\bar{x} \pm$ SEM).

The data were then pooled across all six experiments; the mean number of sperm bound ($\bar{x} \pm$ SEM) at each hour was calculated. For the observations made at 1, 2, 3, 4, 5.5, and 8.5 hours, the respective pooled values were 13.9 ± 6, 33.3 ± 11, 63.5 ± 34, 94.9 ± 49, 88.2 ± 42, and 79.6 ± 40. The calculated 95% confidence interval (13) (two-tailed test, $df = 11$) for the 4-hour data was 60.3 to 128.5 tightly bound sperm. These values compare well with the matching 4-hour confidence interval from our first kinetics study (75.4 to 122.5).

The kinetics of binding for hemizonae which were obtained from ooctyes stored in salt solution (1.5-M MgCl$_2$) for 6, 15, and 30 days were reexamined (6). These data were necessary to validate the use of salt-stored oocytes for the HZA, compared to the original DMSO storage method described above. In each experiment two sperm droplets were prepared under oil. Two matching salt-treated hemizonae were added to one droplet, while two matching hemizonae treated with DMSO were placed in the other sperm drop. The sperm were obtained from two men with normal semen parameters who had both fathered a child naturally. As with the study described above, coincubation was briefly interrupted at the end of 1, 2, 3, 4, and 5.5 hours, with a final reading at 8.5 hours.

The resulting salt-kinetics data are represented in Figure 13.10 (6 days of zona storage), Figure 13.11 (15 days), and Figure 13.12 (30 days). Each curve represents the average number of spermatozoa bound to one of two matching hemizonae from one oocyte, one stored in the salt and one in the DMSO solution. In each kinetic experiment, a nearly linear binding curve was again observed during the first 4 hours of coincubation.

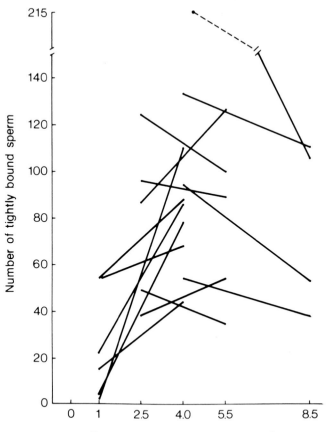

Figure 13.8.   Time-dependent changes in binding of spermatozoa from fertile men when matched hemizonae pairs were evaluated over three intervals in the kinetics study.

Uniformly, binding was maximal after about 4 hours, followed by either a plateau or a slow decline. These results suggest that there was little effect of storage duration (6 to 30 days) on the functioning of the zonae for HZA studies.

Clinical Relevance of HZA Results

BINDING OF SPERMATOZOA FROM PROVEN INFERTILE PATIENTS

Ten experiments were performed comparing the hemizona binding capacity for the sperm of eight known fertile men versus eight husbands who had not achieved fertilization of their wives' eggs during one or more IVF treatments (5). Spermatozoa from the eight infertile men exhibited extremely abnormal morphology (''poor'' prognosis group), as assessed with the highly selective Kruger method detailed in Chapters 4 and 5. The semen from all 16 men had a sperm concentration exceeding 28×10^6/ml. Eleven had a percentage of motility >37%; five of the unsuccessful IVF patients had motility ≤37%. In each experiment one-half of the hemizona pair was placed with the sperm from a fertile man, while the matching hemizona was coincubated with sperm from a previously

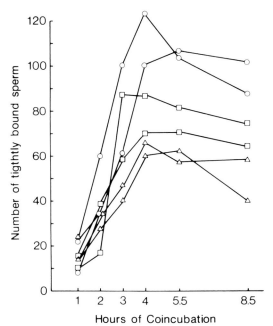

Figure 13.9. Tight sperm binding to matching hemizonae pairs for three fertile males ($\bar{x} \pm$ SEM). In each assay the same hemizona pair was used to evaluate sperm binding at all time points indicated. *Circles*, matching hemizonae for male A. *Boxes*, matching hemizonae for male B. *Triangles*, matching hemizonae for male C.

unsuccessful IVF husband. The standard HZA protocol was followed for zona insemination (0.5×10^6 motile sperm per milliliter), duration of coincubation, and counting of bound spermatozoa.

DEVELOPMENT OF THE HZA INDEX

Within each experiment objective comparisons of the matching hemizona data were made possible by calculating the ratio for the HZA index of tightly bound sperm:

$$\text{HZA index} = \frac{\text{Number of sperm bound from infertile male} \times 100}{\text{Number of sperm bound from fertile male}}$$

Using matched hemizona pairs in all 10 experiments, the spermatozoa from known fertile men bound to the hemizona more efficiently than sperm from IVF husbands who had not achieved fertilization of their wives' eggs in vitro (Table 13.1). For this limited patient group, the mean value for the HZA index was 21 ± 8 ($\bar{x} \pm$ SEM), and 95% of the individual values fell below 62. These preliminary observations are insufficient for the firm identification of an index threshold. However, these data suggested 62 as a tentative threshold, such that lower HZA indices may be prognostic of very low to nil fertilizing potential. The overall number ($\bar{x} \pm$ SEM) of sperm bound was significantly different for the two groups tested (34.0 ± 8.1 (fertile) versus 5.9 ± 2.3 (infertile); $P<0.01$).

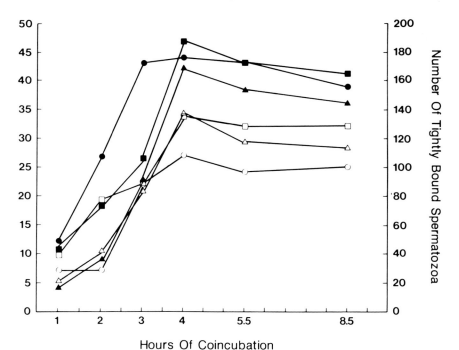

Hours Of Coincubation

Figure 13.10. The number of fertile spermatozoa which bound to hemizonae from oocytes stored in DMSO or stored in salt solution for 6 days. Each curve represents mean binding for two matching hemizonae.

RELATIONSHIP TO NORMAL SPERM MORPHOLOGY

In several of our studies, the influence of sperm morphology on tight zona binding was assessed. In each case the published methods of Kruger were followed for the preparation of slides and subsequent scoring. These methods are presented in detail in Chapters 4 and 5. A brief summary here will indicate the basic methodology we used.

After liquefaction was completed, slides were carefully prepared for later morphological assessment. The slides were stained using Diff Quik (American Scientific Products, McGraw Park, Ill.) according to the technique of Kruger (14). Slides were air-dried at room temperature, fixed for 12 seconds with Diff Quik fixative (1.8 mg/liter triarylmethane in methyl alcohol), then stained with Diff Quik solution number 1 (1g/liter xanthene in a sodium azide-preserved buffer) for 12 seconds. Finally, the slides were exposed for 8 seconds to Diff Quik solution number 2 (0.625 g/liter azure A and 0.625 g/liter methylene blue in buffer). Coverslips were mounted immediately after staining and later scored by the same investigator within each study. Spermatozoa were considered to have perfectly normal morphology when the head shape, head dimensions, acrosomal surface area, and cystoplasmic droplet size all adhered to the published criteria.

Using these strict criteria for normal morphology, all semen samples were assigned to one of three groups: (*a*) the poor morphology group, with <4% normal spermatozoa; (*b*) the borderline morphology group, with 4% to 14% normal spermatozoa; and (*c*) the normal morphology group, with >14% perfectly normal spermatozoa (15).

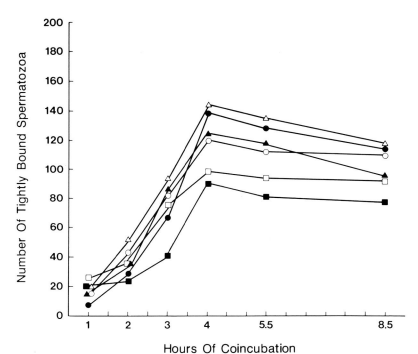

Figure 13.11. The number of fertile spermatozoa which bound to hemizonae from oocytes stored in DMSO or stored in salt solution for 15 days. Each curve represents mean binding for two matching hemizonae.

RELATIONSHIP TO NORMAL SEMEN COMPARED TO SUBNORMAL SEMEN

During an initial investigation of alternative egg storage methods, we compared the HZA data obtained for men with normal semen characteristics to data for patients with semen of subnormal quality. In each experiment one salt-treated oocyte and one DMSO-treated oocyte were used simultaneously.

Subnormal semen was typically characterized by low values for percentage of motility and/or sperm morphology. The first study used the semen of six men in the normal group (two men were used twice) and the semen of eight selected men who comprised the subnormal group. For these two semen groups, the means for sperm concentration were not different ($P > 0.05$). However, the percentage of motile sperm was significantly lower in the subnormal group (22.8% versus 56.6%; $P < 0.001$), as were the percentage of sperm with excellent morphology (7.6% versus 21.8%; $P < 0.01$) and the linear swimming velocity (30.6 versus 39.6 μm/sec; $P < 0.01$).

Matching hemizona pairs were prepared from oocytes that were stored in either DMSO (1 to 6 months) or salt solution (6, 15, and 30 days). Hemizona pairs were obtained from three oocytes stored in salt for 6 days, three oocytes stored for 15 days, and two oocytes stored for 30 days. In each experiment one DMSO-stored oocyte provided a pair of control hemizonae. Thus two dishes were prepared per experiment, one for salt-treated hemizonae and the second for DMSO-treated hemizonae, each containing two sperm droplets (100 μl). After 4 hours the hemizonae were removed and rinsed

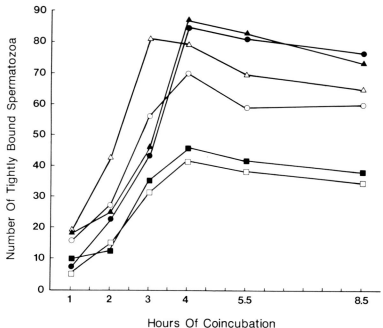

Figure 13.12.   The number of fertile spermatozoa which bound to hemizonae from oocytes stored in DMSO or stored in salt solution for 30 days. Each curve represents mean binding for two matching hemizonae.

before the bound sperm on the outer surface were counted. The same rinsing pipette was used for all hemizonae in a given experiment.

When an index value of 62 is taken as the threshold for identifying patients at risk for IVF failure, only assay number 6 showed discordant index results. In seven of the eight assays, therefore, the salt and DMSO indices were in agreement, either both above

Table 13.1.
Number of Sperm Tightly Bound to Pairs of Matched Hemizonae after 4 Hours of Coincubation: Proven Fertile Men versus Infertile Men

	Number of Tightly Bound Sperm		
Experiment No.	Infertile Men	Fertile Men	HZA Index[a]
1	20	64	31
2	10	16	63
3	0	10	0
4	17	28	61
5	0	17	0
6	3	35	9
7	2	44	5
8	0	90	0
9	4	15	27
10	3	21	14

[a]HZA index = (Infertile × 100)/Fertile.

the 62 threshold or both below it. Statistical comparison of the two sets of index values was carried out by two methods: (*a*) Spearman's rank correlation ($r = 0.88$; $P < 0.001$), and (*b*) the signed rank test ($P < 0.05$). The mean number of bound sperm was significantly higher ($P < 0.01$) for the normal semen group than for the sperm from subnormal semen, regardless of the storage method. The HZA index was also calculated for all matching hemizona pairs. Table 13.2 shows that hemizonae from oocytes stored in salt solution exhibited an equivalent capacity for tight binding of spermatozoa when compared to DMSO-treated hemizonae. The data demonstrate that the hemizonae from salt-stored eggs effectively distinguished between the normal and the subnormal semen samples.

RELATIONSHIP TO IVF RESULTS IN A BLIND STUDY

This study was designed to compare HZA results with IVF outcome. The principal objectives of the study included (*a*) comparing the number of sperm bound to the hemizonae for patients with and without fertilization during IVF; (*b*) examining the influence of sperm morphology on hemizona binding potential; and (*c*) investigating any statistical correlation between zona binding and basic sperm characteristics (seminal sperm concentration, percent of motility, and sperm morphology).

All patients selected for this study had demonstrated a seminal sperm concentration $\geq 20 \times 10^6$/ml, with a percentage of motile sperm ≥ 30. Semen was classified as normal if, in addition, the morphological assessment adhered to the criteria of Kruger (15). Nine other control males were proven fertile, had normal semen parameters, and had been tested previously in the HZA.

Among the 36 IVF patients, seven men had previously shown normal semen profiles; the remaining 29 had teratozoospermia, that is, $< 14\%$ morphologically normal spermatozoa according to the Kruger criteria. All patients exhibited normal plasma endocrine profiles (follicle-stimulating hormone (FSH), luteinizing hormone (LH), prolactin, testosterone, and estradiol). Each IVF couple had also been evaluated for the presence of antisperm antibodies in the semen or in the female serum (16). No patients with immunological problems were included in the study. Data were compiled for preovulatory oocytes only (metaphase I and II); all patients had at least one preovulatory oocyte for insemination. For oocyte insemination a concentration of 500,000 motile spermatozoa per milliliter was used for 17 of the 36 cases. This insemination concentration varied from 0.5×10^6 to 1×10^6 motile spermatozoa per milliliter for the other 19 cases. Seven of these 36 patients had been preselected to serve as controls within the HZA.

All patients were asked to provide a second semen sample for the HZA at 48 hours after insemination of the oocytes. Personnel performing the HZA had no prior knowledge of the patients' clinical history or the IVF outcome. These specimens were analyzed for sperm concentration, percentage of motility, sperm velocity, and percentage of sperm with normal morphology.

Twenty HZAs were performed using sperm from the 36 patients. For each assay one fertile patient with previously normal semen served as the control and was tested against one patient having previously abnormal semen (7). One 50-μl droplet of the sperm suspension (0.5×10^6 motile sperm per milliliter) was placed in a petri dish under oil. In each experiment one hemizona was placed in a droplet with subnormal sperm, while the matching hemizona was incubated with a droplet of control sperm. After 4 hours, rinsing and counting were carried out as normal.

Table 13.2.

Sperm Binding at 4 Hours for Hemizonae from Oocytes Exposed to Two Different Storage Treatments[a]

Assay No.	Salt-Stored			DMSO-Stored		
	Normal (no. bound)	Subnormal (no. bound)	HZA Index[b]	Normal (no. bound)	Subnormal (no. bound)	HZA Index[b]
1[c]	33	32	97	23	32	139
2	49	34	69	30	32	107
3	33	0	0	18	0	0
4[c]	37	10	27	56	5	9
5	118	15	13	120	12	10
6	88	60	68	89	21	24
7[c]	28	18	64	28	26	93
8	46	2	4	29	4	14
Mean ± SEM	$54.0^{d,e} \pm 12.3$	$21.3^{f} \pm 7.6$		$49.1^{d,e} \pm 14.1$	$16.5^{f} \pm 4.9$	

[a]Eight experiments used one salt-stored (6, 15, 30 days) and one DMSO-stored oocyte for simultaneous HZA. In every experiment sperm suspensions from both normal and subnormal semen were incubated with half of a matched hemizona pair.

[b]The correlation coefficient (Spearman's rank) = 0.88 ($P < 0.001$). Also, $P > 0.05$ for the paired signed rank test.

[c]The duration of salt storage was 6 days for oocytes in assays 1–3, 15 days for assays 4–6, and 30 days for assays 7 and 8.

[d]For both treatments, binding of normal sperm was significantly greater than binding of subnormal sperm to the hemizonae ($P < 0.03$).

[e]Mean values were not statistically different ($P = 0.32$; paired T test).

[f]Mean values were not statistically different ($P = 0.37$; paired T test).

The data for sperm binding to the hemizonae were first analyzed after assigning all IVF patients to one of two groups: the IVF fertilization group ($\geq$ one oocyte fertilized) or the IVF failure group (0% fertilization). Spermatozoa from patients in the fertilization group showed an enhanced capacity for tight binding to the hemizonae. The mean number ($\pm$ SEM) of bound sperm was significantly greater ($P < 0.05$) than the mean for the failure group (36.1 $\pm$ 7 versus 10.4 $\pm$ 4, respectively).

The mean percentage for strictly normal morphology (Kruger method) differed significantly ($P < 0.05$) between the two groups (12.7 $\pm$ 1.5 versus 3.2 $\pm$ 0.9; $P < 0.05$). The mean data for sperm concentration and percent of motility showed no significant differences (Table 13.3). However, clearly oligozoospermic or asthenozoospermic patients had already been excluded from this study. For comparison, the corresponding seminal data for the nine proven fertile controls were sperm concentration ($87.2 \times 10^6 \pm 18$ spermatozoa per milliliter), percent of motility (57.3 $\pm$ 4), and percentage of sperm with normal morphology (26.4 $\pm$ 7). None of these fertile control values was statistically greater than the IVF fertilization group data in Table 13.3 ($P > 0.05$).

The data were also analyzed using a second approach, in which the 36 IVF cases were assigned to three new groups according to the percentage of strictly normal spermatozoa in the semen (Kruger method): (a) the normal morphology group ($n = 7$); (b) the borderline morphology group ($n = 14$); and (c) the poor morphology group ($n = 15$). The mean values for these semen parameters are presented in Table 13.4.

Table 13.3.
Number of Sperm Which Bound Tightly to Hemizonae during HZA and Corresponding Semen Parameters[a]: IVF Fertilization Group versus IVF Failure Group

Parameter	Fertilization Group (n = 27)	Failure Group (n = 9)
HZA: no. of tightly bound sperm[b]	36.1 ± 6.8	10.4 ± 3.6[c]
% Normal morphology[d]	12.7 ± 1.5	3.2 ± 0.9[c]
Sperm concentration (× 10^6ml)	74.2 ± 10.0	54.8 ± 7.8
% Motility	45.2 ± 4.0	33.3 ± 6.2

[a]Mean ± SEM.
[b]Based on the method of Burkman (5).
[c]Mean is significantly less than the value for the fertilization group ($P<0.05$).
[d]Based on the method of Kruger (14, 15).

For the nine proven fertile men, tight binding in the HZA was statistically greater ($P<0.05$) than the mean for the poor morphology group (43.8 ± 12 versus 20 ± 7, respectively). However, the value for the proven fertile men did not differ significantly from the mean for either the normal or the borderline morphology group. The borderline group demonstrated an intermediate capacity for binding to the hemizonae; the mean was not significantly different from the data for the two other groups.

Further insight into sperm factors that might be linked to zona binding was sought by evaluation of between-factor correlations. Pearson correlation coefficients were obtained for a matrix with 17 parameters. Significant linear relationships were observed between the number of sperm tightly bound to the hemizona and (a) the percentage of motile sperm in semen ($P<0.0001$); (b) the percentage of seminal sperm with strictly normal morphology ($P<0.001$); and (c) the seminal sperm concentration per milliliter ($P<0.01$). In a second blind study (8), the principal findings above were confirmed when the HZA used control spermatozoa from men who were recent fathers after natural conception. In brief, tight sperm binding to the hemizonae average 64.4 for the controls compared to 57.0 (p>0.05) for IVF patients with normal semen characteristics and 12.8 ($P=0.05$) for IVF patients with subnormal semen. Mean binding was significantly greater (58.6) for IVF cases with ≥75% fertilization of mature oocytes than for those cases with poor or failed fertilization after IVF (mean binding = 6.0; $P<0.05$). Based on the HZA index values for 17 experiments, the HZA accurately predicted IVF results in 13 of 17 cases (three other cases were equivocal, and one gave a false negative result).

Discussion and Future Developments

We have shown that binding of sperm to hemizonae was significantly greater for men who succeeded in fertilization during IVF than in men who did not. Based on the group data, tight binding of spermatozoa to hemizonae correlated well with IVF performance. Our findings demonstrate no significant differences in sperm binding function when using hemizonae that were treated with high salt versus DMSO during storage. Furthermore, the kinetics of sperm binding were essentially the same regardless of the oocyte storage.

Abnormal sperm morphology is known to be a significant factor in failed fertilization. Semen specimens that were classified as morphologically poor by the strict Kruger

Table 13.4.

Number of Sperm Which Bound Tightly to Hemizonae during the HZA and Semen Parameters[a] for Three IVF Patient Groups Classified by Percentage of Sperm with Strictly Defined Morphology

Morphology Group	HZA: No. of Tightly Bound Sperm[b,c]	Concentration ($\times 10^6$ml)	Motility (%)	Percentage of Normal Morphology[d]
Normal[e] ($n = 7$)	$46.4 \pm 11^*$	$108.0 \pm 14^†$	57.0 ± 5	$18.2 \pm 1^{‡,§}$
Borderline[f] ($n = 14$)	31.7 ± 11	$48.0 \pm 9^†$	39.0 ± 7	$8.1 \pm 1^§$
Poor[g] ($n = 15$)	$20.0 \pm 7^*$	74.0 ± 15	37.3 ± 4	$1.4 \pm 0.3^‡$

[a]Mean $\pm$ SEM.
[b]Symbols: *, †, ‡, §. Values carrying the same superscript symbol are significantly different from each other ($P < 0.05$).
[c]Based on the method of Burkman (5).
[d]Based on the method of Kruger (14, 15).
[e]Excellent morphology in $>14\%$ of evaluated spermatozoa.
[f]Percentage of sperm with excellent morphology was $>4\%$ but $<14\%$.
[g]Excellent morphology in $\leq 4\%$ of sperm.

method exhibited a significant impairment of sperm binding to the zona pellucida. Kruger reported that such semen, with $<4\%$ normal forms, was associated with a very low IVF fertilization rate (7.6% per oocyte) when using 0.05×10^6 sperm per milliliter.

Our present observations support the argument that the HZA can identify individual patients who are likely to encounter fertilization difficulties during IVF treatment. A diminished capacity for tight binding to the zona pellucida is implicated as a principal cause of fertilization failure in certain male factor patients.

In summary, the HZA seems to be a useful diagnostic test for estimating the fertilizing potential of human sperm. Although a few studies have been completed and the data summarized here, the HZA will require further evaluation to provide a fuller understanding of its best uses and limitations. Reproducibility in the HZA is presently being examined in two studies: simultaneous testing of a given semen specimen with three pairs of matching hemizonae, and the repeated testing of a given man over several months. An important objective will be the development of a commercial kit that will allow HZA-like tests to be done on a widely available basis.

Other potential applications of HZA include (*a*) sperm injection for fertilization, whereby a sperm attached to the zona pellucida can be picked up into the micropipette (such sperm may be superior to other sperm picked at random, without demonstrated affinity for the zona surface); (*b*) determining whether residual spermatogenesis (induced oligospermia) during male contraceptive therapy (such as gonadotropin-releasing hormone antagonist with testosterone treatment) is likely to lead to unwanted pregnancy; and (*c*) development of contraceptive vaccines, derived from either zona or sperm antigens, that can be titered on the ability to inhibit sperm-egg interaction in the HZA.

References

1. Overstreet JW, Hembree WC: Penetration of zona pellucida of nonliving human oocytes by human spermatozoa in vitro. Fertil Steril 27:815, 1976
2. Bedford JM: Sperm/egg interaction: the specificity of human spermatozoa. Anat Rec 188:477, 1977

3. Overstreet JW, Yanagimachi R, Katz DF, Hayashi K, Hanson FW: Penetration of human spermatozoa into the human zona pellucida and the zona-free hamster egg: a study of fertile donors and infertile patients. Fertil Steril 33:534, 1980

4. Yanagimachi R, Lopata A, Odom CB, Bronson RA, Mahi CA, Nicolson GL: Retention of biologic characteristics of zona pellucida in highly concentrated salt solution: the use of salt-stored eggs for assessing the fertilizing capacity of spermatozoa. Fertil Steril 31:562, 1979

5. Burkman LJ, Coddington CC, Franken DR, Kruger T, Rosenwaks Z, Hodgen G: The hemizona assay (HZA): development of a diagnostic test for the binding of human spermatozoa to human hemizona pellucida to predict fertilization potential. Fertil Steril 49:688, 1988

6. Franken DR, Burkman LJ, Oehninger SC, Veeck LL, Kruger TF, Coddington CC, Hodgen GD: The hemizona assay using salt stored human oocytes: evaluation of zona pellucida capacity for binding human spermatozoa. Gamete Res 22:15, 1989

7. Franken DR, Oehninger S, Burkman LJ, Coddington CC, Kruger TF, Rosenwaks Z, Acosta AA, Hodgen GD: The hemizona assay (HZA): a predictor of human sperm fertilizing potential in in vitro fertilization (IVF) treatment. J In Vitro Fertil Embryo Trans 6:1, 1989

8. Oehninger S, Coddington CC, Scott R, Franken DA, Burkman LJ, Acosta AA, Hodgen GD: Hemizona assay: assessment of sperm dysfunction and prediction of in vitro fertilization outcome. Fertil Steril 51:665, 1989

9. Rosenwaks Z, Muasher SJ: Recruitment of fertilizable eggs. In Jones HW Jr, Jones GS, Hodgen GD, Rosenwaks Z (eds): In Vitro Fertilization—Norfolk. Baltimore: Williams & Wilkins, 1986, p 30

10. Yoshimatsu N, Yanagimachi R, Lopata A: Zonae pellucidae of salt-stored hamster and human eggs: their penetrability by homologous and heterologous spermatozoa. Gamete Res 21:115, 1988

11. McDowell JS: Preparation of spermatozoa for insemination in vitro. In Jones HW Jr, Jones GS, Hodgen GD, Rosenwaks Z (eds): In Vitro Fertilization—Norfolk. Baltimore: Williams & Wilkins, 1986, p 162

12. Ahuja KK, Bolwell GP: Probable asymmetry in the organization of components of the hamster zona pellucida. J Reprod Fertil 69:49, 1983

13. Remington RD, Schork MA: Statistics with Applications to the Biological and Health Sciences. Englewood Cliffs, NJ: Prentice-Hall, 1970, p 152

14. Kruger TF Ackerman SB, Simmons KF, Swanson RJ, Brugo S, Acosta AA: A quick reliable staining technique for sperm morphology. Arch Androl 18:275, 1987

15. Kruger TF, Acosta AA, Simmons KF, Swanson RJ, Matta JF, Oehninger S: Predictive value of abnormal sperm morphology in in vitro fertilization. Fertil Steril 49:112, 1988

16. Acosta AA, van Uem J, Ackerman SB, Mayer JF: Estimation of male fertility by examination and testing of spermatozoa. In Jones HW, Jr, Jones GS, Hodgen GD, Rosenwaks Z (eds): In Vitro Fertilization—Norfolk. Baltimore: Williams & Wilkins, 1986, p 126

Part Three—Flow Cytometry Assay

R. JAMES SWANSON, R.N., PH.D., ANIBAL A. ACOSTA,
M.D., RAMONA AUSTIN, B.S., AND SILVINA BOCCA, M.S.

Analysis of sperm morphology is proving to be one of the most important tools for the evaluation of male fertility. Oehninger (1) has shown a very good correlation between the assessment of human sperm morphology patterns and fertilizing capacity. Important observations have been reported after analysis of sperm morphology with classic cytological staining techniques and light microscopy (1) and after quantitative microscopy of the sperm shape (2, 3). By inducing genetic damage in mouse sperm, Wyrobek (2) demonstrated an increase in the frequency of abnormal sperm morphology. Mouse sperm carrying certain chromosomal translocations which influence head morphology have been distinguished from normal sperm by quantitative microscopy (4). The same phenomenon has been observed in human sperm after chemically induced alterations in spermatogenesis (3).

For fertility counseling and genotoxic screening, more accuracy, sensitivity, objectivity, and reproductibility of the results are needed. Flow cytometry seems to provide these results in cytological studies. Fluorescent-stained sperm from mice, hamsters, rabbits, and bulls screened with slit-scan flow cytometry have given species-characteristic profiles of sperm heads, with heads of similar outline producing comparable fluorescence profiles (4) (Fig. 13.13).

Method

Flow cytometry uses single-cell suspensions to evaluate samples based on size (Ford angle light scatter), granularity (90° light scatter), or fluorescence (red or green). This method permits analysis of each cell within a population. The cell suspensions, produced from various tissues, may be obtained by such methods as mincing, sonication, and enzymatic treatment (5). Since semen is collected as a suspension of fully differentiated single-cell structures, sperm are ideal for analysis by flow cytometry.

After the suspensions have been obtained and stained, if necessary, they are filtered, introduced into the cytometer from a pressurized container, and carried to a flow chamber through a series of tubes (5). In the flow chamber, the sample is surrounded by an isotonic buffered saline sheath. This sheath confines the cells to the center of the stream as it passes through a focused light source, usually an argon laser. This process ensures optimal illumination of cells as they flow one at a time past the light source. As the laser strikes each cell, light is scattered, absorbed, or re-emitted as fluorescence (5). A special optical system filters the light before the photomultiplier tubes measure the intensity. Information from the tubes is sent to a computer, where analog signals are changed into digital signals. The individual cells are counted and indexed according to specific parameters. The laser is capable of separating individual populations based on a charge applied to the cells. Sorting allows for recognition and purification of specific cell

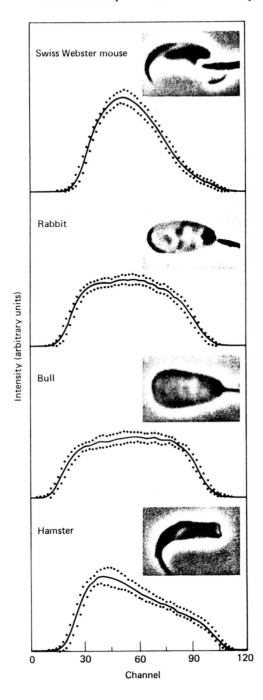

Figure 13.13. Average slit-scan flow cytometric profiles for sperm from four mammals. The *solid line* is a sample average; the *dotted lines* represent 1 SD from the average. Sperm from each animal yield an average profile with a distinct length and shape. (From Gledhill BL: Cytometric analysis of shape and DNA content in mammalian sperm. Ann NY Acad Sci 438:189, 1984.)

subpopulations. Cell distribution is plotted on histograms, which may be single or double parameter (Fig. 13.14**A** and **B**).

Some applications for the flow cytometer include cell surface marking such as antigen-antibody binding, viability, DNA and RNA analysis, or tumor cell identification.

Some fluorescent dyes used in these procedures include fluorescein and phycoerythrin, both of which stain proteins, and propidium iodide and acridine orange, both of which stain DNA and RNA.

Applications

Although current literature on flow cytometry of sperm is limited, important aspects of fertilization physiology can be analyzed by this method. The ability of nuclear sperm chromatin to undergo decondensation in oocyte cytoplasm can be mimicked in an in vitro system. This decondensation has a unique characteristic for all species studied to date (6) and is closely related to the extent and efficiency of sperm nuclear disulfide bonding. Flow cytometric analysis of nitrofurantoin-treated sperm has demonstrated the significance of sulfhydryl oxidation in maintaining the morphology of immature caput epididymal hamster sperm and implies the importance of sulfhydryl oxidation in motility acquired in vivo (7).

Flow cytometry can be used to determine the proportion of X and Y chromosome-bearing sperm, based on the quantitative difference between the sex chromosomes with respect to DNA content (3.4% difference between the X and Y subpopulations of human sperm) (8) and on the differences of DNA base composition (9). Even though the latter method may be time-consuming, it can be magnified by staining techniques that require decondensation with proteolytic enzymes of the highly compact sperm nucleus.

DNA analysis of sperm and testicular tissue includes evaluating the shape and position of the haploid peak in flow cytometer histograms. A typical DNA histogram of human testicular tissue showing normal spermatogenesis is characterized by four peaks (Fig. 13.15). Peak I represents elongated spermatids which do not stain in proportion to their DNA content because of their highly condensed chromatin. Peak II, at 1-c DNA, represents round spermatids. Peak III represents non-germ cells and germ cells with a 2-c DNA content (G_1 spermatogonia, preleptotene, and secondary spermatocytes). Peak IV represents mainly primary spermatocytes plus a small percentage of G_2 and M spermatogonia. Between peaks III and IV, the cells synthesizing DNA are registered (10). Normal sperm samples, with a high percentage of 1-c DNA, should be demonstrated by a narrow, high 1-c peak with a narrow base (Fig. 13.16). A variance from normal positioning or distribution may indicate andrological disease.

Patients with testicular carcinoma have been evaluated by the flow cytometer (11). In this study, acridine orange was used to stain aliquots of fresh or frozen semen from patients and controls. Acridine orange intercalates into the double-helix DNA and fluoresces green, while fluorescing red with single-stranded DNA or RNA (12). After staining, the aliquots may be measured by the cytometer, with the percentage of normal sperm staining (red) determined by computer analysis (11). The staining profile of patients and controls is shown in Figure 13.17. This figure demonstrates the abnormal DNA in a cancer patient compared to normal semen.

A sperm chromatin structure assay has been developed (13) to evaluate the relationship of the susceptibility of nuclear DNA to denaturation in bovine fertility. At low

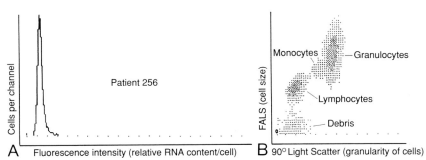

Figure 13.14. **A**, Single-parameter histogram representing RNA values of 10,000 sperm cells. The abscissa indicates the fluorescence intensity which is proportional to the relative RNA content, and the ordinate indicates the number of cells per channel. **B**, Double-parameter histogram representing leukocyte subpopulations. The abscissa indicates increasing granularity of cells, and the ordinate represents increasing cell size.

pH, the DNA that resists denaturation, and remains in its double helix configuration, fluoresces green; single-stranded DNA fluoresces red with acridine orange. This test may prove to be useful in evaluating sperm which tests as normal by present techniques.

Current work in our laboratory includes immunocytochemical analysis of antisperm antibodies in male patients. A swim-up separation is performed on their semen samples,

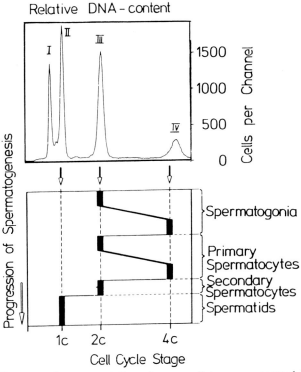

Figure 13.15. Diagrammatic representation of germ cell types represented in a histogram of normal adult human testicular tissue. (From Hacker-Klom U, Ritter J, Kleinhans G: DNA-analysis of human testicular samples by cytofluorometry. Andrologia 18:304, 1986.)

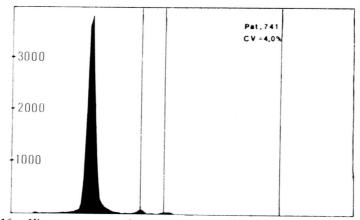

Figure 13.16. Histogram representing normal sperm with characteristic spermiogenesis. The high, narrow peak represents the mature (haploid) spermatozoa.

with each sample then divided between two tubes. To one tube, 50 µl of fluorescein anti-human Fab is added as a 1:20 dilution. To the other tube, 50 µl of phosphate-buffered saline (PBS)-bovine serum albumin (BSA) is added; this is the control tube in each sample. After incubation and subsequent washings, the samples are evaluated by flow cytometry and wet-mount slides. Computer analysis provides comparisons of the anti-human Fab tubes and the control tubes. The results are compared to samples viewed by fluorescent microscopy.

  Further work may include separating normal sperm cells from those with antibodies attached, testing the viability of these cells, and comparing DNA in normal and infertile males.

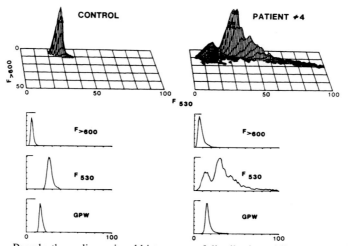

Figure 13.17. Pseudo-three-dimensional histograms of distribution of fluorescence intensities per cell. Cells in normal semen are on the *left;* semen cells from a cancer patient are on the *right.* The cells from the normal (control) sample demonstrate homogeneous acridine orange staining compared to the cancer cells (11).

References

1. Oehninger S, Acosta AA, Morshedi M, Veeck L, Swanson RJ, Simmons K, Rosenwaks Z: Corrective measures and pregnancy outcome in in vitro fertilization in patients with severe sperm morphology abnormalities. Fertil Steril 50:283, 1988
2. Wyrobek AJ, Gordon LA, Burkhart JG, Francis MC, Kapp RW Jr, Letz G, Malling HV, Topham JC, Whorton MD: An evaluation of the mouse sperm morphology test and other sperm tests in nonhuman mammals: a report for the GENE-TOX Program. Mutat Res Rev Genet Toxicol 115:10, 1983
3. Wyrobek AJ, Gordon, LA, Burkhart JG, Francis MC, Kapp, RW Jr, Letz G, Malling HV, Topham JC, Whorton, MD: An evaluation of human sperm as indicators of chemically induced alterations of spermatogenic function: a report for the GENE-TOX Program. Mutat Res Rev Genet Toxicol 115:73, 1983
4. Gledhill BL: Cytometric analysis of shape and DNA content in mammalian sperm. An NY Acad Sci 438:189, 1984
5. Kruth HS: Flow cytometry: rapid biochemical analysis of single cells. Anal Biochem 125:225, 1982
6. Perreault SD, Barbec RR, Epstein KH, Zucker RM, Keefer CL: Interspecies differences in the stability of mammalian sperm nuclei assessed in vivo by sperm microinjection and in vitro by flow cytometry. Biol Reprod 39:157, 1988
7. Cornwall GA, Vindivich D, Tillman S, Chang TSK: The effect of sulfhydryl oxidation on the morphology of immature hamster epididymal spermatozoa induced to acquire motility in vitro. Biol Reprod: 39:141, 1988
8. Otto FJ, Hacker U, Zante J, Schumann J, Gohde W, Meistrich, ML: Flow cytometry of human spermatozoa. Histochemistry 61:249, 1979
9. Pinkel D, Lake S, Gledhill BL, Van Dilla MA, Stephenson D, Watchmaker G: High resolution DNA content measurements of mammalian sperm. Cytometry 3:1, 1982
10. Hacker-Klom U, Ritter J, Kleinhans G: DNA-analysis of human testicular samples by cytofluorometry. Andrologia 18:304, 1986
11. Evenson DP, Klein FA, Whitmore WF, Melamed MR: Flow cytometric evaluation of sperm from patients with testicular carcinoma. J Urol 132:1220, 1984
12. Lerman LS: The structure of the DNA acridine complex. Proc Natl Acad Sci 49:94, 1963
13. Ballachey, BE, Evenson DP, Saacke RG: The sperm chromatin structure assay relationship with alternate tests of semen quality and heterospermic performance of bulls. J Androl 9:109, 1988

Index

Page numbers in *italics* denote figures; those followed by "t" denote tables.

)